# Understanding Health and Social Care

# Understanding Health and Social Care

This Reader forms part of the Open University course *An Introduction to Health and Social Care* (K101), a 60 point first level undergraduate course. K101 is a compulsory course for the Foundation Degree in Health and Social Care; BA/BSc (Hons) Health and Social Care; BA (Hons) Social Work (England), (Wales) and (Scotland). It is also a compulsory component of the following awards: Diploma of Higher Education (Adult Nursing), Diploma of Higher Education (Mental Health Nursing); Diploma of Higher Education (Social Care); Diploma of Higher Education in Social Care (England), (Scotland) and (Wales). Certificate in Health & Social Care; Certificate of Higher Education in Social Care (England), (Scotland) and (Wales); Certificate of Higher Education (Social Care); Certificate of Higher Education (Health Care Practice).

Details of this and other Open University courses can be obtained from the Student Registration and Enquiry Service, The Open University, PO Box 197, Milton Keynes MK7 6BJ, United Kingdom: telephone +44 (0) 845 300 6090, e-mail general enquiries@open.ac.uk Alternatively, you may visit the Open University website at http://www.open.ac.uk where you can learn more about the wide range of courses and packs offered at all levels by The Open University.

# Understanding Health and Social Care

## An Introductory Reader

Second edition

Edited by Julia Johnson and Corinne De Souza

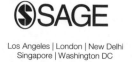

Los Angeles | London | New Delhi
Singapore | Washington DC

The Open University

The Open University
Walton Hall
Milton Keynes
MK7 6AA
United Kingdom
www.open.ac.uk

Editorial arrangement and original material
© Open University 2008

First published 2008

Reprinted 2009 (twice), 2010

SAGE Publications Ltd
1 Oliver's Yard
55 City Road
London EC1Y 1SP

SAGE Publications Inc.
2455 Teller Road
Thousand Oaks, California 91320

SAGE Publications India Pvt Ltd
B 1/I 1 Mohan Cooperative Industrial Area
Mathura Road
New Delhi 110 044

SAGE Publications Asia-Pacific Pte Ltd
33 Pekin Street #02-01
Far East Square
Singapore 048763

**Library of Congress Control Number: 2007941601**

**British Library Cataloguing in Publication data**

A catalogue record for this book is available from the British Library

ISBN 978-1-84787-080-3
ISBN 978-1-84787-081-0 (pbk)

Typeset by C&M Digitals Pvt Ltd., Chennai, India
Printed and bound in Great Britain by
CPI Antony Rowe, Chippenham, Wiltshire
Printed on paper from sustainable resources

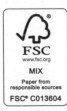

# Contents

# Acknowledgements

Every effort has been made to trace all the copyright holders, but if any have been inadvertently overlooked the publishers will be pleased to make the necessary arrangement at the first opportunity.

Grateful acknowledgement is made to the following sources for permission to reproduce material in this book.

**Chapter 1, 1.1**
Wood, G. and Thompson, P. (1993) *The Nineties: Personal Recollections of the 20th Century*. London: BBC Books. Reprinted by permission of The Random House Group Ltd.

**Chapter 1, 1.2**
Welsh, D. (2005) *Fortress Britain: Working Lives and Trade Unions in World War II*. London: National Pensioners Convention, pp. 77–79. Reproduced with permission.

**Chapter 1, 1.3**
Kramer, A. (2006) *Many Rivers to Cross: The History of the Caribbean Contribution to the NHS*. London: Sugar Media Limited, pp. 90–91. Reproduced under the terms of the Click-Use Licence and by permission of Sugar Media Ltd.

**Chapter 1, 1.4**
Townsend, P. (1957) *The Family Life of Old People*. London: Routledge and Kegan Paul, p. 61. Reproduced with permission.

**Chapter 2**
Bornat, J. (2003) '"Kate": the constant rediscovery of a poem', *Generations*, 27(5): 89–93. Reproduced by permission of the American Society of Aging.

**Chapter 3**
Purves, R. (2004) 'Racist abuse ruined my life', *Nursing Times*, 100(32): 24–25. Reproduced with permission.

**Chapter 4**
Toynbee, P. (2003) 'Portering' in P. Toynbee, *Hard Work*. London: Bloomsbury, pp. 55–83. Copyright © 2003 Polly Toynbee. Reproduced by permission of the author c/o Rogers, Coleridge & White Ltd., 20 Powis Mews, London W11 1JN.

**Chapter 6**
Bibbings, A. (1994) 'Carers and professionals – the carer's viewpoint', in A. Leathard (ed.), *Going Interprofessional*. London: Routledge, pp. 158–171. Copyright © 1994, Routledge. Reproduced by permission of Taylor & Francis Books UK.

**Chapter 7**
Yeandle, S., Escott, K., Grant, L. and Batty, E. (2003) *Women and Men Talking about Poverty*, Working Paper Series No 7. Manchester: Equal Opportunities Commission. Reproduced with permission.

**Chapter 8**
Stainton, T. and Boyce, S. (2004) '"I have got my life back": users' experiences of direct payments', *Disability and Society*, 19(5): 443–454. Reprinted by permission of the publisher (Taylor & Francis Ltd, www.tandf.co.uk/journals).

**Chapter 9, 9.1**
Martin, R. (1995) *Experiencing Home Care*, C743/02/07 (F4935), Tape 5, Side b. British Library Sound Archive. Reproduced with permission.

**Chapter 9, 9.2**
Peace, S., Holland, C. and Kellaher, L. (2006) *Environment and Identity in Later Life*. Milton Keynes: Open University Press, pp. 138–140. Copyright © 2006, Open University Press, reproduced with kind permission of the Open University Press.

**Chapter 9, 9.3**
Bryden, C. (2005) *Dancing with Dementia*. London: Jessica Kingsley, pp. 144–146. Reproduced with permission.

**Chapter 9, 9.4**
The Judith Trust (2004) *Going Home? A Study of Women with Severe Learning Disabilities Moving Out of a Locked Ward*. London: The Judith Trust, St George's Hospital Medical School, University of London. Reproduced with permission.

**Chapter 9, 9.5**
Commission for Architecture & the Built Environment (CABE) (2004) *The Role of Hospital Design in the Recruitment, Retention and Performance of NHS Nurses in England*. Reproduced with permission of CABE (www.cabe.org.uk).

**Chapter 10**
Hanley, L. (2007) *Estates: An Intimate History*. London: Granta Books, pp. 1–15 and 148–183. Reproduced by permission of Granta Publications.

**Chapter 11**
Barnes, C. (2005) 'Independent living, politics and policy in the United Kingdom: a social model account', *Review of Disability Studies*, 1(4): 5–13. Reproduced with permission.

**Chapter 12**
Norman, A. (1980) *Rights and Risk*. London: Centre for Policy on Ageing, pp. 14–19. Reproduced with permission.

**Chapter 13**
Jones, K. and Fowles, A. J. (1984) 'Goffman: the radical', *Ideas on Institutions*. London: Routledge and Kegan Paul, pp. 12–16. Copyright © 1984, reproduced by permission of Taylor and Francis Books UK.

**Chapter 14**
Lee-Treweek, G. (1994) 'Bedroom abuse', *Generations Review*, 4(1): 2–4. Reproduced by kind permission of the author.

**Chapter 15**
Bakardjieva, M. (2005) *Internet Society: The Internet in Everyday Life*. London: SAGE, pp. 169–180. Reproduced with permission.

**Chapter 16, 16.1**
Prynn, B. (2001) 'Growing up alone', *Oral History*, 29(2): 62–72. Reproduced with permission of The Oral History Society (www.oralhistory.org.uk).

**Chapter 16, 16.2**
Vokins, I. (2004/05) Transcript from *Diabetes Stories* (www.diabetes-stories.co.uk/transcript.asp?UID=44) (accessed 15 May 2007). Reproduced with permission.

**Chapter 16, 16.3**
Magee, B. and Milligan, M. (1995) *Sight Unseen: Letters Between Brian Magee and Martin Milligan*. London: Phoenix, pp. 64–69. Originally published in *On Blindness*, 1995, OUP. Reprinted by permission of Oxford University Press.

**Chapter 16, 16.4**
Clark, D., Small, N., Wright, M., Winslow, M. and Hughes, N. (2005) *A Bit of Heaven for the Few? An Oral History of the Modern Hospice Movement in the United Kingdom*. Lancaster: Observatory Publications, pp. 144–148. Reproduced with permission.

**Chapter 16, 16.5**
Denis, P. (2005) *Never Too Small to Remember: Memory Work and Resilience in Times of AIDS*. Pietermarizburg: Cluster Publications, pp. 45–47. Reproduced with permission.

**Chapter 17**
Lawler, J. (1991) *Behind the Screens: Nursing, Somology and the Pattern of the Body*. Melbourne: Churchill, pp. 117–133. Reproduced by kind permission of the author.

**Chapter 18**
McKenna, H. P., Hasson, F. and Keeney, S. (2004) 'Patient safety and quality of care: the role of the health care assistant', *Journal of Nursing Management*, 12(6): 452–459. Reproduced with permission of Wiley-Blackwell Publishing Ltd.

**Chapter 19**
Allandale, E. (1996) 'Working on the front line: risk culture and nursing', *Sociological Review*, 94(3): 416–451. Reproduced with permission of Wiley-Blackwell Publishing Ltd.

**Chapter 20**
Lawton, R. and Parker, D. (1999) 'Procedures and the professional: the case of the NHS', *Social Science and Medicine*, 48: 353–361. Reprinted from *Social Science and Medicine*, vol. 48, Copyright (1999), with permission from Elsevier.

**Chapter 21**
Ziebland, S., Chapple, A., Dumelow, C., Evans, J., Prinjha, S. and Rozmovits, L. (2004) 'How the internet affects patients' experience of cancer: a qualitative study', *British*

*Medical Journal*, 328(7439): 564–569. Reproduced with permission from the BMJ Publishing Group.

**Chapter 22**
Pyper, C., Amery, J., Watson, M. and Crook, C. (2004) 'Patients' experiences of accessing their on-line electronic patient records in primary care', *British Journal of General Practice*, 54(498): 38–53. Reproduced with permission.

**Chapter 23**
Patel, V. K. P. (ed.) 'Positive Action', in *In on the Act: Barnados Projects Implementing the Children (Scotland) Act 1995*. London: Barnados. Reproduced with kind permission of Barnados.

**Chapter 24, 24.1**
Maslow, A. H., Frager, R. D. and Fadiman, J. (1987) *Motivation and Personality*, 3rd Edition. Upper Saddle River, NJ: Pearson, pp. xxxiii–xxxvi. © 1987. Reprinted by permission of Pearson Education, Inc..

**Chapter 24, 24.2**
Bowlby, J. (1969) *Attachment and Loss*. London: Hogarth Press. Reprinted by permission of The Random House Group Ltd.

**Chapter 24, 24.3**
Bowlby, J. (1969) *Attachment and Loss, volume 1: Attachment*. London: Hogarth Press, pp. 266–268 and 304–307. Copyright © Tavistock Institute of Human Relations 1969, 1982. Reprinted by permission of Basic Books, a member of Perseus Books Group.

**Chapter 24, 24.4**
Finch, J. (1984) 'Community care: developing non-sexist alternatives', *Critical Social Policy*, (9): 6–18. Reproduced with permission of SAGE Publications.

**Chapter 24, 24.5**
Finkelstein, V. (2002) 'Whose history???', keynote address at the Disability History Week, 10 June 2002. Reproduced with permission.

**Chapter 25**
'Introduction to the Beveridge Report', in J. Jacobs (ed.), *Beveridge 1942–1992: Papers to Mark the 50th Anniversary of the Beveridge Report*. London: Whiting and Birch Books, pp. 5–19. Reproduced by kind permission of the author.

**Chapter 26**
Symonds, A. and Kelly, A. (eds) (1998) *The Social Construction of Community Care*. Basingstoke: Macmillan, pp. 241–253. Reproduced by permission of Palgrave Macmillan.

**Chapter 27**
Walmsley, J. (2006) 'Organisations, structures and community care, 1971–2001: From community care to citizenship?', in J. Welshman and J. Walmsley (eds), *Community Care*

*in Perspective: Care, Control and Citizenship.* Basingstoke: Palgrave Macmillan, pp. 77–96. Reproduced by permission of Palgrave Macmillan.

## Chapter 28
Kerridge, I., Lowe, M. and Henry, D. (1998) 'Ethics and evidence-based medicine', *British Medical Journal*, 316: 1151–1153. Reproduced with permission from the BMJ Publishing Group.

## Chapter 29
George, V. and Wilding, P. (1985) 'The anti-collectivists', in *Ideology and Social Welfare*. London: Routledge & Kegan Paul, pp. 35–43. Copyright © 1985, Routledge & Kegan Paul. Reproduced by permission of Taylor and Francis Books UK.

## Chapter 30
Coates, D. (2005) *Prolonged Labour: The Slow Birth of New Labour Britain.* Basingstoke: Palgrave Macmillan, pp. 3–20. Reproduced by permission of Palgrave Macmillan.

## Chapter 31
Shaw, M. and Dorling, D. (2004) 'Who cares in England and Wales? The Positive Care Law: cross-sectional study', *British Journal of General Practice*, 54: 899–903. Reproduced with permission.

# Introduction

*Julia Johnson and Corinne De Souza*

We are all involved in health and social care one way or another, be it as informal carers, users of health or social care services or as workers. It is not surprising, therefore, that this topic commands a substantial literature. As pointed out by Celia Davies and Martin Robb in their introduction to the first edition of this reader, there are already a number of books on the financing, organisation and administration of care services and this book does not duplicate them. Rather it juxtaposes the experiences and voices of service users with findings from research and current academic debates, making the links between theory and practice more amenable.

Since the first edition of this book was published in 1998 (Allot and Robb) there have been some substantial developments and changes in health and social care policies. The impact of some of these developments are reflected in the content of this new edition. By the end of its second term, the New Labour government, elected in 1997, had begun to implement a more choice-based approach to both health and social care. Money was to follow patients who would make choices about which hospital or other service provider they preferred; likewise disabled adults and older people were to be given their own budgets to spend on the support services they wished to purchase (Glennerster, 2006). Chapters in this book which reflect these developments include Stainton and Boyce on users and direct payments and Colin Barnes on independent living and the social model of disability. A further development has been devolution in the UK and divergence from the centre in terms of policy. This means that choice-based developments have varied. In Scotland, for example, the uptake of direct payments in no way matches that in England. Another marked development since 1998, reflected in this book, is in the use of the internet. Several chapters address the topic directly and it is through the internet that service users are able to acquire knowledge and, therefore, the power to make informed choices. That said, it is likely that the more advantaged sections of society are those most able to make best use of the opportunities new technology offers. One enduring feature of health and social policy in early 2000s is the persistence of inequalities in health and in care provision. The concluding chapter of this book by Mary Shaw and Danny Dorling provides evidence of this.

## Using the book

This book has been put together so as to attract a variety of readers. Students on undergraduate or pre-degree level courses should find the chapters of great relevance to their studies. Indeed the book is a set text for the Open University first level undergraduate course, K101: *An Introduction to Health and Social Care*. It should also, however, be of interest and use to those working in or providing health and social care services: the variety of paid workers, personal assistants, volunteers, service users and informal carers. The content of the book has been compiled with all these readers in mind.

The contents have been organised into four sections. Each starts with an introduction which takes the reader through some of the underlying themes in the section. These introductions will be of particular use to the reader who wants to work through the book from beginning to end or for those who want to focus on one particular aspect of care provision. The first chapter of each section contains an anthology of personal accounts or commentaries, often historical, of relevance to the section theme. The focus of the first section is on *people* who use and work in health and social care services. It contains accounts from individuals which as a whole provide a diverse range of perspectives on care provision including, for example, those of direct payment users, a black nurse, hospital porters and people experiencing poverty. The second section is organised around different care settings or *places* for care. It starts with an account of council estates but also includes hospitals, care homes, domestic settings and the internet. The third section focuses on *approaches* to care provision or, put another way, how care is provided. This section includes a number of chapters on issues of importance in the early 2000s such as the increasing use of unqualified health care assistants to provide hands-on nursing care, ways in which people use online electronic records and the impact of the internet on people's understanding of health and illness. The final section draws together chapters on some of the *ideas* that underpin health and social care provision in the 21st century and how they evolved. There is, for example, a chapter on the social construction of carers – a concept now central to health and social care – and other chapters which examine some of the political and philosophical ideas underpinning the provision of welfare.

Much of the content of this book has been put forward by members of the course team at the Open University and others involved in the production of K101: *An Introduction to Health and Social Care*. They include Dorothy Atkinson, Ken Blakemore, Joanna Bornat, Hilary Brown, Joyce Cavaye, Roger Gomm, Rebecca Jones, Andy Northedge, Sheila Peace, Jan Walmsley, Naomi Watson and Fran Wiles. As editors, we would like to thank them for their suggestions and their contribution to the editing. We would also like to thank Sarah Wright and Pat Jeal for their help and support in preparing the manuscript. Finally we wish to thank Margaret Allott and Martin Robb, the editors of the first edition of this book for their support and encouragement.

# References

Allot, M. and Robb, M. (eds) (1998) *Understanding Health and Social Care: An Introductory Reader*. London: SAGE.

Glennerster, H. (2006) 'The health and welfare legacy', in A. Seldon and D. Kavanagh (eds), *The Blair Effect 2001–5*. Cambridge, Cambridge University Press, pp. 283–305.

# Section 1
## People

## Introduction

This first section of the book focuses on people in the context of health and social care. Few of us are likely to say that we have never been involved in some kind of caring relationship. Relationships between family members, both intra- and inter-generational, and between friends and neighbours often involve caring 'about' each other and sometimes involve caring 'for', or being cared for by, another. Caring also comes into relationships between people who draw upon health or social care services and those who provide such services. And at some time during our lives, this is most of us. Through the eight chapters in this section we have tried to give voice to some of the diverse range of people engaged in caring relationships.

As with the other three sections in this reader, this section starts with an anthology. It was put together by Joanna Bornat, an oral historian, and Ken Blakemore, a social policy academic. It was assembled so as to capture something of the historical context of today's caring relationships and the people who work in and receive health and social care services. It contains not only accounts from nonagenarians of life before the inception of the post-war welfare state in Britain but also accounts from people who joined the new welfare state workforce, such as doctors from the Caribbean.

The second chapter in this section provides a fascinating account of the origins of the poem 'Kate' or as it is sometimes known 'Crabbit Old Woman' or 'Come closer, see me': a poem that has become iconic amongst many care workers because of the way It brings the dismissal of the lives of, and invisibility of the needs of, older people to the fore. It was supposedly found in the locker of a patient on a geriatric ward after her death but the 'true' story of its origins are revealed in Chapter 2, a story which helps to explain its lasting impact and significance.

Chapter 3 moves to another side of the hospital coin, from being a patient to being a nurse. In this case we have featured racism rather than ageism, that experienced by Rosie Purves when her managers and colleagues colluded in not allowing her to provide care to a white child on the paediatric ward. Chapter 4 focuses on another 'invisible' group of workers, hospital porters, and offers an invaluable insight into the situation of an essential workforce in a service which has now been contracted out to private agencies. Chapter 5 also reflects the experience of a worker, Howard Mitchell, from the now demolished Lennox Castle Hospital in Glasgow where he was born. He conducted some research into the hospital's history and engages us in a discussion of the advantages and disadvantages of being an 'insider researcher', a discussion that is highly pertinent to any practising or aspiring 'practitioner researcher'.

Chapter 6 turns to the situation of informal carers and gives voice to their collective needs. Although this was written some time ago, we have included it again here because the pressures on informal carers in the first decade of the 21st century are increasing and the messages remain important. They are particularly important for people living in poverty who, as the final chapter by Mary Shaw and Danny Dorling in this book indicates, are most likely to be providing informal care services. So, Chapter 7 gives voice to men and women living on low incomes. In particular, it spells out some of the differences for men and for women in experiencing poverty. The final chapter focuses on a group of relationships that are on the borderline of formal and informal, that is the relationship between disabled people and those they are paying to be personal assistants. This chapter illustrates the value of handing over control to service users.

What all these chapters have in common are the often unheard voices of the 'underdog': the not so important patients, the undervalued and sometimes discriminated against or unrecognised front line workers.

# Chapter 1

## Anthology: people

*Compiled by Joanna Bornat and Ken Blakemore*

Each section of this reader begins with a selection of short excerpts from a variety of different sources. Some are from classic books and reports about social care; others are from the pioneers and leaders whose writings and research have proved influential. Others again draw on accounts of practitioners and users of services as they experience different forms of provision. This first selection looks back in time through the words of people who have witnessed tremendous transformations in society during the 20th century. The words and voices of these people show how much has changed, and what has remained the same. They provide eye-witness testimony to how things were in the past. In this way we are better informed when it comes to making choices and plans for today's health and social care, as well as for the future.

## 1.1   Personal recollections of the 20th century

Gloria Wood and Paul Thompson's book *The Nineties*, published in 1993, draws on a series of interviews with people who were aged 90 or more that were conducted for a television series of the same name. The extracts below are taken from four of these interviews. This selection provides some brief but telling insights into what it was like to live through the first decade of the 20th century, before the creation of the welfare state in the 1940s.

### George Walter Cureton

*George Walter Cureton was the son of a policeman who died when George was seven years old. Born in 1901 in Staines, Middlesex, he was one of a close-knit family of three boys and four girls. When he was eight, he was sent away from home to the Police Orphanage at Strawberry Hill, Twickenham, for his education.*

[...]

When my father was alive he was a very, very efficient provider. When he died they cut his allotment into three and gave it to three other fellows. He grew everything he wanted. There was quite a good deal of bartering done in those days. The average copper was able to do a good turn here and a good turn there, get a leg of pork and that sort of thing. And we did very well thank you. He was a very good provider.

When he died, my mother had got nothing. She didn't work. She was an extremely good needlewoman, but she'd got four daughters. The only place in Staines where they could work was the Middlesex and Surrey Laundry, and as in every other place in the world, and definitely in this country, if there was a bountiful supply of labour and not many places to be filled, the wages come down. I believe my sisters got a maximum of about three and six a week for packing in the laundry. The stuff they had to pack was very largely the stuff that came from Buckingham Palace. Every single hamper had to have every layer in perfect order, almost plumb line and spirit level. Each member of the Royal Family had a vast laundry basket of their own and then of course there was an enormous amount of linen for the household. So what with Windsor and Buckingham Palace, that laundry could have managed very well on the royal bounty. But my sisters wouldn't have managed very well on the wages. And my mother couldn't live on it.

You see, in those days there was no widow's allowance, no children's allowance. Mother's main job was to keep the family together, because if they'd have gone in the workhouse, the girls would have gone one way, the boys would have gone another, and we should have been broken up. So mother immediately got herself in gear and did what she could to keep the place going.

Her father, who lived in Birmingham, suggested that the thing to do was to pack all her house up, move up to Birmingham, and he'd find plenty of work for 'em up here. So that's what they did. I was in the orphanage. I was left there while everybody else came up to Birmingham. I suppose they were financially better off, because they could get better jobs, slightly better pay and that sort of thing.

I was nearly fifteen when I left the orphanage, and I was just turned sixteen when I joined the Navy about twelve months later, or fifteen months later. If we remained in the same employment for twelve months after we'd left school we got a whole guinea. But I never got mine. I couldn't stick in the job. So I didn't get my guinea but I got in the Navy instead. Got myself a fourteen-year job.

## Edith Smith

*Edith Smith is the youngest of three children, and was born near the docks in Deptford, London, in 1901. When she was three years old her father, a Scandinavian sea captain, died at sea after a fight on board ship.*

[...]

I must have been eleven or twelve, and things were so tight that she had to apply for me to have meals at school, which if people were very poor, they could have free. I remember the humiliation I felt, going to school to have breakfast. It consisted of two pieces of bread and jam and a cup of cocoa, and the dinner was always a stew of some kind. But I can feel now the humiliation, you know, of all my school friends knowing that my mother was too poor to feed me.

[…]

I loved going to school but I went so very little. I was the one who had to look after the babies, you see, while my mother worked and tried to make more money. When I was thirteen and a half I was offered a job. My mother was working at a tailoring place and they said that I could have a job if I wanted it. And that meant four and sixpence extra a week. So I left school.

[…]

I used to walk to work with a girl, she was a Jewish girl and her father kept a shop. One day she said, 'Would your mother allow you to come out?' Mind you, I was eighteen then. So I said to my mother, 'Could I go out?' and she said 'Well, yes.' She let me go.

Well, the thing is that there used to be a parade, Mare Street, Hackney. All the girls used to parade in pairs, the boys used to parade in pairs. However this particular Saturday night we were walking along, and a couple of boys came towards us. The one on my side was the very fair boy. And the one on her side was the very dark boy. So, you know, with everything being even, I should have gone to the fair boy, and she should have gone to the dark boy. But somehow we crossed over, so that I got the dark boy and she got the fair boy and we were absolute contrasts! Anyway we got chatting about one thing and another and he said, 'Do you like reading?', and I said, 'Oh yes.' I had discovered books when I was quite young and so we talked about books. He wanted to take me out on the holiday Monday – wanted me to go to Epping Forest. I said, 'Oh I don't really know whether I would be allowed to.' So he said, 'Would you ask your parents if you can come out with me?'

Well, it wasn't only a question of going out with him but, you see, we bought our clothes on the 'never never'. We bought the things and paid a shilling a week for them. But in our house, things were so tight, that every Monday morning when I wore my clothes to go to work, my best costume was taken to pawn, to pay the rent, you see. I thought, 'Well, how am I going to get to go out, without my good costume?' And, 'How am I going to ask my mother if I can have my costume on Monday morning, to go out? – even if she'd let me go out with a boy.'

However, I talked to her and I said, 'I've met a very nice boy, I think you would like him.' And I said, 'He lives fairly near.' I said, 'He asked me to go out on Monday. He wants to take me to Epping Forest,' She said, 'Well, I don't like the sound of that.' However, she did let me go and she let me wear my costume. She pawned it on the Tuesday.

[…]

But the place where we lived, I wouldn't never, ever, let him come. I would never ever let him see me home, because it was down a little cutting, down a little alleyway. At the end of this cutting there was a glass-blowers' place, and the loo that we had was out in the yard. As the glass-blowers was warm, they got a lot of cockroaches in there, which used to come into our house. Well, I had no bedroom. I had to sleep in the living room on a little camp bed. And as I went to sleep all these cockroaches used to crawl up the wall. I could hear them all scrabbling about and I used to put my head under the sheets and hope I could go to sleep. And I often wonder whether that was the cause of me not sleeping well, for I was woken up so many times by these things I think being awake became second nature to me. It wasn't very good, wasn't good.

[…]

## Colin Thomson

*Colin Thomson was born in Dublin in September 1900, but was brought up in the north-east of Scotland. He came from an army background: his father was a major in the Scottish Highlanders. [...] He went to medical school in Edinburgh in 1917 and because he was a student he missed action in the First World War. When he qualified in 1922, he would have preferred to be a surgeon, but ended up as assistant to a GP in Rotherham, a poor industrial steel town in Yorkshire.*

I had an appointment with the Poor Law Authority as a medical officer and the result was I had to look after the, well, lower third of humanity you might say.

In those days rickets was very common, particularly in the big cities – in Glasgow particularly, it was full of rickets. The typical rickety person had a big head – a head like a philosopher, a chest like a whippet, a belly like a poisoned pup and legs like a grand piano. That was the description of the ultimate in rickets. But of course we've no rickets any longer because people don't live in those terrible tenements any more. They never saw the light of day, and they never got proper food.

Rotherham – it grieved me. I used to see these poor children, and it was a thing that got me down quite a lot. But it didn't mean that I wanted to get out of medicine. I saw one child with a septic meningitis in its ear, and it was going to die, and I knew it was going to die. And I actually cried. Which is very foolish: you know you shouldn't do that sort of thing.

To tell you one of the most harrowing experiences, a woman came into the surgery one day with a little girl, in a blanket. When I pulled the blanket apart, there was the poor little mite, desperately ill. She was breathing very rapidly, and I had an idea what was wrong. When I looked in the child's mouth I was absolutely appalled, because the whole of the back of the throat, and the palate as well, was full of pus, and a dirty great white membrane was stuck across the whole of the back of the throat. And the poor child's neck was swollen right to the chin. Now, I knew what this was. The smell, which was characteristic of diphtheria, clinched the whole thing. She was so ill she couldn't cry. I had to send her to the fever hospital and the poor little mite – died – the same afternoon. Now, that's – a picture – of the sort of terrible disease – it should never be – it was the most harrowing thing I've ever had in my life. I'll never forget it.

Tuberculosis, particularly pulmonary tuberculosis, was another big killer. It used to come often in young people, adolescents, people in their early twenties. It was very common then. Now some got very ill and ultimately developed what was called a hectic fever. You recognised it. It presaged the end of the poor soul. The strange thing about these sick young people was that they developed a terrific optimism during this period. It was – pitiful to see it, because you knew they were going to die; yet they would have a superlative optimism. They would talk about what they were going to do, and where they were going and who they'll do it with and all this sort of thing. It was given a special name: it was called Spes Phthisica. Now *spes* is the Latin for hope and *phthisica* was the name of pulmonary tuberculosis in the olden days. Hence the name 'Spes Phthisica'. Ultimately, of course, tuberculosis was banished from this country with antibiotics. The sanitoria were all closed and gone. Unfortunately I believe it's coming back again.

[...]

## David Taylor

*David Taylor was born in 1898, the youngest of three, in the slums of Manchester, where his father worked in a local slaughterhouse. When he was small both his parents drank and both were violent, and the family slept on top of egg-boxes, all five in one room. Instead of a toilet they had to use a common earth closet in the yard.*

[...]

We were all lousy, every one of us. We'd have to use a small tooth-comb to get the lice out of us heads every day. We used to borrow the tray, after one had finished, put in on your knee and scrape your scalp with a small tooth-comb and the lice'd come out, you see. Poor old dad, I can see him now, when he was doing it, he'd be cracking 'em all down – we used to kill 'em all wi' our thumb as they come out of our head. We were all lousy, and yet we tried to keep clean. You could go out in the street and it was a common thing for to just take one off you and put your foot on it. It was thought nothing to have bugs, you know. And the wallpaper's there, if you peel it off you'd find it's infested with bugs, infested with 'em. So, although you had your bug bites they didn't seem to do you any harm. We all did it, see.

Scarlet fever and diphtheria were common. There was always the yellow van coming down from Monsal Fever Hospital carting them away. I think it was the hygiene conditions, why there was such a lot of diphtheria and the other ailments. And the death rate was very, very high with children.

It was a common saying that 'you're never a mother until you've lost one,' see. I should think that nearly every woman in those days lost one. They just had the ordinary rough midwife come to them, and she used to do the job, and if it wasn't done proper the mother died or the child died. My mother lost two but I think it was probably over-laying. When a child was born, you see, they had to put it somewhere, and of course it was a common thing to put it in the bed between man and wife. Perhaps the poor woman used to welcome the child in there to keep her husband from lusting after her, you see. Well, you see what happened. You only needed to pull the sheet over your head and the poor little child, it couldn't breathe. And they called it 'over-laying', overlie.

If you got sick, you used to lie on the sofa and perhaps have some lemonade; we used to think it helped us get better. We used to lie and work it off. Of course, if you got too sick you could go to the doctor, but you had no money to pay him. He would come around on a Friday night, have you down for how much you owed him, try and get his money back. There was the Hulme Dispensary on Stratford Road; you could get a bottle of medicine and perhaps a little bit of treatment there. But you didn't get anything for nothing – you had to pay for everything. There were no special services to help you out a bit, no health service or anything like that.

We used to be hungry and we'd go the soup kitchen, a gang of us, as soon as we came out of school. We used to line up, and on the other side would be Irish navvies that couldn't get work. They were really hungry. If you were out of work your family had to try and keep you some way or other. If you couldn't be kept you were put on Parish Relief. The Relief Officer used to come round and give you so much for your rent and so much for your food. It might be only about fifteen shillings. Well if the rent was, say, seven shillings – it was a struggle to keep the whole lot of you on. Every so often they used to stop that and put the husband in the workhouse, more or less deliberately to penalise him, if he couldn't get work. They would send him in there for about six weeks.

*Source*: G. Wood and P. Thompson (1993) *The Nineties – Personal Recollections of the 20ᵗʰ Century*. London: BBC Books, pp. 26–60.

## 1.2    Working on 'The Home Front'

Flip Thornett-Roston was a nurse at St Mary Abbot's Hospital in London. She was interviewed for a project which marked the contribution of Home Front workers at the 60th anniversary of the Second World War in 2005. Funded by the Big Lottery, the 'Home Front Recall' project was launched by the National Pensioners Convention and the TUC. By the end, 105 interviews were collected and recorded, drawing on pensioner and older people's organisations for contacts and volunteers. This excerpt appears in a book which includes a selection from the interviews.

Well, it was a general hospital in those days, so you were supposed to be orientated from surgical, to medical, to geriatric to children's, to get experience of them all. But I didn't get on very well with the night Sister who seemed to think that she could tell me what I could do when I was off duty, like turning up on the steps of the church, which I didn't want to do. It was an old hospital and we had quite a lot of disasters with staff. There were twenty-two of us and I think only three finished the training actually. It was four years training. And we had one girl, because we had to go on night duty across the grounds, and there was a pond in the middle, and nobody thought to put white paint around the edges, and she fell in! And she was only found because her white apron showed up in the dark, but she was permanently damaged. Another girl was permanently damaged because we had these underground corridors and they were very badly lit. There was a bulb missing somewhere. It had a direct hit. A ward, the children's ward, which was supposed to have been closed years ago because it was architecturally, or structurally, unsound, was still in use. So some children got killed and about five staff got killed as well. These beams that crossed over. They were very beautiful. You could hear the shrapnel falling all around you. It was like hail coming down. If you didn't get hit, that was just luck. Everybody must have played a part, in London. There were lots of fires from incendiary bombs. Quite often followed up by high explosive bombs. It was all fire, lit up. People swept up the streets in the morning and just carried on. We all did. A big fire I do remember, because at that stage I was living in Highgate and you could see the whole of London silhouetted against this enormous fire. And you could read a newspaper up in Highgate by this fire from down there. We had to live in, yes.

The nurses' home was very interesting. We had a very old nurses' home where I lived, and then later on by some mistake somebody put me into the new nurses' home, which was beautiful. It had a kitchen each end of the corridor. I think it had two or three stairways. But we weren't allowed to use the kitchens! I remember fusing all the lights on one occasion because I had an iron. And there were no ironing facilities for us, as such, so I plugged it into the light outlet. And all the lights went. Yes, it was very primitive. The food was absolutely appaling. We reckoned that they bought a shipload of mouldy semolina because we got it three days running for lunch and supper. And it was revolting. And throughout the war we never saw a raw egg. We got this powdered egg which was like carpet, actually. The food was diabolical, and as a result I got very ill. I developed a lung abscess. It was pre-penicillin days. I was ill for six months. They got a surgeon over from the Brompton who opened my chest up under a local anaesthetic because I was too ill to have a general anaesthetic. When they got me out of bed after about six months, I couldn't walk any longer. I was really ill. So I got bunged up to North Wales for three months with some women from the East End of London. These women had no money. Any money they had they would spend on their children and their husbands. I also remember children with mouths full of black stubs that didn't have teeth. These are real memories that I can still see in my mind and will never forget. And then of course, '48 came and we got the National Health Service, which was wonderful.

*Source*: D. Welsh (2005) *Fortress Britain: working lives and trade unions in World War II*. London: National Pensioners Convention.

# 1.3    The Caribbean contribution to the NHS

The doctors included in this excerpt were interviewed by Abigail Bernard for a Department of Health project which sought to mark the contribution of people from the Caribbean to the National Health Service. Following the Second World War, thousands of people from across the Caribbean were recruited to work in the NHS. By 2006, men and women from black and minority ethnic backgrounds comprised 14 per cent of the 1.3 million NHS staff, yet few reach the highest levels of the organisation.

[...]
Dr Moonsawmy was advised to emigrate but, having married, he decided to go into general practice in the UK. Of that time [1973] he says: 'there were a lot of stories in tabloid newspapers about foreign doctors in Britain often in a stereotypical, rather derogatory way ... Most of us had to go into single-handed practice which was much more strenuous and much more difficult but enjoyable at the same time. That is how I ended up a single-handed practitioner since 1973 to the present time ... In this area of Edinburgh, there were no non-white consultants at all when I was a student and young doctor, and the first non-white student appointed in Edinburgh had to be in the specialities where white doctors did not want to go into, such as the venereal diseases clinic, psychiatry or geriatrics. None of these attracted me as I wanted to specialise in respiratory diseases.

I ended up in a village just on the edge of Edinburgh, which was a mining community ... I did encounter problems in my first one or two years here ... Quite a few of my patients heard that it was a foreign doctor and disappeared completely by registering with other practices. So that meant I had to inherit a practice with less patients and therefore of course with less income, but over the years I've built it up and won the respect of the local population by hard work, extremely excellent work and the word spreads around very quickly in communities if you set certain very high standards and you keep to them. Difficult at times, but one has learnt how to survive.'

Dr. Franklyn Jacobs had always intended to return to the Caribbean. 'I was offered a partnership at every practice where I worked. My answers were always the same: "No, I will be going back home." That was, until I was "bitten" by a surgery in Hornsey Road, North London, not too far away from here. In fact, I have never roamed far and Hornsey has remained my medical constituency. The principal of the surgery where I did locum work had advertised for a partner. He indicated [that] he was interested in me applying. I gave my usual spiel that I was heading home back to the Caribbean [and] he encouraged me to speak with my father [who] was, at the time, a practising GP in Bradford ... When given the details of the offer my father had no hesitation in convincing me to stay remarking that the offer of a partnership and the terms were excellent. I remember him saying "You're a very lucky boy" ... I remember being totally undecided and having a headache over the enormity of the effect of my decision. My whole life was about to change. Needless to say, I succumbed and accepted his offer. I officially began working as a partner within the National Health Service on 1 April 1977. April Fools' Day! And so, here I was, a foreigner, a West Indian, working within a predominantly Greek surgery where most of the patients and all of the staff were of Greek or Greek Cypriot descent. As such, it was necessary for me to have an interpreter with me during my consultations. It was a truly exciting time, which I enjoyed immensely. About 18 months after officially joining the practice, I remember looking at myself in the car mirror while driving to work one morning and thinking "My God! I'm really enjoying my work. I was born to be a GP." I have enjoyed my work ever since.'

*Source*: A. Kramer (2006) *Many Rivers to Cross: the history of the Caribbean contribution to the NHS*. London: Sugar Media.

# 1.4    The family system of care

In 1957, Peter Townsend, a young researcher (now Centennial Professor of Social Policy at the London School of Economics and Professor Emeritus at the University of Bristol), published his seminal study of the family life of old people living in Bethnal Green in the East End of London. In this short extract from Chapter 5 of the book he describes the family system of care and the importance of inter-generational reciprocity.

When there were several children the main burden of care often fell on the daughter who lived nearest, but she usually had some support from her brothers and sisters. The following is fairly typical of what happened in large families.

Mrs. Bliss was first interviewed a year before her final illness, and visited briefly many times. In her late seventies, she had five surviving sons and four daughters, all married. All except the youngest daughter and youngest son were living outside the borough. These two were both in the same block of flats, but she and her husband lived alone. When first interviewed she was still fairly well. Her youngest daughter did much of her cleaning and washing, and during a previous illness lasting ten weeks had left work to look after her. Her youngest son did various odd jobs for her. Her remaining children, whom she saw once a week or once a fortnight, did no regular jobs for her, but brought gifts and most gave her 2s. 6d. or 5s. when they came. When Mrs. Bliss had a succession of strokes her doctor tried to persuade her to go to hospital. She was very weak indeed. She and her family pleaded against this and her children organised a night-watching service for several weeks. On several occasions I saw a makeshift bed her son had put in her room. Her youngest son and daughter took it in turns to sit up with her for about two nights in three, but the other children gave them a break the remaining nights of the week. All the children visited her much more frequently and news was passed on daily from one telephone box to another. The youngest daughter left her work and the youngest son for a time too. Between them they did all the shopping and cleaning. The son lifted his mother when necessary and the daughter prepared meals and washed her. The husband, now very infirm, attended to some personal needs. On every visit I saw evidence – food, vases of flowers, sheets and blankets – of the devotion of her family.

Old people themselves were sometimes under considerable strain in caring for their husbands or wives or other relatives. In the care of their spouse 22% of the married people were experiencing strain at the time of the interview (6% severe and the rest moderate or slight). In the care of relatives other than a spouse, usually children or grandchildren, a few of whom were crippled or mentally defective, 12% experienced strain, none of it severe, however.

We started this chapter by examining the three types of family home, three, two and one generation, as a first step in finding how domestic affairs and illness were managed in old age. We found that one person in one dwelling was rarely living alone in any real sense. The domestic unit was generally spread over two or more households in proximity. We found old people getting a great deal of help, regularly and in emergencies, from their female relatives, particularly their daughters, living nearby. The remarkable thing was how often this help was reciprocated—through the provision of meals, the care of grandchildren and in other ways. The traffic was not all one way. This exchange of services seemed to be an essential feature of the relationship between the generations; this is one of the main conclusions of the book. The family system of care was mainly organised around female relatives, with an old grandmother at its centre. To find that there were limits to what it could do for old people, that it sometimes produced strain and that a minority of people fell outside its scope, simply because they had few or no surviving relatives, modifies, but does not alter, this conclusion.

*Source*: P. Townsend (1957) *The Family Life of Old People*. London: Routledge & Kegan Paul, pp. 59–61 [abridged].

# Chapter 2

## 'Kate': the constant rediscovery of a poem

*Joanna Bornat*

## 'Kate'

What do you see nurses
　　What do you see?
Are you thinking
　　when you are looking at me
A crabbit old woman
　　not very wise,
Uncertain of habit
　　with far-away eyes,
Who dribbles her food
　　and makes no reply,
When you say in a loud voice
　　'I do wish you'd try'.
Who seems not to notice
　　the things that you do,
And forever is losing
　　a stocking or shoe,

Who unresisting or not
　　lets you do as you will
With bathing and feeding
　　the long day to fill,
Is this what you're thinking,
　　is this what you see?
Then open your eyes nurse,
　　You're not looking at me.
I'll tell you who I am
　　as I sit here so still,
As I use at your bidding
　　as I eat at your will.
I'm a small child of ten
　　with a father and mother,
Brothers and sisters who
　　love one another,

This chapter is a revised and updated version of a paper that was originally published in *Generations* (2003), 27(5): 89–93.

A young girl of sixteen
　　with wings on her feet,
Dreaming that soon now
　　a lover she'll meet:
A bride soon at twenty,
　　my heart gives a leap,
Remembering the vows
　　that I promised to keep:
At twenty-five now
　　I have young of my own
Who need me to build
　　a secure happy home.
A young woman of thirty
　　my young now grow fast,
Bound to each other
　　with ties that should last:
At forty my young ones
　　now grown will soon be gone,
But my man stays beside me
　　to see I don't mourn:
At fifty once more
　　babies play round my knee,
Again we know children
　　my loved one and me.
Dark days are upon me,
　　my husband is dead,
I look at the future
　　I shudder with dread,

For my young are all busy
　　rearing young of their own,
And I think of the years
　　and the love I have known.
I'm an old woman now
　　and nature is cruel
'Tis her jest to make
　　old age look like a fool.
The body it crumbles,
　　grace and vigour depart,
There now is a stone
　　Where I once had a heart:
But inside this old carcass
　　a young girl still dwells,
And now and again
　　my battered heart swells,
I remember the joys,
　　I remember the pain,
And I'm loving and living
　　life over again,
I think of the years
　　all too few – gone too fast,
And accept the stark fact
　　that nothing can last.
So open your eyes nurses,
　　Open and see,
Not a crabbit old woman
　　look closer – see ME.

'Kate', or 'Crabbit old woman' or 'Open your eyes' – the lines come with different titles – is a poem which has become iconic within care delivery settings, training programmes and more generally in the UK. It is one of those few poems which has developed from its apparently humble vernacular and non-literary origins to be included in the curriculum for national exams for school students, to feature in a cinema advert for a national ageing charity and to be a typical example, 'canonised by public choice', of the nation's repertoire of memorable poems (*Guardian*, 1998).

The poem on its own might be considered remarkable enough to command such special attention but what provides it with a unique quality is the story of its origins. Each time the poem is presented as being 'discovered', in Scotland, Ireland or England, it is accompanied by the same account. The poem was found in the locker of a frail old woman who had been living on a hospital ward who was unable to speak but did occasionally write. After her death, when someone was sorting through her possessions the poem was found. This is the account given on first publication and, with a few variations, it has remained the standard story (Searle, 1973: 6–9).

I am not someone who has literary training so cannot really claim to make an informed judgement about the quality of the poem's language, style and meaning. However, I have always wondered about the story of the poem's origins and resisted its powers to seduce me into feeling guilty and unknowing. I wondered if others also were secretly ambivalent about what might be the true history of this poem.

# Finding 'Kate'

I decided to carry out a small piece of research by placing a letter in the magazine of the British Society of Gerontology, *Generations Review*, and in the Geriatric Nursing Newsletter of the Royal College of Nursing. I invited people to let me know when they first remembered reading the poem and also when they had most recently seen it published or referred to in any way. In all I received sixteen replies, one from as far away as Brisbane in Australia. Not surprisingly, most of the respondents were people working in nursing contexts or who had retired from nursing. Since then, and as people have come to know that I am interested in 'sightings' of the poem, I have continued to receive copies of documents such as church magazines and training materials where 'Kate' has appeared.

Amongst the responses I received two seem to me to be characteristically polarised. One was a true fan:

> This poem is one of those 'Do you remember where you were when you heard that Kennedy had died?' experiences for me! It was late autumn 1986, I was on a one year postgraduate CQSW [social work qualification] and I was reading an OU [Open University] reader about older people ... in the university library. 'Kate' was at the front of the book. The university library is a crowded and busy place and not one where you want to be seen with tears streaming down your face, so I remember snuffling into my handkerchief and feeling pretty self-conscious! However, whenever I come across the poem, the effect is the same. I guess I could be rational and put it down to sentimentality, but I prefer to think it's because, for me, it epitomises much of the truly shameful treatment of older people in many spheres of life, not least by services supposedly designed for them and probably some guilt for my own shortcomings (at least before I was more aware of them)!

Another sent me a contrasting account of her reactions:

> The first time I heard this was as a student nurse in 1977/8ish. It was given to us on a handout – photocopied from a nursing text (?). The last time was about two weeks ago [1998] on an early

morning Radio 4 programme – I think 'Something understood' at around 6.30am. In the intervening years it has appeared with monotonous regularity in any education/training programme for nurses related to care of older people ... Its popularity perhaps peaked at a time (late '70s and early 1980s) when there was a big emphasis on 'wrong' attitudes being at the root of all that was inadequate in hospital care of older people. I must say I got heartily sick of it and its sentimentality became increasingly cloying ...

People were able to tell me about the many different contexts in which they had seen the poem over the years. Apart from its contribution to their own training, they had seen it displayed in hospital wards, residential and nursing homes. As one retired officer-in-charge put it, 'I honestly don't believe until you know how it "feels" to be older and needing help you cannot work effectively with/for the elderly. "Look Closer" [sic] hits you right between the eyes, and I believe it says it all. I personally gave each of my staff a copy. They in turn told me that, yes, it did make a difference, it was like caring with older and wider eyes!!' One correspondent told me that she had seen 'Kate' included in a GCSE poetry reader as part of her English syllabus.

Gerontologists who were also educationalists had from an early stage identified the potential of 'Kate' as a means to induce reflection and empathy amongst students and colleagues. After first publication the poem went on to appear in other anthologies and eventually took its place in the gerontological curriculum, making its own contribution to the development of a biographical approach to work with older people both in academic and practice settings. Gerontological education in the UK has, since its early days, identified biography as a strongly enabling perspective, recognizing its potential for empathy and individualised care planning (Johnson, 1976; Carver and Liddiard, 1978; Bornat, 1989).

# Exploring its origins

So much for the feelings the poem evokes and its power to inform and educate, but what about its origins? I wanted to know more from the person who had first published it, what he thought about its literary and substantive provenance and how he had come by the poem. 'Kate' first appeared in a pamphlet of poetry, titled *Elders* written by older people, published in 1973 by Chris Searle, a radical writer and teacher. I interviewed him at Goldsmiths College, University of London in 1999, where he was then lecturing in educational studies. Chris Searle's view is that 'Kate' has 'a universality and a directness which penetrated deeply into young minds'(Searle, 1998: 44). He talked to me about the poem's achievement in terms of 'imaginative empathy' which he explains as 'using the imagination as a source of bonding and human connection'. He spoke of the poem as being enduringly powerful, a text which he has used with all sorts of groups, old, young and with children from quite diverse backgrounds: 'Pakistani, Yemeni, Caribbean children and they can all identify with it'.

'Kate' has powerful messages relating to gender and life meanings, he argues:

... it's a kind of 'everywoman' poem ... I remember when I read it feeling that there was an allegory within it of a person's life and the structure of a person's life, and a suggestion that she wasn't 'everywoman'. But at the same time it came back for me to the old kind of Solomon

Grundy myth, you know about 'born on a Monday, married on a Thursday' – you know, the whole notion that life is a narrative, from birth to death. And all the parts of living in between. It's an extraordinary poem.

As someone who was familiar with older people's long-term care, one of my reservations about 'Kate' was my inability to imagine how such a poem could come to be written by someone living on a continuing care ward. Lack of privacy, personal frailty and the imposition of routines do not create opportunities for creative activity, but Chris Searle was not fazed by this:

I don't think we'll ever know. I mean, I accepted it as authentic. And you know it could have been that it was a concoction by a nurse, or a relative, or by somebody who was masquerading as an old person. I find that difficult to believe, because it's got the – it's stacked with life experience, which I think is one reason why it's had a kind of mythical status since then. And it's also, because of its traditional form, it's a ballad. It has all the features of a ballad: the versification of a ballad, some of the stock images, like the wings on her feet, you know I mean they're clichés, but they're also the stock images of romantic ballads. And the fact that it uses life itself as its structure, again is you know something that you might encounter in Africa, in various parts of the world, which gives it that kind of universality... and the fact that it's an old woman speaking – you know, the notion of an old person reflecting, going back over their life, almost like a wise woman ... The whole issue is that Kate is determined that she's not going to be reified. You know, she's not going to be considered a 'thing'  ...she's human being. And it's a shout for humanity. That's what gives it its enormous power.

There seems to be no question as to the poem's literary merit, its powers to connect universally and its political messages. Does that make the question about its origins less relevant? Chris Searle had been the person who had first encountered 'Kate'. He explained how this came about:

Well it goes back to 1971 when I was a teacher in the East End, in Stepney. ... I was also involved at that time with a group called the London Old Age Pensioner's Trade Union Committee ... it was a kind of liaison committee of different trade union representatives who were campaigning for higher pensions ... we had a number of events. We had a poetry reading ... and invited a number of poets who were into their later years, but also young poets who were writing about the experience of age and trying to empathise with it and understand it. And...out of this came this anthology called Elders.

... the actual poetry that was being used was the poetry of the experience of elderly people. And there were some beautiful poems in the book, very stark, very moving. One of the poems that was sent to us was Kate's poem. Because I remember we left adverts in the local press, Left press, I think some of the pensioners' organisations, that we were looking for poems. And I got a poem sent to me, this poem, Kate's poem, from a nurse. And she'd typed this poem out and she said that this was a poem by this patient of hers who was – who appeared to be a mute – didn't speak at all. But constantly asked for pen and paper. I suppose through some kind of sign, or however she asked for it. And was seen to be writing on this paper in a shaky hand ... but didn't say anything to the nurse. And the nurse obviously cared for her and looked after her.

Chris Searle provides an expressive and historical account of 'Kate's' origins, enabling us to situate the poem's genesis at a particular point in political time when organisations of older people were developing more openly campaigning policies (Bornat, 1998).

Chris Searle's commitment to the story of 'Kate's' origins is convincing; however, amongst the correspondence I received, following my appeal, was a press cutting from the *Daily Mail*. Under the title, 'Poet was too shy for fame' and in answer to a reader's question about the origin of the poem, was a letter from Michael McCormack, who explained:

> My mother, Phyllis McCormack, wrote this poem in the early Sixties when she was a nurse at Sunnyside Hospital in Montrose.

> Originally entitled Look Closer Nurse, the poem was written for a small magazine for Sunnyside only Phyllis was very shy and submitted her work anonymously.

> A copy of the magazine was lent to a patient at Ashludie Hospital, Dundee, who copied it in her own handwriting and kept it in her bedside locker. When she died, the copy was found and submitted to the Sunday Post newspaper, attributed to the Ashludie patient.

> Since my mother's death in 1994 her work has travelled all over the world ... (*Daily Mail*, 1998)

This was fascinating and might have been the end of the story, but a more recent encounter with Michael McCormack suggests an added twist. Though Phyllis McCormack depicts the family-centred life of 'everywoman' it seems her own early life did not match up to this ideal. As her son explains, 'sadly Mum's life was nothing like as secure as ... Her mother died in 1916 when she was three years old and from then it seems as if she was passed, like the proverbial parcel, from home to home. ... she was very reticent about that part of her life so much of it is guesswork based on things she said at different times to different people over a long period of time. However it is pretty safe to say that Kate's life could well be the one she wished she'd had' (Personal communication, 18 September 2007). He remembers her writing the poem in the early 1960s and he thinks something had upset her and, because what she wrote sounded critical of colleagues, she wanted the poem to be published anonymously.

Whatever provoked Phyllis McCormack to write when she did, it is perhaps ironic that her own early identity is apparently so shrouded in mystery, though her own feelings about this may have contributed to the emotions she sought to convey in the poem.

# Reflecting on 'Kate'

It seems, if this really is the end to the quest, that the answer to the mystery of its origins was there all the time. Does it matter the 'Kate's' origins are less remarkable than we had thought, and, thirty years on, does 'Kate' speak in the same way to younger and older people? We may still need to be reminded of those silenced lived and hidden identities. However, times have changed, those impulses which drove Phyllis McCormack to write and Chris Searle to publish may still be there but do we read the poem differently? Biographical approaches to understanding ageing are now well accepted; does this therefore give the poem greater stature or perhaps make it more open to critical and more discerning analysis?

Perhaps the poem can be said to have continuing relevance if it enables us to evaluate critically those practices and attitudes which characterise care and support for frail older people. Indeed, with the advent of community care policies and the closure of so many long term care hospital wards 'Kate's' care is now everyone's responsibility, not just hospital nurses'.

However, a more critical approach to the poem might argue that it serves to distract us from the present person and their current needs by celebrating youthful vigour and reinforcing a view of ageing as loss and decline. Does it promote a particular normative and conforming type of biography in its formulation of everywoman's story while denying some of those positive and informative socio-cultural understandings of ageing which more recently gerontologists have come to identify in the lives of older women, and men? For example, Tom Kitwood's emphasis on 'personhood' in care work with people with dementia draws attention to the need to identify the human qualities of each individual (Kitwood, 1997), while Peter Coleman has identified the significance and content of meaning amongst frail people in late life (Coleman et al., 1998). At the same time the vocabularies of embodiment (Gubrium and Holstein, 1999) and well-being (Strawbridge et al., 2002) have also become part of our repertoire of recognition of each individual aged person. And, with her rather conventionally described life stages, are we led to believe that Kate in late life was without friendship (Jerrome, 1993), or opportunities for sociability and socialising in institutional settings (Adams et al., 1998; Hubbard et al., 2003) or the support offered by inter-generational ties (Wenger, 2001)? Her narrative offers us none of these insights.

That 'Kate' raises questions is confirmation that the poem still has a role to play, however often rediscovered, in informing, critiquing and theorising policy formation and practice relating to late old age. Although we might now question some of the meanings, hidden and not so hidden, and even accept that the story of 'Kate's' creation is a myth, it does mean that those of us who spend less time with art in our daily teaching and research may have to acknowledge that in provoking debate and emotions a poem can affect us directly, and powerfully, in ways that any number of academic presentations fail to achieve.

# References

Adams, J., Bornat, J. and Prickett, M. (1998) 'Discovering the present in stories about the past', in A. Brechin, J. Walmsley, J. Katz and S. Peace (eds), *Care Matters: Concepts, Practice and Research in Health and Social Care*. London: SAGE, pp. 27–41.

Bornat, J. (1989) 'Oral history as a social movement: reminiscence and older people', *Oral History*, 17(2): 16–24.

Bornat, J. (1998) 'Pensioners organise: hearing the voice of older people', in M. Bernard and J. Phillips (eds), *The Social Policy of Old Age: Moving into the 21st Century*. London: Centre for Policy on Ageing, pp. 183–199.

Carver, V. and Liddiard, P. (eds) (1978) *An Ageing Population: A Reader and Sourcebook*. London: Hodder & Stoughton, pp. ix–x.

*Daily Mail* (1998) 12 March, p. 56.

Coleman, P. G., Ivani-Chalian, C. and Robinson, M. (1998) 'The story continues: persistence of life themes in old age', *Ageing and Society*, 18(4): 389–419.

Gubrium, J. F. and Holstein, J. A. (1999) 'The nursing home as a discursive anchor for the ageing body', *Ageing and Society*, 19(5): 519–538.

Hubbard, G., Tester, S. and Downs, M. G. (2003) 'Meaningful social interactions between older people in institutional care settings', *Ageing and Society*, 23(1): 99–114.

Jerrome, D. (1993) 'Intimacy and sexuality amongst older women', in M. Bernard and K. Meade (eds), *Women Come of Age: Perspectives on the Lives of Older Women*. London: Edward Arnold, pp. 85–105.

Johnson, M. (1976) 'That was your life: a biographical approach to later life', in J. M. A. Munnichs and W. J. A. van den Heuvel (eds), *Dependency and Interdependency in Old Age*. The Hague, Netherlands: Martinus Nijhoff, pp. 147–161.

Kitwood, T. (1997) *Dementia Reconsidered: The Person Comes First*. Buckingham: Open University Press.

Searle, C. (ed.) (1973) *Elders*. London: Reality Press.

Searle, C. (1998) *None But Our Words: Critical Literacy in Classroom and Community*. Buckingham: Open University Press.

Strawbridge, W. J., Wallhagen, M. I. and Cohen, R. D. (2002) 'Successful aging and well-being: Self-Rated compared with Rowe & Kahn', *The Gerontologist*, 42(6): 727–733.

Wenger, G. C. (2001) 'Introduction: intergenerational relationships in rural areas', *Ageing and Society*, 21(5): 537–545.

# Acknowledgements

I would like to thank Chris Searle, Michael McCormack and Julia Johnson for their help as I wrote this chapter.

# Chapter 3

## 'Racist abuse ruined my life'

*Rosie Purves*

Rosie Purves, a black nurse who was prevented from looking after a white baby, won a racial discrimination claim against her employer in May this year. Ms Purves was awarded £10,000 – the highest payout possible for her type of claim after an employment tribunal ruled that Southampton University Hospitals NHS Trust was 'effectively silent and complicit' in the racist demands made by a woman who did not want her baby treated by black staff. Here Ms Purves tells *Nursing Times* her harrowing story of how for seven years she suffered this abuse in silence.

'I've been nursing since 1964 and have worked at Southampton University Hospitals Trust for nearly 30 years as a staff nurse in paediatrics. I've always loved my job. There has never been anything else I wanted to do. I love working with children. It is where I felt I could serve people best.

'But I've always had to prove myself – and if you talk to many black nurses they will also say they have had to prove that they are up to the job. I feel that because of my race I have to be even better, to work harder. It becomes normal – which doesn't make it right. It's only recently people are saying it's wrong and I don't think hundreds of us [black nurses] can misread a situation.

'The abuse started when a consultant in paediatrics told me that a mother didn't want me, or any other black person, looking after her child. I was horrified. It was nothing I could argue about. I am a good fighter and I don't keep quiet about most things, but I was ashamed that people could treat me like this. I didn't tell anybody.

'Over the years as a nurse I've looked after many of my children's friends. And many of their parents have said, "If it wasn't for your mum, our child wouldn't be here". My family had always regarded it as being great that I was a nurse. I felt I'd let them down in some way [when I was stopped from looking after the child]. Logic didn't come into it.

'Nobody at the hospital apologised. The priority was the child, according to the consultant. The team was saying, "We don't see you as being black" but they were still prepared to move the child. I went along with it.

'I work weekends mainly, so if the child came into hospital, by Friday the mum would ask for the child to be moved so that they would not be on the side of the ward I

Originally published in the *Nursing Times* (2004) 100(32): 24–25.

was working on. The child had a long-term condition so was regularly in hospital. At least three times a year I was put through this for two or three weeks at a time. Most of my colleagues went along with it. It was an unspoken thing.

'I felt alone. I felt there was no one there for me really but I had to keep my chin up. I thought everyone was colluding with the mother to keep themselves safe. I feel that by moving the baby the other staff were sending out the message that it was OK to be racist. Then for two years I had a break from the situation when the child went to another hospital in 1997. The mother and child came back in 2000 and it started all over again.

'I put a brave face on at work, then I would come home and dissolve into tears at night. People said, "What's the matter with Rosie, she's so quiet at work?" It was affecting me – I was getting depressed. I thought about it all the time. I would be at a child's bedside and the pleasure in my work would come back. But I was always frightened they [the mother and child] would come in.

'In 2002 the mother got a second mum involved. She was also bringing her child to the hospital the two mothers had become friends. The second mother started to abuse me. She said to my face, "Don't go anywhere near my f**king child, I don't want people like you looking after my child, and that is my right".

'I decided that after seven years of silence I had to tell someone. I then went to the manager of the paediatric unit and told her what was going on. They asked me to put it in writing and to attend a meeting. I thought, "I'm not going to a meeting on my own" and I got my union [the Transport and General Workers Union] involved. They attended all the meetings about my case with me.

'At this time I was also attending as a Nurse at a special needs school. The second mother had a sister who attended the school. I started getting abuse there as well from the sister who would talk about "black jelly babies". I thought, "I can't take this any more".

'I went to the head of department at the school and said that I couldn't cope any more. He called the family in straightaway for a meeting. He was very stern and said if there was any more abuse at the school the child would be asked to leave. So the school took action but the hospital did not.

'One day my manager [at the hospital] rang my son and said, "I think you better go home and see your mum" and that's who told my family what was going on. My family was upset and angry but very supportive. All those years when I never told them, I felt that I had to protect them somehow. I was protecting a lot of people apart from myself.

'In the end I had to go to occupational health. I told them the whole story and they wrote a letter to my doctor asking for me to be signed off work. I was off work between September 2003 and February 2004 I went for counselling but I knew what the problem was. I was so desperate – I had had enough and I wanted somebody to listen to me.

'The union was very supportive and said, "let's take it to a tribunal". The trust cancelled the first appointment for the tribunal, which was set for July last year. Eventually it was held in April this year.

'One brave nurse who attended the tribunal gave a statement on my behalf. She said that everyone knew about it [the mother refusing to let Ms Purves treat her child] and that's what we had to do. She said that she was asked one day to move a child and when asked why, was told, "Because mum doesn't want Rosie or any black person to look after their child." She said she realised she should have challenged this but didn't.

'The chairman of the tribunal went in my favour and accused the trust of being "silently complicit" and awarded me £20,000 in compensation. The trust has since moved both mothers to another hospital. I returned to work from sick leave just before the tribunal. I don't want to be there but I feel I've started something I need to finish. I know the trust has brought in nurses from the Philippines, Africa, India. I've got to give them voice. It's too late for me but this mustn't happen to anyone else.

'I'm relieved about the verdict but this whole experience has knocked my confidence. It has made me self-conscious. I'm in a turmoil when meeting new parents – I wonder, will they accept me?

'Then I feel guilty and think why did I mistrust them?

'Since winning the tribunal, other people from all over the country have contacted me and have told me they have experienced similar abusive situations – one man was even in tears on the phone to me about the verbal abuse he was suffering at work.

'Racist abuse ruined my life. If I could put the clock back I would put my pride aside and speak up. Verbal abuse needs to be tackled. As nurses we accept patient anxiety, but we don't have to put up with abuse – not verbal, not racist, not any form of abuse. Management has got to respond to the problem.

'I'd like to see verbal abuse wiped out. I'd like to see posters go up to make patients and relatives aware of it – that verbal abuse will not be tolerated, that if they are abusive they will be asked to leave. Nurses should have the right to refuse treatment. I really do believe that.

'Winning the tribunal was not about the money. I've been asked, "How are you going to spend it?" But it's not happy money. When I do feel happy about the money I shall do something nice with the kids – but not until this feeling of sadness about what has happened to me has gone.'

# Chapter 4

## Portering

*Polly Toynbee*

*In the early 2000s,* Guardian *journalist, Polly Toynbee, decided to find out what living on the minimum wage was like. She moved into a council flat in Clapham Park, London and took up whatever work was on offer at the job centre. This included being a dinner lady and a cleaner, working in a call centre, a cake factory and a care home. She wrote about her experiences in her book* Hard Work: Life in Low-pay Britain. *In this extract from the book, she describes being sent by an agency to work as a porter at the Chelsea and Westminster Hospital.*

[...]

I arrived at the hospital, hoping my makeshift second-hand uniform would do, exactly a quarter of an hour early for the shift, as required. That extra unpaid hour and quarter a week was something demanded in every job I did. In each job I always had to be ready in uniform in some distant part of the building well before the official paid start of the shift. I found the porters' room in the basement at the back of the hospital in a far underground recess, a tiny cramped space where two controllers were sitting in front of computers and telephones. They were taking orders from all the wards and clinics in the building, logging the jobs on to computer worksheets and then assigning them to porters in rotation through their radios.

'Is this the porters' lodge?' I asked a thin, grey-haired Asian man, as he put down the telephone and looked me up and down.

'What can I do for you?' he asked politely.

'I'm the new porter, from Grange Executives.'

'You!' he said. I panicked at once – wrong age, wrong clothes, wrong demeanour, something wrong altogether?

'You weren't expecting me?' I asked.

'We never know what to expect from agencies,' he said with a deep sigh. Then he put his head back and laughed. The other controller looked at me and laughed too. I felt terrible. 'Whatever next!' he said and I thought they might send me away. Seeing my embarrassment, he learned forward and patted my arm kindly. 'No offence. We just had your surname but we were not expecting a lady. We never had a lady porter before.'

From P. Toynbee (2003) *Hard Work: Life in Low-pay Britain*. London: Bloomsbury, pp. 57–72.

'That's what I said at the agency. I asked if this wasn't a man's job, but they said no. Is it very heavy lifting? Is it something a woman can't do?'

The controller was at once contrite and friendly. 'Not at all, not at all! Of course there's no reason why you can't. We shall be very pleased. It just took us by surprise, you see?'

Mr Patel, known as Mr P, turned out to be a gentle man, quietly elegant and courteous, a porter for twenty-eight years, first in the old hospital, now in the new one.

'No, no, we give you a very big welcome and of course I am sure you can do the job very well. But people will be a little bit surprised to see a lady porter, you see? But no problem, no problem at all!'

After that, he was unfailingly kind. Everyone liked him.

Next door was the small porters' rest-room with chairs and a table grouped round the television alongside a microwave, a fridge and a hot-water urn. Mr P introduced me to the men getting ready for their shift and jaws dropped with a bit of sniggering banter about a woman porter. But soon most were friendly enough. My age was not the problem I thought it would be – some of them were older than me. One night porter I met had retired and then unretired again at seventy, finding himself too short of money. As for my general demeanour, I don't know what they thought but I soon discovered that a curious array of people from all kinds of backgrounds fetch up here and in most low-paid jobs, for any number of reasons. This I found time and again: there is a conspiratorial democracy in minimum-wage jobs, everyone levelled down by the lowness of the wage that binds people together. A middle-class accent is an irrelevance down in the fraternity of low pay.

Here many of the porters saw themselves as either on the way up or having fallen down: few regarded these jobs as their natural lot in life. Many had stories they were eager to tell of more prosperous days, of having tumbled down to this level from better lives in the past. Others, the younger ones, lived with their dreams of what was still to come, of somehow working their way up. But most were family men, just earning a living as best they could, working as many shifts as they could manage, some with second jobs elsewhere. I fitted in well enough, once they got used to a woman.

Most porters were dressed in smart white shirts with plum-coloured company ties and navy V-necks emblazoned with Carillion, the logo of the company that employs all the non-medical staff. Whatever else, private companies are good at eye-catching uniforms, branding their employees all over, offering a reassuring appearance of confidence and affluence whatever the reality beneath the logos. In the hospital now everyone below the rank of nurse – all the cleaning, catering, portering, technical and other non-medical staff – work for Carillion not the NHS. Or at least they work for Carillion in principle but in practice, as I soon discovered, many of those wearing the Carillion colours were, like me, employed by agencies, working for the proliferating array of agencies around the fringes of London. I was working not at one but at two removes from the national health service, lower paid and more insecure than even the Carillion workers, who were themselves lower paid and more insecure with worse pensions than thirty years ago.

Hanging my coat on a corner peg, I was put with Samuel for the morning. Samuel was a Jamaican in his forties who had worked in the hospital since he arrived in England some years ago. Like many of the others, he said he was not planning to stay much longer, eager to get back to Kingston, Jamaica and set up his own taxi firm again. His 'useless' brother had driven the last one into the ground. In his head he was not a hospital porter at all but a small businessman. He had two children in school in London, and he worried about them. Would they get on, do well, pass exams? He worked exceptionally long shifts to pay for his family, while his wife worked as a cook. 'You can't survive, not with a family, unless you do the long, long hours, unless you both work all the hours there are,' he said. He was concerned about his children being left alone too long, because of the combined working hours of him and his wife. I witnessed this frequently: good parents who earn so little they are reluctantly forced to become bad parents by working overlong hours to make ends meet. Many said they would work shorter hours if they could find higher-paid jobs.

One porter had been a high-earning, self-employed electrician on building sites until he had a heart attack and had to take a less stressful job. 'The walking all day here is very good for me, the doctor says. But my standard of living fell through the floor since I got sick.' There was an accountant from Russia whose English was execrable: he read the encyclopaedia every night in his bedsit to try to improve it, hoping to be able to move up into an accounting department of the hospital one day. But there was no ladder up, no encouragement. In some hospitals the union, Unison, runs English language courses for foreign staff. It would not cost much for the NHS or for the contractors to run on-site basic literacy and numeracy classes everywhere. Another porter, Olly, ran an elaborate and incomprehensible Irish social security scam from his farm in Ireland, with its sixty sheep and twenty-four cows. It somehow concerned the fact he looked exactly like his brother. There was Francisco from the Philippines who had been an embassy butler for twenty years, until he took to the bottle. Anyway, he said, the money in butlering was just as bad and the hours far worse: he was full of horror stories of how badly he had been treated, working from dawn until the small hours with no overtime pay. Most people had their own private explanations for why they had ended up in a dead-end job: desire to work in the health service for the greater good of public service was not at the top of their list. But then no one had ever suggested to them that they were an integral and valued part of the institution or that they could contribute more.

Samuel was a good explainer and guide, for at first this huge place was a daunting maze. Maybe it was a test, but during my time at the hospital the only heavy lifting job I was given was the first one that morning. We were sent to collect hefty tables from the Hospital Friends Library to set up in the main atrium for a sale of toys and books the Friends held every day to raise money. An old lady Friend who ran the library gave us each a Kit Kat. 'She always does that,' Samuel said. 'That's why we are desirous to do this particular job in the mornings.' He had that West Indian-educated use of a wide and flowery vocabulary from a good old-fashioned schooling, spoken in a strong accent.

I had to learn not just the names and locations of thirty-two wards spread across the top four floors (which, confusingly, were not numbered but named), but also myriad clinics, X-ray departments, CT, MRI, haematology, pathology, various out-patient departments, the many mansions within A & E and all the specialist labs with their own acronyms and abbreviations. It needed a taxi-driver's brain to absorb maybe a hundred locations. Messages would come through on the radio; 'Samuel and Olly, go to Adele Dixon and take Kamal Abdullah on a bed to OP3.' Moving patients in beds was a two-porter job and Samuel showed me how to fix the bed's brakes, pump up the height, watch out for the weights if patients were in traction and trundle them down the long walkways to the lifts, find the right clinic, park them in the passage and hand in their notes at the clinic desk. This we did all morning, wheeling beds up and down and in and out of clinics and wards, the old, the young, the unconscious and the snoring, patients with drips and oxygen, patients who moaned, others who were embarrassed at these very public bed-journeys in nightdresses and hospital gowns, naked down the back.

By the afternoon I was given a radio, a map and a list of locations to find my own way around. There were too few leather pouches for carrying the heavy radios so porters hoarded them jealously, hiding them in secret places for their next shift. That meant I had to carry mine in my hand all the time while pushing people in wheelchairs. Next day I brought in a black leather belt-bag from home that just about fitted the radio, plus an essential notebook ready to take down the details of each job. In my second-hand black trousers, jumper and white polo shirt (of which more later), I did not look as smart as the men with their neat leather pouches and Carillion ties, but the belt-bag worked and left both hands free for wheeling. How important small irritations are at work, when repeated all day long. Enough radio pouches for all porters was just the kind of niggling request Carillion ignored. 'We ask, we keep asking, nothing happens,' Samuel said with a shrug. 'It is always the same thing.'

Once alone, I was often lost, wheeling people up and down, in and out, and sometimes round and round hoping they didn't notice us passing the same spot twice looking for the George Watts Dermatology Clinic or the Physio Gym. The radio messages were hard to hear. The various controllers all had their own accents, some so strong the porters often asked to have messages repeated. Porters from all nationalities, some speaking little English, were trying to understand English spoken in a variety of ways, from Mr P's Indian accent to another's Filipino, to thick Scots and other less identifiable accents all calling out names of wards and patients over the crackling airwaves. It meant much guesswork, writing down the sounds and hoping for the best. As you arrived in a ward with a half-heard, half-guessed genderless name of a patient, the nastier nurses would often give a snort and say tartly, 'No, no one here of that name!' In several wards there were running battles between porters and nurses who liked to chide and sneer at us. Sometimes you would stand at the nursing desk for five minutes waiting for one of them to deign to break off to speak to you. In other wards, kindly nurses went out of their way to avoid wasting your time.

Then there was the wheelchair problem: there were never enough of them. Often I spent twenty minutes searching every ward and corridor, hunting through out-patient departments and occasionally finding a secret trove piled up on the ground floor at the patient transport exit. Fifteen minutes was assigned to every wheelchair job, twenty minutes to a bed journey, so failing to find chairs was a cause for anxiety. Sometimes porters would try to hide a spare one in a back lift area or behind a door, but usually another porter would find it and whisk it away. The wheelchair hunt was a constant source of irritation among porters, another of those petty meannesses that cost a great deal of time. Worse, some of the wheelchairs had wheels as bad as broken supermarket trolleys, some had jammed brakes, so that dragging a patient backwards was the only way to go. Complaints had been made many times, but to no avail.

On the notice board in the porters' rest-room minutes of the last Carillion Staff Forum registered yet another complaint about wheelchair shortages that nothing had been done about. These minutes were revealing of what was happening in other departments, too. A cleaner had raised the issues of mops: 'Mops were being shared and the same mop was being used to clean the toilets and wards. She (the complainant) added that she even had to buy a dustpan and brush from her own money.' Another complaint came from the staff on the front desk who 'raised the issue that there were still no seats on reception and that the heated floor was causing them to go home with swollen ankles. Quesioning why the staff couldn't sit down, the reply was that they were not allowed to sit behind the counter.' Another complaint was of 'a general lack of equipment in the hospital in both the portering and estates department'. All these and more complaints were handled within Carillion between managers and workers of the company, nothing to do with the NHS management who had effectively lost control. These were not, after all, NHS staff any longer.

If it wasn't for the miserable pay, however, this could have been a good and satisfying job. Although it meant walking all day on an eight-hour shift with only a half-hour break for lunch, it was a pleasing building and a purposeful job. Trundling along, waiting for lifts, patients liked to chat and tell their operation stories, worrying about what was happening next, confiding about their families or the doctors and nurses they liked or feared. The porters seemed like the life-blood of the place or perhaps like the engine oil that greased the system, fetching and carrying, finding out everything that was happening, well-conversant with the pleasant and unpleasant staff in different locations. We knew the snappy receptionists in some clinics, the downright rude nurses in some wards, the very friendly ones elsewhere, the places where nurses would let you stop for a quick coffee, other kitchens where you would be chased away. An arrogant male staff nurse was the worst, 'You, porter person, come here!' he snapped at me my first day with deep disdain, as if he hadn't also crossed a traditional gender line. Nurses complained porters were bone idle, porters complained nurses did nothing all day but chat. Neither was often true. It was ever thus, the notch above in the hierarchy is always the class in any workplace that gives you a hard time, the kulaks, the foremen.

This was hospital life from the underside, where the passing doctors belonged in another universe, even the young medical students. (They never held the door open for a porter with a patient, letting it swing without acknowledgement.) The nurses straddled the two worlds, snooty ones pointedly placing themselves beyond communication with porters or cleaners, the nice ones helpful and welcoming. You could bet those who were nice to porters were nice to patients too. But there was no predicting, no useful stereotype – neither age, gender, race nor nationality predisposed good or bad nature. There were friendly Africans and surly angry ones, cheerful Australians and grudging ones, older nurses who might be abrupt or warmly helpful.

One thing became clear: people are recognised more by their status than by their face. I was now a porter first, myself second. Passing by in the corridors and in the wards, I saw several consultants I had interviewed in the past; one whom I knew quite well had treated both my daughter and myself. Once I saw a patient I knew. But porters are part of the invisible below-stairs world, the great unnoticed. No one ever recognised me.

Desperately anxious to please in my first days, I worried about being late or lost or having no wheelchair for a job. So I scuttled furiously from place to place, eager to radio in the moment a job was done, with a breathless 'Job completed!' like a kind of Joyce Grenfell on speed. The number of jobs each of us completed per day was listed on the computer worksheets and I feared falling behind the others. As the only woman porter, I had something to prove. But on the second day Samuel said to me, 'Cool it, chill out, man.' He tugged me into the back area by the service lifts where several porters were leaning against the wall for a few minutes' rest where they couldn't be seen by Big John, the boss, if he happened to pass by on the prowl. I didn't meet Big John for days but watched out warily for anyone who might be him, well warned by the others. We perched on an old upturned shelf behind the door near out-patients, eking out any spare time, making sure each job was checked in at fifteen minutes, never less.

Some jobs took longer because a patient was not ready or took time to shift into a chair. Sometimes a patient would be surrounded by a doctor and his entourage and we had to wait at a respectful distance. Sometimes a patient was still very slowly eating lunch, not to be rushed. Some patients were just bloody-minded and refused to move. There was the mountainous woman with terrible sores on her legs, a job everyone dreaded because she was bossy and bad-tempered, obviously in great pain. She needed the Fat Boy, a special extra-wide wheelchair that had to be collected from the basement, and she took a long time to manoeuvre into it. Jobs took longer when a lift was out of order: waiting for lifts wasted as much time as hunting for wheelchairs. So jobs could take longer than their allotted time but the porters' private code said a job should never, ever, take less than fifteen minutes. 'Why are you scurrying around like a mad rabbit?' Samuel said. 'Wait a bit. Take it easy, pace yourself.' It was good advice. I realised that in my anxiety I had got ahead of the others in jobs checked into the computer.

When the hospital services were first privatised, Carillion (then called Tarmac) had the first contract and cut back many jobs, including porters. 'How else do you think they were going to make their money?' Samuel said. Later Carillion cut staff numbers again. Mr P described how they had started with sixteen porters before privatisation but were now cut down to eleven, although the numbers of jobs grew all the time with an ever-faster throughput of patients. 'They promised no cuts when they privatised but of course we could all see this would happen, and it did. Now they are talking of cutting two more. How, I ask you, are we to get the work done?' That Saturday, there had been just one porter on duty who had complained vigorously that the workload was impossible. That pattern, I later discovered, exactly mirrored what happened everywhere after contracting-out began. Every report and study records how pay and conditions were cut and work was made harsher as staff were shed. It goes on still, this paring down to the bone, cutting right into the bone at times.

So if we lingered by the lifts to ensure no job was ever done in under fifteen minutes, there was a purpose. These men had learned through experience to give no inch because, every time they did, it was taken advantage of. If the time-and-motion men studying our computer printouts saw that some jobs were done faster, they would never understand why other jobs took so much longer. They would assume we could work all the time at the speed of the fastest jobs. They would never take account of the mountainous lady with the seeping legs or the old woman who cried for ten minutes about her dog before I could coax her into the wheelchair, or the time I stayed with a frightened woman gripping my hand while she waited for her X-ray when I should have been off calling back to base.

Being nice to patients was not designed into the job; quite the contrary. Samuel explained, 'Never touch a patient. That is the company rule. Touching patients, helping them into wheelchairs, is nurses' work, not ours. We have been told never to touch a patient even just on the arm because if they fall they might sue Carillion.' By then I had heaved countless patients in and out of wheelchairs when there was no nurse in sight to help. Very frail old people slowly edging out of their chairs at risk of tumbling and breaking bones needed an arm. I had thought portering meant, well, portering, carrying things and especially people if need be. That was certainly the case thirty years ago when the porters always helped the nurses to carry patients. But since the work has been contracted out, that kindly part of the job appears to have been written out of the contract specification altogether. Whatever is not specified in cold contractual print does not happen.

'We are not trained in lifting so the company tell us never to lift people,' another porter said, too. This was lunchtime, sitting round in the porters' room, and the others joined in. Yes, definitely, absolutely, only nurses were allowed to touch patients. Yes, they agreed, as a result diminutive nurses heaved about hulking great patients while porters had to stand by with their arms crossed because that is what Carillion declared. The nurses were not Carillion and they were covered by NHS hospital insurance if they harmed themselves or a patient sued, so it was OK for them. Insurance matters more than anything, never mind the nonsense of able-bodied porters standing there watching nurses struggle unaided.

That was just another unintended consequence of privatisation. Most of the porters were decent people, not really jobsworths, and I saw them lending a hand more often than not. I often saw them help out with patients in ways that were not in their job description. But they said they could be disciplined if found physically aiding patients, though yes, many of them said, of course it should be part of their job. Osman, a suave Iranian porter, said a patient had fallen yesterday when she stood up to get into his wheelchair. He did lift her up because he couldn't just leave her lying there, whatever Carillion said. 'But maybe the company could be sued.' The effect of the litigation mentality that now poisons many aspects of NHS life is exacerbated by private companies' over-anxiety to protect themselves.

Worse was the lack of any idea that we should play a part in caring for the patients. We would park them in corridors and outpatient queues, many of them old, confused, frightened and needing a friend. Although mostly the system worked well and they didn't wait too long before being taken back to the wards, there were plenty of days when people in distress or pain, lost and dumped, begged me to take them back to their wards. 'You brought me down, can't you just take me back?' they would cry out as I hurried by.

One woman was in tears because her friend was waiting for her upstairs and, although her X-ray had been done two hours ago, she was still waiting to be wheeled back again. It would not have taken long, I wanted to do it for her, but no, I could not, it was more than my job was worth. I did, nervously, ask the particularly brusque ward clerk in X-ray if he could call my controller and request a porter, then I might be assigned the job to take her back. The ward clerk barked out an unsympathetic answer, rightly taking it as a personal criticism that he had left a plainly distressed woman sitting there in front of his nose for so long. All the same, out of his earshot I also called my controller to ask if I could take her, but he said firmly the job had to wait to come up in its turn. So I had to leave her there. No initiative was permitted, no extra kindness nor any chance to step in and put right something that had gone wrong. Just follow instructions, that was all the company required. In the end that lack of initiative is what makes any job unbearable.

Big John was a powerful man. I felt his unseen hand long before I came across him, for he set the rota and said yea or nay to requests for shift changes. (His answer to my request for a shift change had been relayed back as a nay.) He was short and rotund, black, with the officious air of managerial importance that came with his Carillion blazer. 'So you are the new woman porter?' he said to me suddenly one day as I was walking out of A & E. 'How do you like the job?'

I said I liked it fine.

'You think you will stay?'

I said I was thinking about it. The job was fine – which it was – but the problem was the pay.

'Maybe you will become permanent when you have worked out your time with the agency,' he said. Maybe, I replied, but the money would still be a problem. 'You would move up to £4.85 an hour then,' he said. He was having difficulty with the high turnover of staff which the other porters said was getting worse month by month, with more agency workers and more people passing through for a short time.

Now I had the chance, I asked what the prospects were for some kind of training to get a better job later on? He thought about it and suggested, 'You could do training in restraint and calming methods. That gives you a certificate so you could work in security.' A security job would be no better paid with no better prospects than portering. Otherwise it seemed that Carillion was offering no inducements with any vision of a path upwards to a better career in the hospital some time in the future. Growing and developing staff was probably not high on Carillion's agenda for staff at the bottom. Big John looked at his watch and said, 'I hope you decide to stay,' which was gratifying, and he glided away on his rounds.

I had my doubts about how long it would be before I might be made permanent if I did stay on. In theory, after three months I would be free of the agency and allowed to apply for an interview to be taken on by Carillion with all the rights and conditions of a member of their staff. It seemed to make sense that Carillion should want to take on any agency workers as soon as possible. After all, they were paying some £7–8 an hour to these agencies to employ people who only received £4.35 of that. Why shouldn't the company want to end this waste as soon as possible? But it didn't work that way, either deliberately or out of managerial inefficiency.

A good example came from Winston, an earnest young black porter who talked about his working conditions while we were waiting together for a patient outside A & E. Although he was wearing the smart Carillion uniform, he said he was still trapped working with his agency in Catford after a year of portering in the hospital. He was given the Carillion uniform because his working life was so complicated he often couldn't get home to change his clothes. He lived in Edmonton, took a course in IT in central London and often did double shifts to cut down on his travelling time. His journey from home to the hospital took him two hours by train and two buses and cost him £74 a month. 'I have filled out the application form to be taken on by Carillion so I can move up to the £4.85 rate. I keep asking for an interview with Big John but they keep putting it off. They say yes, I will get an interview, then nothing happens. I keep asking, but I just get excuses. I don't know what else to do now. One porter filled out the Carillion application three times; they kept doing nothing about it and then he started to get angry. He started coming in late and answering back, then they told him to go. I know how he felt.'

It would make a big difference to Winston's pay. It was not just the job security and the extra rights; it was not just the extra 50p an hour. If he was taken on to the staff, he explained, he would get time and half for his overtime and double time for Sundays. As I knew, because I had signed the same terms and conditions, any overtime for agency staff was paid at the regular flat rate. 'I worked twenty-one hours in a row last week,' he said. 'That would be a lot of overtime money if I was staff. But they just won't give me that interview. It costs them too much.' There were other staff perks too. One of the older porters who had stayed on from the old hospital told me the Carillion staff got a £180 a month Inner London weighting allowance, plus a £180 a month bonus. This was on top of a £4.55 an hour pay rate, plus overtime. Why £4.55? He didn't know.

The pay structure was Byzantine because everyone I asked (they were all quite happy to discuss their payslips) came up with slightly different sums per hour or different bonuses for reasons they could not really explain. £4.85 was the highest hourly rate I encountered, while the bonus had no clarity about it, either in who got it or what exactly it was a bonus for. (Later a union official explained why employers prefer adding bonuses: if they raise the base rate it would also raise the time-and-a-half overtime rates.) Porters who rotated at the controllers' desk, operating the telephones and computers, were paid a little more for those shifts, but not enough for many of them to strive for that job. Many preferred the freedom of walking the hospital to sitting in this poky underground dungeon all day with the added anxiety in busy times of hot pressure when nurses and clinics were shouting for porters and couldn't get through on the telephones. Often by the time they did get through they were already angry at the shortage of porters.

Winston blamed Big John personally for refusing to give him the interview to transfer him from the agency on to the Carillion books but it was far more likely to be company policy higher up the line. Big John, for all his airs, was only a small jump up from the rest of the porters. Winston was particularly gloomy that day: 'You can try really hard at this job, like I do, but you just get nowhere. I work and work, I never hang about, I try to get noticed so they will transfer me. But in the end I can see I will get like some of the old ones, the ones who keep telling you to slow down all the time. That's the way it is, no reward for hard work here.' If he could only pass his IT qualifications, he would be off and away but he said his hard working life with its gruelling and expensive travelling made getting to his IT classes increasingly difficult and he wasn't sure he would make it to the end of the course. He wanted to get married, but life was just too hard at the moment.

Later that day Winston and I were talking to Steve, a dapper porter in his thirties with a grey-streaked quiff. 'You ask Steve,' Winston said. 'He's in the same position as me.' Steve nodded and said, 'I don't know if it's something I do or if maybe they don't like my face, my face don't fit or something, you know what I mean? Why is it I fill out the Carillion application form three times and three times I ask for an interview, but they will not give me it. I cannot get this transfer from the agency to the company. I wait, wait, wait, but nothing happens.' His wife was a cleaner in the hospital, and they worked alternate shifts so they could take it in turns to be home for their children. The result was that they rarely saw one another.

Winston was right about one or two of the older ones who were not paragons of porterly virtue. Irish Olly was the most adamant member of the 'slow-down' faction. He was as idle as he could manage, skulking about, stirring up trouble wherever he could. He picked arguments, teased and bullied in surreptitious ways but, when I turned on him once, he just waved his hands in the air and said, 'No harm meant. Just joking! You've got to have a laugh, haven't you now?' in a thicker than usual Irish brogue, as if blarney would always get him out of it, but he lacked charm. You had to watch out for him as he picked on newcomers to torment. He would mock and mimic foreign accents or small things people got wrong, as when I reported through my radio 'Job finished' on my first day and he made fun of me for not saying 'Job completed, over and out', like the others. Once I saw him hold on to the back of the Hospital Friends' trolley so that the elderly volunteer wheeling along her array of Lucozade, knitting wools, newspapers, sweets and Kleenex tugged and pulled but couldn't understand why the thing wouldn't budge.

He had strong dislikes and deliberately got me into trouble on my first day with another porter who was his old enemy. A Malaysian porter had stopped to talk to someone in one room, foolishly leaving his empty wheelchair outside in the corridor. 'Take that one!' Olly hissed at me. In all innocence I did as he said and he told me to hurry, hurry away with it to the lift. By the time the Malaysian came out I was wheeling it down the walkway and he shook a very angry but safely distant fist at me, cursing under his breath, giving me black looks thereafter. Olly, of course, had nipped out of sight, leaving me to take the blame. Dull jobs breed petty rows and rivalries that reminded me of school. Olly was keen to confide in me, tell me the wheezes and ways round things but I avoided being taken under his wing.

Winston and Olly were from opposite ends of the public-service spectrum. I saw them as the two distant poles, North and South, that represented political perceptions of the public sector and its workers. If Tony Blair and most of his ministers are ambivalent about public servants, it is because they have both Winston and Olly in mind. One day there will be fulsome political praise for the hard work, devotion, enthusiasm and determination to get trained and move up of a Winston. Thinking of the Winstons ministers will talk of the need for more money, more training, more support and even more pay for public-sector workers. Then in the same breath they will spoil it all by remembering the Ollys and talk threateningly of the need for 'reform' to go hand in hand with any extra money. The code is well-understood. It means no more money for the Ollys unless they show better spirit, harder work with more motivation, more flexibility in working practices and willingness to take on other tasks. Fair enough – but this carrot-and-stick language is desperately wrong-headed. To be sure, every workplace has its Olly quota of shirkers and grumblers but in this hospital, among the porters, nurses and clinic staff, the enthusiastic, well-motivated Winstons I came across outnumbered the Ollys ten to one.

# Chapter 5

## The insider researcher

*Howard Mitchell*

As a novice, starting project work for the first time, my concept of academic research included the assumption that a necessarily detached standpoint was required in the search for objective truths. Like many, I had some hazy image of research which was based on the natural sciences; the laboratory, the white coat, the breakthrough. With the social sciences, fieldwork replaced the laboratory, but for many years the methodologies of the more established and higher-status sciences provided the template for research. With this template came the associated premise: knowledge is a neutral portrayal of fact achieved through impartial collection and analysis of data. […]

My initial grasp of research and the little I had discovered of methodological theory provided me with problems concerning the area that I wanted to do my own research in.

I was no 'outsider' and I did not want to describe any 'otherness'. I was an insider to the subject area and many of the people and practices I wished to investigate. Could I be 'scientific' and objective with a subject I was so familiar with and just where and how would I address this or even acknowledge this in my work? I had no theoretical framework to apply.

## My insider status

I was born in Lennox Castle Hospital in 1955. For 23 years, several of the wards which were purpose built for patients with a mental deficiency were converted for use as a maternity unit. I grew up in the village of Lennoxtown, living 400 metres from the hospital entrance. My family were in the minority in our street in that none of us worked in 'The Castle' at that time. I could not help but be aware of the institution throughout my childhood. Sunday walks were often along the hospital drive and around part of the grounds and the staff housing. We would usually be engaged in conversation by some of the patients and the redbrick villa where I was born was pointed out.

This chapter was commissioned for the first edition where it first appeared.

In our block of terraced council housing the three other families consisted of:

> husband and wife, both nurses at Lennox Castle;
> mother, son and daughter, all Castle nurses and the father, latterly boiler room
>    worker;
> father (Castle van driver) and daughter (domestic worker).

This was typical of Lennox Road. If there was a house where no member of the family had some attachment to the hospital then it was unusual. Irate nightshift workers regularly interrupted my football training regimes as I curled free kicks against their bedroom walls.

The children from the staff houses went to a one-room school in nearby Campsie Glen along with those from outlying farms and communities and joined the rest of us in Lennoxtown primary in primary five. I became close friends with one of the 'Castle kids' and spent a few years of my adolescence around the Oval. I became party to some of the lore surrounding the hospital and thoroughly explored the large grounds. There were no frightening or threatening connotations attached to the place at all for me. I would regularly cycle home from my friend's house in the dark, through the grounds, when I was 12 and 13, with little trepidation. Major preoccupations at the time were, who was allowed to play in the Oval – the children jealously guarded their swings from anybody from Lennoxtown – and who owned the hospital.

My recollection of any kind of view I had about the patients who inhabited Lennox Castle is hazy. Certainly news of escaped patients seemed to filter down to us as children but there was no attempt in my family to use the hospital or the patients as a means of control – no bogeyman stories. I grew up with a benign acceptance. From any dealings I had with the patients I took them to be talkative and amusing. There were several individuals in the village who were recognized as 'simple'. They stayed with their families and were subjected to varying degrees of intolerance. I did not equate them with patients from the Castle.

For my first 19 years I lived adjacent to the institution, had been aware of the part it played in employment for much of Lennoxtown, had seen the separate community that was the staff housing, had had limited contact with some of the patients, but I had little idea what happened inside the wards. I benignly accepted the existence of the hospital and can recall little curiosity.

Unemployed, a friend and I were ushered into starting as nursing assistants in Lennox Castle by a friend of our families who was senior tutor there. We commenced on the same ward on the same day and were orientated by a nurse who was my next-door neighbour. Adjusting to working with the range of patients we encountered was challenging. There were some with gross physical deformities, some tiny people, some huge. From these bodies some would scream or grunt all day and some would hold interesting conversations with us. Some patients would tear all their clothes off, break windows and try to run away. Some would try to sell us TVs or tape recorders they had acquired while out on pass in Glasgow. Some appeared sensible and wise. It took me many months before I had any clear idea of what mental deficiency, as it was called then, was.

Adjusting to the range of staff who we worked with was also challenging. Some seemed cruel and indifferent to the patients but most were caring and giving. All were welcoming to us initiates in their own ways. The personnel all seemed slightly eccentric in one form or other but were full of personality.

It was a culture totally different from anything that I had encountered before. I had worked in various jobs and had grown up in close proximity to the hospital and knew many of the people associated with it but the inside environment was still totally unexpected. It was shocking in many ways but also exciting and embracing. The sheer novelty of such a range of characters – both patients and staff – and the lively social life surrounding the workplace was intoxicating.

I took nurse training there and was a charge nurse for a year before leaving to do general nurse training and eventually attend university. Over the five-year period that I worked in Lennox Castle my feelings and opinions inevitably shifted. The stimulation of many new and odd acquaintances was to be replaced with a far more questioning attitude towards their behaviours and practices. I had witnessed and indulged in conduct which I was later ashamed of and was determined not to repeat or allow to be repeated.

My concerns became more focused on the needs and rights of people with learning disabilities and towards creating an environment in which these could be best met and maintained. As such I regarded the Castle as anachronistic and many of its practices and personnel corrupt. However at this point in the late 1970s it was also obvious that institutional care of this group had suffered and was suffering from gross and chronic lack of provision and recognition. Many attempts at progressive measures from well-motivated and far-sighted staff and management seemed to be met with indifference from higher levels. There was a feeling of powerlessness among the nursing staff together with a perception that there was little understanding or appreciation of their work. National press coverage of conditions and criticism of several incidents at Lennox Castle had created a poor image of the institution. Staff in the hospital felt they were more aware than anyone else of the shortcomings but were unable to change them. A group of workers who were suspicious of comment or criticism from outsiders was the result. They reasoned that only those who worked in the place could understand it.

I left with a great deal of ambivalence. I felt that perhaps the only solution to the problems of the hospital would be closure and relocation of the residents. But there remained with me a large degree of affection and respect for many of the nurses and patients. I particularly had a lot of time for some of the older men and women who had worked there for a long number of years. Their attitudes by the standards of the time were certainly out of date but this was understandable, coming from a very different era, and some of their stories about 'the old days' in the hospital were fascinating and illuminating.

# Research strategy

As an undergraduate I was familiar with the work of Paul Thompson and Trevor Lummis and was attracted to the concept of oral history providing a forum for the voices of people who had been neglected, disadvantaged or discriminated against. For postgraduate research I considered concentrating on patients who had lived in long-term institutional care, a group whose voices had rarely been heard. However, several depictions of life within these hospitals which I read all portrayed the patients as victims and the nursing staff as perpetrators of various forms of abuse and neglect. I recognized these depictions as being truthful and accurate for I had witnessed similar actions. I also knew that the total truth was not being represented. While I myself felt critical of the actions of many

nursing staff and the whole concept of institutional care for those with learning disabilities, I still experienced a residual defensive stance to criticism from outsiders 'who don't
understand'.

Nursing staff were seen as perpetrators but they also suffered from a lack of representation and voice. The patients were seen as victims but the nurses were in many ways victims
also: victims of established practices, difficult conditions and a powerful medical presence.
I did not want to be in any way an apologist for those who practised mistreatment but I did
want to encompass some kind of balanced account and explore the understanding that *both*
groups had of their experiences.

By concentrating on the relationship between the patients and the nurses and researching and analysing the factors which made up their separate but parallel communities and
cultures I hoped to illuminate what I believe to be the core of life in the institution: the
interface between the two groups. This would hopefully lend some under-standing to the
nature of this particular institution, and to institutions for people with learning disabilities
in general.

As can be seen, I was very intimate with and emotionally attached to my area of
research. This gave me many worries as to the value of the work I was doing. Was it 'real'
research? Was I in some way cheating by having all this pre-knowledge and therefore pre-
judgement? And how could I represent the involvement that I had experienced? Would I
just ignore it and present my data and analysis from an outsider's standpoint like a proper
researcher? These thoughts all clouded my early work but I got on with the task of my
research processes and put these awkward bits to the side.

## Insider advantages

While the theoretical concepts of being an insider continued to cause me angst, I was experiencing some practical advantages. I was not coming cold to the subject of learning
difficulties in general and had a fair knowledge of their history and related social, medical
and parliamentary milestones and watersheds, and so had a fair start in background reading. Researching the local environment was also helped by the fact that I had known the
librarian in Lennoxtown for a long number of years.

Possibly the area where I was most at an advantage was with informants. I started interviewing nurses whom I had known when I worked in the hospital and who were retired. I
simply phoned them up, told them what I was doing and asked if I could interview them.
With this group I was always made very welcome. Another set of people I interviewed
were those who had worked at Lennox Castle at the same time as myself, were retired but
who did not know me. I turned up at their doors and explained who I was and that I had
worked in the hospital at the same time as them and again, they were all very co-operative.
A third group were those who had retired before I started work and whom I did not know.
They were suggested by some of the other informants. Again I knocked at their doors and
explained what I was doing and told them who I was personally as well as professionally,
i.e. who my mother and granny were. They were all familiar with my family, who had lived
in Lennoxtown for generations. These work and family familiarities certainly eased my
way into people's homes to record and set up an initial trust in me. I do not suggest that it
would have been impossible for an outsider to record some of these people, but I am fairly

sure that some others would not have co-operated at all. Latterly, as word circulated in the community, I was being approached in pubs by nursing staff and offered interviews.

To interview people with learning disabilities, I started in a community unit in Glasgow where ex-residents from Lennox Castle were living. I knew the nurse who was manager there personally. After obtaining consent from any relatives through the unit, I visited the residents, most of whom I knew and who knew me, and recorded the interviews on videotape.

It was only at this stage that I contacted Lennox Castle Hospital itself and asked to interview residents there and have access to documentary material. I had been reluctant to do this initially as I anticipated a rejection, probably based on my perceptions of the institution from the past. I could not have been more wrong. The hospital manager had been my immediate line manager when I worked there and he was enthusiastic and helpful. The management team and medical consultants gave me permission to interview, within the wards, residents and staff, providing they consented of course. I was also given access to hospital documentation and ledgers which were kept on site and various old documents and artefacts which were offered by various individuals. There was an obvious interest in the work that I was doing from the manager and various other staff, based, I think, on the fact that someone was acknowledging the institution and themselves as being of some social and historical significance.

Whether I would have encountered a similar attitude had I not been known, I am not sure. I suspect that there was a large degree of personal trust shown again. I should probably ask. When the manager retired he was succeeded by another acquaintance who had been brought up round the corner from me and she was equally co-operative and interested in the research. […] Probably the least I can conclude is that the accommodating and supportive climate I encountered from the hospital management was partly due to my insider status and that this certainly eased and simplified my work. As an academic attached to a university, in pursuit of a legitimate research topic, I had been granted access to Greater Glasgow Health Board archives and would have expected access to any local archive material as well, but assistance, thankfully went far beyond that.

This was well illustrated when I attempted to seek permission to interview Margaret Scally. She was living in a community house after leaving Lennox Castle and the suspicion, obstruction and lack of help I initially encountered from the management of the agency responsible for her residence, brought home the difficulties that an outsider might experience.

Nursing is a profession, like others such as medicine, law or the police force, where confidentiality is instilled as part of the training and carried on in day-to-day work. Institutions for people with learning disabilities were held in very low esteem, particularly Lennox Castle which had generated criticism from many areas. People who worked there were touchy. These factors may have provided a barrier first of all to access to a nurse informant and secondly within the interview itself if there had been no shared background. I was able to gain rapport and trust through many shared factors: community, class, workplace, language – not only dialect but the language of the hospital – and certain attitudes. I was able to interview people in their own homes, which is usually conductive to a more relaxing and rewarding encounter. The questions I asked within fairly open-style interviews would be relevant, informed and sensitive given my familiarity with the subject.

When interviewing informants with learning difficulties, again I knew many of them personally from the past. I knew something of their day-to-day lives, environment, habits, preoccupations and sensitivities and the network of peers and members of staff who they were familiar with. I was used to talking to and interacting with people with disabilities, some of whom present special problems in communication and temperament. Some were shy and some were overbearing but they all, apart from one, were aware of the background that I shared with them.

## Insider disadvantages

Trust opened many doors for me as an insider. People trusted me as one of them, from the hospital management to the nursing informants. They welcomed me into their homes and workplaces partly because they knew me or my background and had confidence in me. This was a double-edged sword. What did they trust me to do and did I have a duty towards them because they had shown trust in and friendliness towards me? Would this influence me to present my data and draw conclusions in a more sympathetic manner, first of all because it was expected of me and secondly because I was aware that many of my inform-ants wanted to read what I wrote?

My data, however, had been influenced by my insider status from the beginning. I selected who I was going to interview according to my preconceptions and contacts and while I was attempting to portray a representative cross-section of the nursing community over time there is no doubt I could have obtained a very different picture by interviewing different personnel.

While I may have gained initial rapport in my interviews and felt confident in directing informants into relevant areas, these had their downsides also. There is always a danger that an informant will fill in little detail of a subject or incident if they are aware the inter-viewer has similar knowledge. I found this most prevalent in trying to establish the daily routines of the nurses who usually started off describing this fine then soon said something like, 'Och you'll know yourself.' There were also many times, on reflection, when I did not ask for more detail when I should have, as I knew about what was being described or alluded to, but most would not. Perhaps sometimes I was so confident about the facets that I wanted to touch on that I did not allow the interviewee to establish the things that were most important to him or her.

Similar critical points can be made about my interviews with residents and ex-residents of Lennox Castle but further, there is the factor of my nurse–patient relationship with them. As mentioned above, many had known me in the role of nurse and all of the others except one were aware of my status. This must have influenced them in their contributions in the interviews. I would certainly have been perceived as a representatives of established author-ity and, given the effects of years of institutionalization, their conversations might have been quite different with someone without my connotations. This factor may be partly responsi-ble for the fact that the most free and lurid criticism of the hospital and nurses that I recorded was from an ex-patient who did not seem to grasp that I had worked there myself.

## Ethical considerations

I first interviewed three residents in one ward in Lennox Castle and went to the duty room to thank the nursing staff and say goodbye. Unexpectedly they had laid out the three sets of case notes for me to read and left me to it. I did read them and was impressed by the corroboration of accuracy of incidents and dates mentioned in the interviews. However this raised the question of whether I should make any use of the material in these notes that were available to me. Reasoning that the relationship I had formed with these people with learning difficulties as a researcher and interviewer would he challenged if I did this, I decided against it. I felt I would be going behind their backs. I also had no similar recourse to check on any of the nurses I had interviewed. This may have been poor research verification technique but I was certainly happier that way.

I also felt some uncertainty over the issue of informed consent. I had gone through 'the proper channels' in my interviews with ex- and current residents of the hospital, but many of the group were so used to accommodating requests from authority figures that there could hardly have been any refusal.

I was not particularly comfortable that some of my nurse informants wanted to and would read what I had written about them and the hospital. This was ameliorated by the knowledge that at least they would experience something tangible in return for giving their time and experience even if they might disagree with the picture I had painted and the conclusions I came to. However, the same could not be said for those with learning difficulties whom I had interviewed. I questioned if I was exploiting them and my position, as it is so easy to do, and offering them nothing in return.

# Theoretical framework

When I began research work I could not have contemplated writing the above. I would have regarded these issues as subjective, unscientific, peripheral and self-indulgent. However, along the way I did manage to discover methodological frameworks and theories which allowed me to address concerns which I initially felt would cloud and restrict the subject. In fact a burgeoning literature on the relationships between researcher and researched has placed this dynamic at the center of the research process and raises many theoretical and ethical questions.

Facts and data are seen as only one half of a complete picture and 'the other half – how ethnography comes about as a process of perception and writing – deserves to be analysed' (Lonnqvist, 1990: 22). The 'self' has been recognized as the research instrument, dictating which research problem to tackle, which framework to utilize, what informants to give emphasis to and, as such, what goes on inside the researcher has become of the utmost importance.

> The 'self' may be 'simultaneously enabling and disabling' [...] but this means we have two good reasons for paying it due attention rather than dismissing it as an unfortunate, complicating factor in our work. In any case, since we cannot shed the self, we must give it a focal point in our writings. (Crick, 1992: 175)

An awareness of who reads what we write is also to the forefront. No longer can the audience be considered as fellow academics and both the subjects we research and the press have to be considered as readers, and readers who will have a reaction.

The authors collectively ask us to re-evaluate the viability of a distinction between 'insider' and 'outsider.' They examine further the issues of ethnographic authority and the politics of representation, and demonstrate how they personally have dealt with the challenges to authority and interpretation that they have faced either during the process of field work or after the publication of the results of their research. (Brettell, 1993: 22)

Different forms of research text have also been explored and co-operative manuscripts, written by informants and researchers together, are a variation on the conventional productions. I might have attempted this with some of the interviewees with learning disabilities, had I been familiar with the concept at the time, to allow them to experience some autonomy and return.

# Conclusion

The fact that I was so much an insider initially gave me great problems in my approach to the research, although I recognized certain advantages and disadvantages which it generated. One of the biggest disadvantages which I perceived initially was how to communicate my own past experiences and address their effect on my research processes. I came to understand that, far from being a confusing problem, the discussion of my status as an insider should be central to any analysis and that this lent clarity rather than confusion to my work.

# References

Brettell, C. B. (ed.) (1993) *When They Read What We Write: the Politics of Ethnography*. Westport, CT: Bergin & Garvey.
Crick, M. (1992) 'Ali and me: an essay on street-corner anthropology', in J. Okely and H. Callaway (eds), *Anthropology and Autobiography*. London: Routledge.
Lönnqvist, B. (1990) 'Remembering and forgetting. Recording for posterity', *Ethnologia Scandinavica*, 20: 19–30.

# Chapter 6

## Carers and professionals – the carer's viewpoint

*Annie Bibbings*

I see so few people that if the world outside went away in the night, I would not notice it. (Husband caring for wife)

Although all carers have some needs in common, their circumstances can vary enormously. The reasons for this are the nature of the disability of the person cared for and the fact that 'informal caring' takes place within an existing relationship unlike other forms of care provided by nurses, doctors, etc. The person needing care may be a frail elderly mother, a physically disabled husband, a son who has learning difficulties or a friend experiencing mental illness. On the whole, carers are poorly prepared for the task they face. Whatever their circumstances, there are few carers who do not need some help.

This chapter looks at the difficulties experienced by carers, the assumptions and contradictions surrounding their role as both care providers and users, and the support they want from service providers. The chapter concludes by looking at some implications for inter-professional work in the context of working towards partnership in caring. [...]

## Needs of carers

It is not difficult to sit down with any group of people – service providers, social workers, district nurses, carers themselves – and quickly reach agreement about what should be done to help carers. Broadly, this will consist of: more recognition; providing better financial, practical and emotional support; improving access to information; increasing the opportunities to combine paid work and caring; and developing better awareness of the problems that carers face.

---

Originally published in A. Leathard (ed.) *Going Interprofessional*. London: Routledge, pp. 158–171 [abridged].

## More recognition – 'I'm a daughter, not a carer'

Now my task is complete and she is at rest. I have no regrets. I would do it all over again for her. She never in words expressed her appreciation until a few days before her death when she said, 'You're a good daughter; no one but me knows what a good daughter you've been'. (Daughter recently caring for mother)

Many carers, particularly women, do not identify themselves as carers but see their role as a natural extension of family obligations. Carers' own expectations combined with the expectations of the cared-for person, other family members, peers and professionals can make it difficult for carers to feel that they have any control over whether they take on (or continue) the caring role or not.

Once a carer is able to identify herself as such and say 'I'm a daughter and a carer' this may often be the first step in recognizing that she too has needs and that it is quite legitimate to ask for help and support. It is therefore essential that proactive and energetic approaches are developed to help carers identify themselves early on in their caring role and before a crisis is reached.

The attitudes of and assumptions made by professionals can also make it difficult for carers to ask for help. Usually the presence of a carer in a household is the signal for service providers to breathe a sigh of relief and think that this is one problem they can ignore, 'Is there a daughter?' being one of the first questions to cross the lips of many a consultant, doctor or social worker when faced with the problem of needing to organize community care for a patient or client. The aim should be for carers and professionals to work towards partnership in caring, with the carer being seen as at least an equal partner and not just a passive recipient.

## More money

I gave up my job at 60. I now have a reduced occupational pension because of early retirement – one-third of my salary. The hot water tank went and that cost £200. I lost an income of £9,000 a year. (Husband caring for wife)

The financial effects of providing care can be devastating. Extra heating, washing, special food and equipment, transport and substitute care all put a huge strain on household budgets. Additionally, many carers may have given up a paid job and therefore suffer not only the loss of income but also the loss of future promotion and pension income. State benefits are grossly inadequate and unavailable to most carers anyway. Invalid Care Allowance, the only specific benefit for carers, is so tied up with restrictions that of the 6.8 million carers, only about 170,000 actually receive this allowance.

## More practical help

You've got to remember that if you have flu, you can't go to bed – so you just add depression to your physical problems. (A carer)

A major survey of nearly 3,000 carers carried out by the Carers National Association (1992), as part of its Listen to Carers campaign, showed that 65 per cent of carers said that caring had affected their health. The reasons for this are twofold: first, caring is hard work. It consists in many cases of a great deal of lifting and handling which is usually undertaken single handedly, and without any training. Many carers injure themselves in the course of their caring. Secondly, there are insufficient or inappropriate services to enable them to seek health care when they are injured or become ill. For example, a back injury cannot be rested. A hernia cannot be repaired if there is no one to take over the caring while the carer goes into hospital. Caring is often undertaken by the least fit members of the community.

## More emotional and moral support

I found that there was a complete assumption that, because I was the wife, I would take on the total care. I found this amazing and later realized how angry this assumption made me feel. I would have liked to have been *asked* and there to have been *some* discussion as to whether I could manage and what help and support would be available. There are times when I feel like nothing more than a housekeeper, cook, nurse, gardener, shopper and organizer. I often feel like a widow but without the freedom. Tiredness also plays a large part. In addition to all the practical problems, the fact that we no longer have a sexual relationship has an enormous impact and puts a great strain on our marriage. I feel it would be so helpful if my husband and I, jointly and separately, had someone to talk to who was experienced in spinal injury or perhaps in sexual counselling. The physical care that my husband received was outstanding but our emotional problems have been ignored and neglected. (Wife caring for husband with spinal injuries)

Although the physical burden can be heavy, many carers would say that their worst problems are of an emotional nature. Carers feel isolated. They may also feel angry, resentful and embarrassed by the tasks they have to perform; they often feel a sense of loss for the person for whom they are caring, and in addition they feel guilty for having these feelings in the first place. Having someone to talk to, whether a friend, relative or sympathetic professional, can be of immense help to carers as can opportunities to engage in social activities. Carers' support groups can play an invaluable role here in providing moral support, social contact and information.

The total subordination of one's own needs and preferences to those of another – together with the feeling of being out of control of one's own life – are major causes of depression in carers. This depression can make every day an eternity and in extreme cases can result in suicide or physical violence.

Old age abuse, or indeed abuse of a dependant of any age, is only one way in which some carers try to establish some control over a situation which is running away with them. Research carried out by Homer and Gilleard (1990) shows that households particularly at risk are those that are socially or geographically isolated with a carer who is also suffering from significant illness and depression. Other significant risk factors are alcohol consumption by the carer, a poor pre-existing relationship with the cared-for person and a history of abuse over many years.

# More information

I only recently found out about Attendance Allowance by accident after caring for my mother full time for over ten years. I had been ill and arrangements were being made for Mother to go away for two weeks so that I could have a break. An independent doctor arrived to make an assessment for a suitable place for her to go. He finished the assessment and asked, 'Of course, she is getting the Attendance Allowance.' Attendance Allowance, what's that? said I, whereupon I thought he ws going to shoot up to the ceiling with annoyance. He told me to go to the local Social Security office for a form. I did not need telling twice! (Daughter caring for mother)

Carers need information about services available in their area, about the benefits to which they are entitled, about being a carer, about changes in legislation which will affect them and about the condition of the person for whom they are caring. The problem for carers is that over half of them are not in touch with any support service except their family practitioner. While much information does exist, these carers do not have access to it. GPs therefore form the only common link for these hidden carers and their surgeries are the place where such carers are most likely to go. A good GP can transform a carer's life simply by putting him or her in touch with support. However, all too often carers say of their GPs, 'He isn't interested in *me*' or 'She doesn't know anything.' It is hoped that this situation will improve as GPs are now obliged under the terms of their 1990 contract to give advice 'to enable patients to avail themselves of services provided by a local social services authority.'

In order to ensure that carers obtain the information they need, a 'saturation' policy is necessary. Carers' handbooks, factsheets, newsletters and information packs are useful but great care must be taken not to use professional jargon and also to provide multilingual leaflets where appropriate. Nor should information be confined to written material as many people are more likely to obtain their information by word of mouth or through the media. Carers' groups can be vital in passing on information and are particularly useful in persuading carers that a benefit or service might be available to them and indeed that they might even be entitled to it. It should be recognized that a major part of the job of all professionals must be to provide information to carers or at least to steer them to appropriate sources of help.

# More respite care

I have to prepare Dad for days before he goes into the local nursing home and he has tantrums when he comes back. He makes our life hell – so I ask myself, 'Is it worth it?' (A carer)

There is an urgent need for more or different respite care to give carers both short but regular as well as longer breaks from caring. There is a wide variety of need, so there must be a wide variety of provision. The key requirements are the flexibility of the relief care offered and its acceptability to both the carer and the cared-for person. Some people want respite care provided in the home, some want it provided in a residential setting, and some want a mixture of both, including good day-care facilities. The high demand for home care attendants and sitters reflects in part the unwillingness of some frail elderly and disabled people to travel away from home. In addition, carers and users are sometimes unhappy about the quality of hospital and Social Services respite care provision which then puts them off using the service a second time. Another form of respite care, a lifeline to carers of children with special needs, is summer and holiday play schemes. These can be vital if there are other children in the family.

## More employment opportunities

It has been universally assumed that I can cope, that I will cope, that I will continue to cope. This includes the assumption that I can take time off work to take Mother to various medical appointments, to be present when various professional helpers wish to call. I have tried to explain my position at work and my own health problems. Ignored! (Daughter caring for mother)

Trying to combine paid work and care can cause immense difficulties for carers in terms of stress, strain and loss of work opportunities. In a survey of full-time carers undertaken by Opportunities for Women (1990) 55 per cent of carers said that they had to give up their job because of caring responsibilities, 5 per cent took early retirement, 16 per cent decided to work fewer hours, and 7 per cent were working from home. The same survey interviewed a cross-section of people in work and found that 17 per cent of employees had major caring responsibilities for an adult or elderly person. Carers also reported that they felt that their caring responsibilities affected their ability to apply for promotion, seek a new job or relocate to a better job within the same company. There are also considerable difficulties for carers returning to work after they cease caring. 'I had to go straight from the graveside to the Job Centre, only to be told I wasn't qualified for anything and what had I really been doing for the last ten years.' This is how one carer described the experience. Much could be done to help carers combine caring with paid employment. This includes: reinstating the right to unemployment benefit after caring has ceased; increasing the amount that carers can earn before losing state benefits; setting up support schemes that will allow people to combine paid work and caring; setting up workplace carers' groups to provide advice and information to employees with caring responsibilities.

## Young carers

The nine-year-old was no help, but the four-year-old was a great help. (From hospital case note)

My one regret is that I have been robbed of my youth. The past five years have been traumatic; I have had to become an adult before my time. I often say I'm 19 going on 40. (Young carer)

Estimates based on survey work in Tameside and Sandwell (Page, 1988) suggest that nationwide there are well over 10,000 children acting as primary carers. Usually, they are from single-parent families in which a parent develops a disabling illness. There are also an unknown number of children living with an elderly relative, who are providing emotional or practical stability in a family that is experiencing mental distress. Older children are also often needed to help out with a disabled youngster.

Scarce resources and lack of information mean that there is little incentive for families to ask for help. In addition, the fear – real or perceived – that statutory intervention will result in the removal of parent or child (or both) into care is all-pervasive. The media view which paints these children as 'angels' or 'victims' reinforces the pressure felt by disabled parents when appropriate support is not available or is denied. Clearly, there is the problem for professionals of striking a balance between accepting the role of young people helping out with the care of a relative and advocating their rights as children – rights to leisure and uninterrupted education. Children should have the right not to be carers but when they *are* they must be consulted and their role valued. Research carried out by Bilsborrow (1992) shows an urgent need for services and further research into this area. The report, the first to focus on the quality of life for young carers, looks at the views of 11 youngsters aged between 9 and 21. They were caring for relatives with a variety of disabling conditions including arthritis, multiple sclerosis and tranquillizer addiction. Researchers also spoke to a variety of professional groups about their knowledge of the number of young carers in their area and their needs. Not surprisingly, the researchers found that most professionals knew little about young carers and focused attention on the relative being cared for. The problem was one of double invisibility: families were reluctant to ask for assistance because there were few support services available and families feared being labelled as 'problem families'. The Carers National Association young carers project wants to see local authorities:

- include young carers within the 'children in need' priorities for implementing the Children's Act 1989;
- set up a process for multidisciplinary collaboration and planning and delivery of services;
- take steps to combat the stigma felt by families who ask for services; and
- address the particular needs of different racial groups.

## More equality

When this project started not one family was claiming Invalid Care Allowance. No one had told them they were eligible. (Worker in a project for Asian parents of severely disabled children)

Carers face discrimination in many areas of their lives – from employment through to opportunities for leisure and recreation. Without sufficient private income carers have few meaningful choices as they have no automatic rights to services, training or an adequate income. The discretionary nature of service allocation means that decisions about 'who gets what' are often influenced by the attitude of a particular professional towards a particular carer or are based on unspoken assumptions.

Much also depends on the carers' attitudes, how good carers are at articulating their own needs and their skills in negotiating. Research (Charlesworth et al., 1984) indicates that issues of age, class, gender, race and cultural expectations all play a significant part in determining who is likely to receive services. Under-representation of black and ethnic minority carers receiving services suggests that they are a particularly vulnerable and disadvantaged group. Service providers need to be aware of the additional obstacles that such carers face. Time and resources must be spent on training staff in statutory and voluntary organizations to understand the various cultures and religions of their area;

providing multilingual information and interpreting services; and undertaking outreach work with ethnic communities so that their views can be properly taken into account in community care planning […]

# Conflict and contradictions

If you are not confused about community care policies you are not thinking clearly! (Department of Health official)

The question remains that if the needs of carers are now generally better understood, why is it still so difficult for carers to obtain the help and support they need? Part of the answer is to be found in the conflicts and contradictions that exist in the way in which policy-makers, service providers and carers themselves see their respective roles.

## Conflict for the carer

Carers have the difficult job of trying to balance their own needs with the needs of the person they care for, often at a time when the relationship between them is at its most intense and fragile. Deep feelings of love and responsibility may be mixed with feelings of bereavement, resentment and anger. The huge amount of guilt that many carers feel can make it almost impossible for them to feel able to ask for help or indeed to accept it when it is offered.

## Conflict for the cared-for person

There is a natural desire in people to maintain their own independence and not be 'a burden' on others. This is combined with a strong British tradition of 'keep it in the family', 'we can manage' and, for some cared-for people, a strong message to their carer that 'only you can do it'. The result is that some frail, elderly and disabled people are unhappy about accepting help with daily living and personal care tasks from anyone other than a close family member. On the other hand, some disabled people dislike the term 'carer' as they feel it perpetuates the idea that disability means dependency. They don't want to be 'looked after' by their relatives, but want the right to access to resources to enable them to appoint their own personal assistants or helpers. Thus, not only is there a wide range of views among people with disabilities themselves about who should be providing them with assistance, but there are often areas of conflict between the person needing care and the carer about choices and needs. Service providers need to recognize and address the complexities of this situation and attempt to mediate and balance the interests of both parties whenever possible.

## Conflict for professionals

Carers often praise the help that they receive from the caring professions but some also complain bitterly about 'being taken for granted' or not understood. Usually, this is not intentional. It is simply that the training of professionals has not taught them to recognize the needs of the carer. Another reason for ignoring carers is fear – fear which often stems from an awareness of a lack of resources. If carers' needs *are* identified, service providers often fear that they will be unable to meet them, leaving them feeling inadequate and guilty. This lack of resources is, of course, a reality and many members of the public seeking assistance for themselves or their relatives are likely to be caught in the care vacuum. As a consequence, many professionals see increasing the expectation of carers for more help as something to be avoided. The way that carers and professionals perceive each other can also give rise to conflict. Many carers express the view that they feel in awe of professionals and are intimidated by them. These perceptions may have more to do with what people in particular professions are expected to be like than with the actual people involved. Similarly, professionals may regard a carer as some kind of 'selfless angel' and this makes it hard for carers to confess their anxieties and fears in case they disillusion the professionals. Alternatively, professionals may regard a carer as someone who is too deeply involved in a mutually dependent relationship to be able to think rationally and in the best interest of the patient or client. By describing four models of caring – carers as a resource, as co-workers, as co-clients and superseded carers – Twigg and Aitken (1991) provide a helpful framework for understanding the ambiguous situation that carers occupy in relation to service providers.

Seeing carers as *resources* reflects the way that carers are perceived as 'free' community care providers or cheap labour. The aim, if services are provided at all, is to keep the carer caring but at minimal cost. Describing carers as *co-workers* is where service providers aim to work in close collaboration with carers and there is recognition of the importance of the carer's morale and support in the rehabilitation of the client. Carers as *co-clients* is where service providers see carers as having needs in their own right. The fourth model of the *superseded* carer usually applies to parents who have sons or daughters with special needs. Here the aim of services is to move the client away from support provided by family carers into 'independent living'.

## Conflict for policy-makers

The different ways in which carers are seen and defined makes it difficult for policy in relation to carers to be consistent and specific in terms of service provision, eligibility and allocation. A great deal of 'paper' recognition is given to carers and warm sentiments are expressed about the valuable job they do. However, there is still little real commitment in terms of resources to translate these good intentions into practical action. Conflicts also arise between different areas of government policies. For example, women are encouraged back into paid employment, while in reality many women carers are unable to take up paid employment as no affordable relief care is available.

## Conflict for society

Whatever the uncertainty about resources, it is clear that over the next decade, owing to demographic and medical advances, there is going to be an increase in the number of people living at home and needing care with a corresponding decline in the number of carers available. The impact of changes in marriage patterns – more divorce and remarriage and more single-parent families – is not yet clear but it seems likely that, in the long term, they could lead to a lessening of the moral imperatives and the close family obligations which give rise to caring. We may not feel the same love or duty to our ex in-laws or to our step-siblings as we do to closer family, and indeed may even lose touch with them completely. In addition, a single parent with children to care for as well as a job is unlikely to have the time to care for an elderly relative.

There are also fewer single women, who have in the past traditionally been those most likely to become carers. There are fewer children in most families, family members live further apart and the proportion of childless marriages is growing. More elderly people will therefore have no immediate kin to care for them. Lastly, since being a carer can isolate you from your community and from the rest of your family, it may mean that carers themselves are deprived of the opportunity to build up the kind of social networks which give rise to caring. Neither will they have much opportunity to build up any financial reserves. Who will care for them? The world is changing and, like it or not, professionals, carers and users are going to have to learn to understand each other and work together better.

# Working towards partnership in caring

[...]

Carers need opportunities to engage in debate with both service providers and with the politicians who control the resources for the services they need. To achieve this, consultation and participation with carers in community care planning should become an integral part of every element in the work of local and health authorities, family health service authorities, housing authorities, voluntary organizations and other bodies providing community services. Consultation should be shaped to suit the needs and culture of an area and encourage maximum participation from all members of the community. There can be no single, neat definition for consultation, but it should encompass a wide range of activities which together constitute the process of listening to carers.

It is vital that carers know about their right to ask for an assessment of their own needs and a confidential interview should always be offered. Honesty about what is on offer and what is not is essential too. Without a designated care manager, many carers are left with the impossible task of trying to co-ordinate their own care arrangements across a variety of occupational groups and organizations. When problems do occur (e.g. a home care assistant does not turn up or day centre hours are cut) carers and users are frequently told, 'It's not our problem – it's Social Services' responsibility' or 'We have to give priority to elderly people living alone.'

Carers, therefore, report that they spend a great deal of their energy and time trying to understand who is supposed to be responsible for doing what and in plugging the gaps in communication and co-ordination between professional groups.

The experience of the Carers National Association, which is a national charity for all carers, has shown that, in order to get better support and more choice for carers, it is essential for them to have a 'collective voice' at both local and national levels. As part of the Association's Listen to Carers campaign, carers were asked what they felt was the most important piece of advice that they could give other carers. Overwhelmingly, most respondents gave advice on the theme of making yourself heard and being recognized. Their comments included:

> 'Speak up, speak out and keep doing it.'
> 'Shout and keep shouting.'
> 'Keep shouting and don't be shy.'
> 'Ask and keep asking.'
> 'Shout and push – it's an uphill battle but I won eventually.'

Perhaps only by carers speaking up, and speaking out, will enough influence be brought to bear on policy-makers, service providers and professionals to ensure that carers have a better deal. But, like Oliver Twist, it cannot just be up to the disadvantaged and vulnerable to 'keep asking for more'! Professionals must become effective advocates and allies of carers too.

# References

Bilsborrow, S. (1992) *Young Carers on Merseyside*. London: Barnardos.

Carers National Association (1992) *Speak Up, Speak Out*. London: Carers National Association.

Charlesworth, A., Wilkin, D. and Durie, A. (1984) *Carers and Services: A Comparison of Men and Women Caring for Dependent Elderly People*. Manchester: Equal Opportunities Commission.

Homer, A. and Gilleard, C. (1990) 'Abuse of elderly people by their carers', *British Medical Journal*, 30: 1359–1362.

Opportunities for Women (1990) *Carers at Work*. London: OFW.

Page, R.W. (1988) 'Report on the initial survey investigation, the number of young carers in Sandwell secondary schools', *Social Services Research*, 6: 31–36.

Twigg, J. and Aitken, K. (1991) *Evaluating Support to Informal Carers*. York: Social Policy Research Unit, University of York.

# Chapter 7

## Women and men talking about poverty

*Sue Yeandle, Karen Escott, Linda Grant and Elaine Batty*

[O]ne significant missing area in our knowledge of gender and poverty concerns the differential experience and aspirations of poor men and poor women. [...] The study reported here is based on data obtained from focus groups of women and of men, of different ages and of different ethnic origins.

[...]

Participants came from one of three groups: those in Middlesbrough were young people aged 16–18; in Sandwell (West Midlands) they were members of the Bangladeshi community; whilst those in Sheffield were parents, living with their dependent children and a partner. [...]

All were on low incomes, i.e. were living in households below average income (HBAI). Most were not themselves in employment although there were some exceptions: one of the Sheffield mothers who had a part-time job; two of the Bangladeshi men who were in employment; and about half of the young people in Middlesbrough – although it should be noted that most of these were working part-time. [...]

[...]

## Budgeting on a low income

Managing the limited budget available was central to the participants' everyday lives. Many spoke of 'thinking about money all the time', worrying about money a lot, learning to manage money, and having to plan their spending carefully.

From S. Yeandle, K. Escott, L. Grant and E. Batty (2003), Working Paper Series No.7, Equal Opportunities Commission, Manchester [Selected extracts].

I write down what I need to pay. Shopping is always last on the list, the bills come first.

I had to learn to budget, I couldn't budget at first.
(Young women, Middlesbrough)

You have to think about what you buy and set a budget first. The bills come first, and then food.

We can just about maintain our basic needs – we cannot afford leisure costs.
(Bangladeshi men, Sandwell)

We have no peace of mind.

We talk about it all the time.

It is in your head all the time.
(Bangladeshi women, Sandwell)

We go and price things up before we buy.

We are always close to budget.

You can save money by shopping around.

We don't have the money to worry about it.

We have worried for so long that it goes straight over your head.
(Fathers, Sheffield)

Managing money is a way of life.

A lot of money goes out, but not much comes in.
(Mothers, Sheffield)

There was widespread agreement that it was essential to prioritise certain budget items. Parents (of both sexes, white parents in Sheffield and Bangladeshi parents in Sandwell) were very conscious of the essential costs of children. They mentioned the expense of baby milk and of nappies, and of food. In addition, all these parents struggled to limit their children's expectations in the face of peer pressure and extensive advertising. The Sheffield parents, interviewed in early January, were very conscious of the struggle they had just been through to find some way of buying Christmas gifts for their children, and ensuring that:

They will not be disappointed about everything.
(Father, Sheffield)

Mothers in Sheffield emphasised that they had worked hard to reduce children's aspirations. One said her children now understood that they had to choose the cheapest trainers on offer, when shopping, and had learnt 'not to ask for anything'. Even so it could be very difficult to deal with teenagers, who did not always understand the family's financial circumstances. One Sheffield father told us that he only bought clothes for himself at Oxfam, in order to be able to buy new clothes for his son in shops where his friends bought theirs.

Bangladeshi parents faced a similar situation. They stressed the need constantly to be making choices between the things they needed:

> We cannot fulfil the demands placed on us by family and children.
>
> If I buy a jacket I can't eat, if I eat I can't buy a jacket – so I have to make a choice.
> (Bangladeshi men, Sandwell)
>
> We are just about surviving on benefits – food comes first. It's not what you want, it's what you need.
> (Bangladeshi woman, Sandwell)

[…]

Sheffield women told us they concealed bills and debts from their men, to avoid arguments and to give them time to work out what to do. One woman accompanied her husband to the cash point machine at 5am on a Friday morning (the first point in the week when he could draw his wages) to ensure she had adequate housekeeping.

> I'm in control of my bit. Every week's the same. I know, every Friday morning, how much I take off him. And that's it. I don't get any more. Because, like, he ain't got no more. I mean. I've got to let him have a bit for himself.
> (Mother, Sheffield)

Although they controlled the spending, the women also said that they often went without, to ensure men and children had what they needed for clothes, food and essential items, and that they gave men their weekly spending money. (The Sheffield fathers told us they had £5 for this, only getting more if there was 'any left').

> I'll tell you another thing you tend to do as well. You make sure your husband gets a good meal, and your kids get a good meal, – and you'll have a sandwich. You think, 'He's been at work all day, I've got to give him a good meal.'
>
> Men can't make budgets.
> (Mothers, Sheffield)
>
> I leave it to the wife, as she can manage it. She has her head screwed on.
> (Father, Sheffield)

Paying for heating, lighting and fuel took a large amount of the weekly budget for those living in supported housing. Those young people living with their parents had to pay 'lodge', which generally comprised £20 per week, to cover household costs and food. Some spent their remaining money on 'treats', such as favourite foods.

[…]

# Social isolation

One important aspect of the lives of the people interviewed was their isolation: geographically, culturally and socially. Respondents described this as an outcome of living on a low income. People lived out their lives in an enclosed world, largely defined by the immediate neighbourhood. 'We don't go very far' was a common phrase.

The costs of travel, even to travel just beyond the immediate neighbourhood, were regarded as too great, and this restricted lives to a small geographical area. For many respondents travel outside of the city or town, or outside of the country, were unthinkable luxuries.

Holidays were either bargain options or simply did not take place. One respondent had not had a holiday for 15 years, others for 5 or more years. None of the Bangladeshi men or women took holidays, even though they hoped that, one day, they could visit relatives in Bangladesh.

> It takes time to save.

> We can't afford the tickets, as they cost between £2,000 and £2,500.
> (Bangladeshi women, Sandwell)

For the white mothers who took holidays, these were chosen on the basis of cost. They were booked in the 'cheaper' periods, during term time, or at less expensive locations, such as Butlins or caravan parks. Some of the young respondents had been on trips with a local community organization and, for them, leisure time away from home took the form of day trips rather than holidays.

The lack of money for leisure activities was also a common theme. One woman commented, 'We don't even think to go out'. Few could afford to go to the cinema, take the children swimming or go to restaurants. Women's leisure activities were particularly limited. One woman went to Bingo, another to karate once a week – but even this was restricted:

> Karate – I only go once a week, because otherwise it'll cost me £3 if I go on a Tuesday and a Friday. So I only go on a Friday. I'd like to go twice, because I've been going since I was about 9, and I've worked myself up to a blue belt. But now, because I've got kids and I can't afford to go twice – there's no point in going in fact. I only go to keep fit.
> (Mother, Sheffield)

Indeed some of the Sheffield women described smoking as their only pleasure, even though they felt guilty about spending money on cigarettes.

> It's a vicious circle, isn't it? You can't afford to smoke, but because we haven't got any money, I think it forces you to smoke, doesn't it? It eases the stress a bit.
> (Mother, Sheffield)

The young women tended to stay in and watch TV, or they walked the streets with friends. Only one young woman was engaged in sports activities – she attended a gym. For this group, even visiting family was considered too expensive. Although they were trying to retain social contact with their families, financially this was a struggle. The young women's social isolation and lack of a social life left them feeling bored and dissatisfied:

> We would like to visit relatives but we can't afford the bus fares.

> I get fed up with the four walls. It makes you feel down.
> (Young women, Middlesbrough)

For the young male group, leisure activities were slightly more varied and the young men tended to go out more. Some of the young white male respondents went to see films, and the younger Bangladeshi men 'did go out a little bit'. Many of the young men in Middlesbrough spent their leisure time playing computer games on the TV, although none had computers in their own homes. They also participated in sports activities, in particular football in local parks, and some used local leisure facilities where costs for young people were subsidised.

For the Sheffield fathers, the lack of holidays and other leisure activities was in contrast to their earlier lives and the experience of their friends.

> When pals go away, such as to Tenerife in a group, we can't go.
> (Father, Sheffield)

Some men had had to give up activities that they had enjoyed whilst working in the past, like drinks in the pub or fishing. And in this group the inability to take children to the countryside as often as they would like was commented upon. There was a sense of anger amongst the Sheffield men about the limitations on their social life.

> When you've been in a rut it becomes a way of life ... it would drive you mad if you didn't put these feelings to one side.
> (Father, Sheffield)

The men described a shrinking social world. As one man commented about the impact of low income:

> It limits the friends you have.
> (Father, Sheffield)

And there was agreement amongst the Sheffield fathers that even members of their family did not come and visit them as much as they used to. Nevertheless, this narrowing of the social world was also sometimes a choice, albeit one which stemmed from a depressing lack of opportunity and the absence of sufficient money to genuinely enjoy a social life with friends.

> Can't be bothered to go out, I don't want to go out.
> (Young man, Middlesbrough)

The inability to afford holidays, to take part in social or cultural life or to travel beyond their immediate neighbourhood, alongside the way in which people began to distance themselves from a social context, were striking examples of the social isolation of poor people.
[...]

# Social relationships

In the discussions, some of the shared experiences associated with living on a low income were a source of amusement. For example, the strategies employed to try to avoid creditors (who were also family members) – 'if you see them coming you take another route' – were common experiences and made everyone laugh. However, no-one described their social context as supportive, and the negative impact of poverty on social relationships was a more prominent feature of discussion.

For the respondents with young children, poverty was a significant element of their day-to-day relationships with their children. The difficulty of meeting the demands of children was a source of sadness, and generated a sense of failure and of guilt. For example, parents' relationship with children involved concern that their children would suffer at school if they didn't have the 'right' clothes or even that they wouldn't go to school. All the parents were aware of the desire amongst children for 'designer' clothes, but meeting these expectations was very difficult on a low income.

> We try and give the kids the clothes they want to go to school in, as they don't want to go to school otherwise.
> (Bangladeshi woman, Sandwell)

When this wasn't possible, parents felt 'sad' and children's disappointment was reflected back on to their parents.

> If my child wants something and I can't afford it, it gets to you.

> The children are not happy because they can't have the things they want and therefore you're not happy.
> (Bangladeshi women, Sandwell)

All the respondents referred to the ways in which poverty created tensions at home. There were frequent arguments between husbands and wives about money, although some had learned to try to avoid these.

> We argue all the time about money.

> We used to argue about money, but now we say, what's the point? We haven't got it, we can't have it. It's not going to change anything. We can stand there arguing for half an hour, we still ain't got any money.
> (Mother, Sheffield)

[…]

In order to avoid arguments about this, the women tended to conceal the real financial situation from their husbands and tried their best to sort finances out without discussing it with their husbands.

> I jump up before my partner gets up, to hide the bills. It avoids arguments.

> I find myself (lying to my husband about money) when I've bought something for the kids. Say I've spent £15 on their shoes, instead of £10. I'll say to him, "They only came to £10" and I won't tell him I spent an extra £5 on the kids. 'Cause he sees spending money like that on the kids as a waste.
> (Mothers, Sheffield)

Men also described the tensions at home caused by a lack of money, but they had a tendency to refer to this in a context of their own inability to provide for the family.

> If you haven't got enough money you can't put food on the table, you can't look after the family ... so the kids get stressed to the mother and the mother gets stressed to the husband.
> (Bangladeshi man, Sandwell)

A further cause of tension within social relationships resulted from debt. While the process of borrowing and lending money was unavoidable, it nevertheless distorted relationships and undermined friendships.

> If you borrow some money from a friend and you can't give it back in time and he might need it, then that affects your friendship. And then, sometimes, if I see a friend who owes me money and I think he's got the money but he's not giving it to me, he doesn't want to give it to me. That causes problems. You start thinking negative inside.
> (Bangladeshi man, Sandwell)

In general, respondents expressed concern about the negative impact of their low income on their social relationships. They explained that friends with money might offer to cover the cost of a few drinks or a night out, but said they were reluctant to take up these kinds of offers. Some found such gestures humiliating; others were worried that they may not be able to pay them back.

> It makes you feel like a charity case.
> (Young woman, Middlesbrough)

> We want to be able to stand our own corner.
> (Father, Sheffield)

[...]

# Locality and neighbourhood

All six focus groups raised important issues about their neighbourhoods, issues which are well known in the literature on deprived communities and the work of the Government's Neighbourhood Renewal Unit. These included poor housing conditions, lack of employment opportunities, educational underachievement, expensive public transport, and worrying levels of crime. The general view was that problems had worsened over the last decade, and that a sense of community had been lost. Participants indicated that where they lived meant that they were discriminated against, in terms of both employment and car insurance.

Many felt trapped in their neighbourhood, partly by the increasing cost of bus services, and said this exacerbated their sense of isolation and alienation. They felt that the condition of their housing was poor and that their neighbourhoods were blighted by vandalism, dirty streets, and crime.

This was particularly true for most of the young people in Middlesbrough, who were not happy with the location of their housing. A perception that there was increasing drug dealing and prostitution in their areas made the respondents fearful:

I feel locked in, stuck in the house all the time.
(Young woman, Middlesbrough)

The young women described feeling intimidated by children hanging around shops in large gangs. They felt that the street crime in the area was mainly used to pay for drugs. None of the young women went out at night.

There are smack heads about and loads of fighting. I don't go out when it's dark.
(Young woman, Middlesbrough)

[…]

The Bangladeshi women in Sandwell agreed that everyone in their area was in the same predicament, and that they had no money. They were especially concerned about the lack of facilities for children in the area, such as play areas and other activities for school holidays.

[…]

Although the focus groups were not directly asked about social divisions and tensions, several important issues were raised during the discussions. Racism was highlighted in Middlesbrough, and was a worrying feature of the young people's discourse on poverty and deprivation. Some blamed minority groups for some of their problems, and had developed a perception that other racial groups have more support than them.

# Health

There was a general awareness that low income directly affected health through stress, poor diet, lack of exercise and fresh air. Many participants and their families (in Sheffield and in Middlesbrough) were heavy smokers, but were also concerned about the cost of their smoking and the health problems this may cause. Whilst many were aware of a lack of fresh fruit and vegetables in their diet (one Sheffield mother commenting that she could only afford fresh fruit and vegetables once a week), all felt restricted in their purchase of fresh foods. As one put it,

We can't afford to go healthy, can we?
(Mother, Sheffield)

There was less recognition of the longer-term implications of a poor diet, often heavily reliant on high fat, frozen food, particularly amongst the young respondents.

Mothers in Sheffield described feelings of low level depression and reported now, or in the past, taking prescribed anti-depressants. The Sandwell participants felt that stress led to health problems for them. Many of the men suffered from high blood pressure, which they associated with the constant tension they were experiencing. All felt they lacked adequate fruit and vegetables in their diet, and some suffered from a loss of appetite.

> You don't feel like eating. Your appetite just goes away.
> (Bangladeshi man, Sandwell)

Most of the women in Sandwell felt they could not relax. The older two women suffered from heart problems and headaches.

> We can't sleep ... we have no peace of mind.
> (Bangladeshi woman, Sandwell)

They were always worrying about money and about what they could not afford, especially major items such as carpets. The Sheffield group of men felt they did not get enough fresh air, and commented that they tended to sit in the house all the time, getting very little exercise.

> We sit in with the windows shut and the fire on.
> (Father, Sheffield)

Another health problem identified by the focus groups was the lack of good quality GP services. The women in Sandwell shared this view, mentioning long waiting lists and, as one woman pointed out, the 'GPs are not nice'. This view was echoed by the Sheffield mothers, who complained that their GPs 'just gave out tablets' and did not offer any constructive help with their problems, beyond referral to the psychiatric nurse at the hospital.

Whilst all the young people said they felt healthy, the young women felt lonely and isolated because they had no job and lived in isolated circumstances:

> We have no friends to talk about girly things.
> (Young woman, Middlesbrough)

By contrast, the young men tended to participate in more sporting activities and felt this was a good way of keeping fit. Most of the young people in the focus groups were smokers, as were their families, spending a substantial proportion of their limited income on cigatettes.

[...]

# Shared features of women's and men's experiences of poverty

For all groups, 'poverty' was a stigmatising term. Participants disliked the word and the connotations that it held and preferred to be thought of as 'living on a low income'. For both women and men, living for an extended period on a low income restricted social activity, caused stress and difficulty in personal and familial relationships, and had become a dominating feature of everyday life from which it was difficult to escape. Everyone spoke of limitations on travel, leisure, food/eating and dress. The experience of being unable to afford basic items or to participate in everyday activities was contributing to their social isolation.

## Gender differences

Among the young people, it was especially women who spoke of feeling confined to the home, and of being denied participation in cultural pursuits and practices which support women's friendship networks and participation in wider society. Young men were comparatively free in their access to leisure in public spaces, such as parks and football fields, whereas women often feared such spaces and felt unsafe in their own communities after dark.

Women who were mothers wanted to access employment, but felt the very limited opportunities they could see in low-paid, low-status work would exacerbate the strains already in their lives. Their main concerns were the need for low cost and available childcare which would improve their access to employment and training alike, and how they could manage the type of employment available alongside their parental responsibilities. In contrast, the fathers did not mention childcare as a barrier to employment and those interviewed in Sheffield had experienced comparatively well paid employment in the past. Their experience of impoverished circumstances was therefore compared unfavourably to a more satisfactory past.

In Sheffield, it was women who carried the daily burden of financial management, which men often left to their wives or partners in the belief that they were better managers. These women spoke of allocating limited resources, for both food and clothes, to their children and menfolk first, putting themselves last when there was not enough to go round. Young people in Middlesbrough also mentioned this factor as characteristic of their experience with the family.

[…]

# Chapter 8

## Users' experiences of direct payments

*Tim Stainton and Steve Boyce*

After years of activism by disabled people's organizations, the Community Care (Direct Payments) Act 1996 made Direct Payment (DP) schemes a reality. Proponents of DP argue that it allows greater freedom and control for those people using it, but as these programmes only came into effect in 1997, few studies have tried to substantiate these claims. This paper reports on a two-year evaluation of two DP schemes in Wales. Using primarily users' feedback the paper focuses on the effects of DP and difficulties encountered, as well as why people chose—or did not choose—DP in the first place. User responses indicate a broad range of beneficial outcomes, including improved self-esteem, increased control over lives, deeper and more lasting relationships, and new interpersonal, vocational and lifestyle opportunities, as a result of the greater flexibility and freedom of choice enabled by DP. Family carers expressed similar satisfaction with DP schemes, also citing greater freedoms as a result of increased flexibility. While some potential users expressed concern over the administration of a DP scheme, users found that, with support from a user driven Independent Living Scheme, the administrative burden was manageable, and that ultimately the DP scheme was a welcome approach to support.

[…]

## Outcomes for users of DP

The user interviews yielded a large amount of information on the benefits and pitfalls of DP and for most interviewees the experience had been overwhelmingly positive. Only one of the thirty-five interviewees felt that direct payments had been inappropriate for her circumstances. Particularly striking were the ways in which the positive effects of DP had permeated aspects of the lives of many users well beyond the direct influence of their care

From T. Stainton and S. Boyce (2004) '"I have got my life back": users' experience of direct payments', *Disability & Society*, 19(5): 443–454 (abridged).

package. Specifically, DP had benefited users by enabling them to exercise choice and control over the nature and timing of their assistance.

Without exception, all interviewees placed great emphasis on the importance of being able to choose their own staff; this capability was the single most important benefit of direct payments for most users. More than half the interviewees had known their staff prior to employing them, either as agency or local authority carers or as friends or neighbours, and there is some evidence that service users are tapping into existing social networks to employ staff who have never previously worked as personal assistants, carers or in related occupations. Many interviewees spoke about the importance of familiarity and empathy in the relationship, and, for some people, the emotional support a PA [Personal Assistant] could provide when coming to terms with illness or impairment was as important as the physical assistance they provided.

> It really is the best thing since sliced bread. I am totally in control. No matter what happens to me with my help I know I have got people beside me and they will go on walking beside me. Every one of them they would stay no matter what happens. This year has been very very difficult health-wise and they have stayed there. Although its been frightening for them sometimes they are still here. They want to go on being here and they are so very very supportive. (V7F)

For those who employed friends or, in one case, relatives, paying wages made them feel more comfortable about asking for things to be done, and several were glad to be giving something back to people who had provided unpaid care in the past. Although people may initially have felt some unease at formalising the arrangement, there was a sense that a clear definition of when and how much assistance was being provided, with payment for the work, had made the relationship more enduring.

For other users, although happy with the much better relationship they enjoyed with staff since using direct payments, there was a feeling that boundaries between work and friendship needed to be clear. Some people had experienced problems where staff had not respected this.

The ability to control the timing and pattern of care provision had also had a positive impact on the lives of users, opening the door to a lifestyle much less constrained by the need to adhere to externally imposed routines. The opportunities for overseeing the tasks that staff carried out were also broadened by the absence of pre-defined working practices and restrictions on what staff were permitted to do.

Most interviewees reported a much greater degree of independence as a result of using DP. On a practical level, the flexible nature of DP care and the control users exercised over its delivery created possibilities for much greater involvement in the tasks of everyday life and in activities to facilitate personal development and involvement in the wider community.

> The advantages are that you can start to relive your life in the way that you want to. You can, say, pick your own clothes, where when you have got an agency you can't do that; you are in a wheelchair and you are messed up in your brain. You get a lot of companionship. You get a lot of understanding. I found girls that work for me far more understanding. I have got freedom now which I felt for years I didn't have. I have got control. I can control my own life now. I have got the biggest say in it as I used to have before, and that is all so positive. (V7F)

A number of interviewees were engaged in voluntary work, often for organisations which support disabled people or campaign for the interests of disabled people. In each case, the level of involvement they have attained would at best have been difficult and at worst impossible without the flexible care arrangements offered by DP.

Several interviewees were attending vocational courses and one individual used personal assistance when at work. Users were able to participate in social, work and educational activities by virtue of the timing and nature of their personal assistance since flexible routines were possible.

> I've got to learn how to master the computer and learn to do what I want to do on it ... so yes again, the flexibility of the ILS will enable me to go off on a day (to take a training course). (V18F)

However, the flexibility of times and routines was not the only way in which a broader range of activities were facilitated. Some users felt that such activities had been made possible by the skills and enthusiasm of their PAs. Some felt comfortable leaving their PAs to work in the home while they were out, reflecting a measure of trust rarely possible with frequently changing agency and social services staff.

There are, therefore, a number of features of DP, in particular the flexibility and control they give users, which allow a much broader range of activities to be undertaken than with conventional services. However, also striking are the psychological benefits for people who use DP, as has been identified in other studies (Glendinning et al., 2000). Many interviewees spoke about feeling more confident, optimistic and positive about their lives, and of feeling motivated to explore new avenues in ways that hadn't seemed possible before.

> It's built up my self esteem, given me a lot more confidence, made me feel I'm part of the real world, not just a drag on it, financially and physically ... I feel now my horizons are limitless. (V5F)

> I have got my life back. I have got people around me that are so supportive and every time I achieve something no matter how little 'oh great', and its not condescending and they are really thrilled that I can achieve something. We go out, we are good friends, nothing is too much trouble for them. Well I am laughing all the time now you know like Nicki and I are going to Cardiff next week we are going to go shopping. Me and Teresa and Lagite took the dogs out yesterday we had a lovely morning ... They encourage me so much and I am living a life and they are going to take me to the institute to learn how to use this voice control and the girls will be with me. They will be learning alongside me. I have got a life. I have got choice. I can do things. If I want to go to the pub for a drink I could go. No such word as can't or no or you shouldn't. (V7F)

Some reported that the burden of poor, sometimes worsening health had been lightened. Some experienced fluctuating conditions and others had suffered the trauma of an accident or amputation or a sudden onset of debilitating illness. For these interviewees, the presence of trustworthy, sympathetic, dependable staff played a major role in helping them to come to terms with and manage their illness. Having staff that were familiar with their condition and assistance requirements, and who did not need to have the issues explained anew each time, was highly valued.

It's finding a person who understands the disability as well. And there are so many different disabilities and they obviously can't learn about every disability they can only learn I suppose by you telling them about what you need which is something that I always do anyway but you know I always let them know what my needs are and that my needs may be different from what they are used to. I used to say that if there is anything you are not happy about please say now so that we can get it sorted, but that's why I guess I like having Babs so much—because I knew her as home help and a good friend because I had to use her as my personal carer. (C8I)

Feeling confident that their personal assistance was dependable and within their control had removed a source of stress and anxiety for many users, allowing them to focus more energy on healthcare and therapeutic regimes to ameliorate the effects of illness or impairments. One person was able to attend a pain management course as a result of employing PAs whom she felt able to trust to look after her children, and this arrangement had dramatically improved her quality of life. The positive impact of DP on parenting for disabled people has been noted in previous research (Social Services Inspectorate, 2000; Wates, 2003).

It's changed my life being able to go out and it's made me accept things the way that they are a lot better than sitting in dwelling on it, you know. (C15F)

Interviewees reported no significant change in use of health services arising from their use of DP. One user reported that the district health nurse had suggested that the PA could do the tasks they currently carried out, but the user chose to continue using the district nurse and there was no suggestion, at the time of interview, that this service would be withdrawn now that an alternative was available. For most users, there appears to be a clear distinction between personal assistance and health care, which is at variance with other research on DPs that found many users disinclined to distinguish between the two (Glendinning et al., 2000). A number of users attended appointments at specialist outpatient services, sometimes at a considerable distance from home, and there were clear benefits from using DP for these users in terms of flexible times and assistance in attending appointments.

# Effects of using DP on other members of the family

Most of those interviewed depended to a greater or lesser extent on other members of their families for some assistance. For some family carers, the burden of care remains heavy even with DPs, and users reported a strain on relationships and on the health of carers since care packages were too small to reduce the burden substantially. However, family carers enjoyed many of the same benefits as users from DP. The increased flexibility of the new arrangements had allowed some to continue shift working, which would not have been possible using Social Services Department, and the dependability of PAs had reduced the number of crises requiring intervention by family members when agency/SSD staff had been unavailable.

In the case of one family with a daughter with a learning disability, the confidence and comfort in having control over who provided respite support was, as they put it, 'like light on a cold dark day':

> The respite care was the problem, that was the big thing. We could overcome everything else but it was very difficult to overcome that, not having relatives or friends or anybody close who would have her, so it was marvellous, it was like a light on a cold dark day, it really was. So far I know we have only been a part of it for less than 12 months but so far it's been absolutely brilliant. (M6F)

> Diane takes a long time to build her trust up in … this lady knows Diane as well as I know her, she knows her likes, her dislikes, what pleases her, what upsets her and not only is there that, looking at it from my point of view, I can let Diane go on respite care without a worry in the world. I can have complete and utter freedom without any worry because I do worry about it but I don't when she is on her respite care because I know that she's home from home and she's being looked after as I would want her to be looked after. (M6F)

The greatest benefits to other family members were in the positive relationships people had with their PAs and the much greater confidence they felt in the care they were receiving. Family members who provide care were more likely to be able to take an evening off by virtue of the flexibility of DP, and sometimes reported feeling more able to 'let go' a little, knowing that their disabled relative was receiving high quality assistance. Knowing this often had a positive effect on the disabled person as well.

> He's a person in his own right, and I lost sight of that for a long time—I was so wrapped up in my own [needs] …

> I've really learnt now, that for every half an hour that somebody else does, it's something that he doesn't have to do … (C11F)

# Conclusion

The nature of much personal support work is such that people need to receive their support from others who they trust, feel comfortable with and to whom they can relate. These criteria are not easily achieved through large bureaucracies, and the evidence above certainly indicates widespread dissatisfaction with traditional methods of providing support. However, the evidence also suggests that they can be achieved when individuals are in control of their own staff. The evidence above suggests that DP can help create an environment where a service user is in control, is confident and it treated with respect by those hired to provide support.

> I would advise anyone to go for it, no matter how apprehensive they may be. If they get the right help and the right encouragement, I would say go for it because you start to live your life again. I was disabled suddenly in a wheelchair over night. I had no working up to it, and no matter what your disability is, how long you have had it or whatever, go for it. It really brings your life back in perspective again. You have got the say and you have got the driving seat. If you

work it properly, it does work. Like I don't have to worry about the girls upstairs. They are getting on. They are doing the lunch, they are doing dinner for tonight. One has been doing ironing. That's without me asking they just look and see what needs doing. I would say grab it with both hands and do it. It won't be easy the first six months but you can do it and that goes also for mentally disabled people because they are quite capable of doing this and administering this; all they need is help. No matter what your disability is, all you need is help and the will to want to improve things. Whoever thought up the idea needs a medal. (V7F)

Our study suggests that DP can facilitate a broad range of beneficial outcomes for users confirming the anecdotal and research evidence (see Dawson, 2000; Glasby and Littlechild, 2002). While the administration and management demands were not inconsequential, as the quote above suggests, they are not seen by disabled people as a significant barrier to using DP. It should be remembered, however, that the participants in this study had access to a high quality support service run by a disabled people's organization. While the current study cannot 'prove' the necessity of this factor, users certainly indicated its positive benefits, as is consistent with other findings (Dawson, 2000; Lord and Hutchison, 2003).

Participants in the study identified increased control over their lives, improved self-esteem, deeper and more rewarding relationships with other people, and a range of new interpersonal, vocational and lifestyle opportunities as key outcomes of direct payments. In some cases, these contributed to improved health and healthcare as well as educational opportunities. There was also an indication that this 'new found freedom' extended to other family members as well.

Ultimately, this notion of freedom and independence underlies the most profound aspects of the experience of users. The use of emancipatory language was common, as others have found (Dawson, 2000), and emancipation has been suggested as a key goal of DP as a policy (Pearson, 2000; Stainton, 2002). The users in this study would confirm this.

I have got freedom now which I felt for years I didn't have. I have got control. I can control my own life now. (V7F)

# References

Dawson, C. (2000) *Independent Successes: Implementing Direct Payments.* York: Joseph Rowntree Foundation.

Glasby, J. and Littlechild, R. (2002) *Social Work and Direct Payments.* Bristol: Policy Press.

Glendinning, C., Halliwell, S., Jacobs, S., Rurnmery, K. and Tyrer, J. (2000) *Buying Independence: using Direct Payments to Integrate Health and Social Services.* Bristol: Policy Press.

Lord, J. and Hutchison, P. (2003) 'Individualized support and funding: building blocks for capacity building and inclusion', *Disability & Society,* 18(1): 71–86.

Pearson, C. (2000) 'Money talks? Competing discourses in the implementation of direct payments', *Critical Social Policy,* 20(4): 459–477.

Social Services Inspectorate [SSI] (2000) *A Jigsaw of Services.* London: Department of Health.

Stainton, T. (2002) 'Taking rights structurally: rights, disability and social worker responses to Direct Payments', *British Journal of Social Work,* 32: 751–763.

Wates, M. (2003) *It Shouldn't be Down to Luck: Report on a Consultation with Disabled Parents for Disabled Parents Network.* Available online at: www.DisabledParentsNetwork.org.uk (accessed July 21, 2004).

# Section 2
## Places

## Introduction

This second section focuses on where care takes place and how this affects the experience of caring for both the receivers and the providers of care. The importance attached to home and homeliness and the associated notions of autonomy, independence and control are recurring themes in many of the chapters in this section.

The opening anthology chapter – put together by Sheila Peace, a geographer and gerontologist, and Dorothy Atkinson, a historian with a particular interest in the histories of people with learning difficulties – provides a variety of perspectives on places for care. While giving voice to people receiving care and support in their own homes, it also considers a diverse range of issues related to design and adaptation which enable people to sustain their independence and workers to perform more effectively. The last extract, for example, is taken from a report about the role of hospital design in the recruitment, retention and performance of nurses.

The following chapters in this section focus on specific places and spaces. Chapter 10 is extracted from Lynsey Hanley's book on council estates. As someone brought up on a large estate, she provides an insider account of the relationship between environment and identity and makes some telling suggestions about the future direction of social housing. Housing and the relationship between housing policy and community are relatively neglected topics in the health and social care literature. It has generally been the case that health and social care work and education have a tendency to focus on individuals and particular professional interventions, overlooking the broader contextual and structural factors that lead to disadvantage and inequality in the first place. This chapter makes quite clear the connection between structural factors and individual chances and is, therefore, an important contribution to general debates on health and social care and to discussions about how best to regenerate communities.

In the remaining chapters, the focus is more upon specific contexts for care and support. In Chapter 11, Colin Barnes discusses the notion of 'independent living' within the framework of the social model of disability. Chapter 12, taken from Alison Norman's classic book *Rights and Risk*, persuasively describes what happens to people, in this case older people, when they lose their independence through enforced relocation. She argues that the consequence of losing your home is a risk that should be weighed up when considering the advantages and disadvantages of being relocated to a safe environment, such as a residential care home. Chapter 13 moves on to the institutional environment and its features. It outlines Erving Goffman's seminal work on what he conceptualised as 'total institutions', such as prisons, boarding schools or mental asylums. His observations have had a lasting impact on our views of and understanding of how institutions operate. At a more detailed level and picking up on Goffman's work, Chapter 14, by Geraldine Lee-Treweek describes research she undertook in a residential care home for older people. In particular, her focus is on what happens in spaces hidden from public view – bedrooms. She examines the contradiction between bedrooms as places of privacy but also as workplaces where body work is performed or, in Goffman's terms, where the 'backstage' work takes place.

The final chapter in this section returns to a broader spatial context, the internet. It is taken from Maria Bakardjieva's book, *Internet Society*, where she describes researching how people make use of the internet in their own homes. She asked people about what they used the internet for, who they met online and whether or not all this changed their lives. This chapter features chat rooms and, in the context of health and social support needs, considers their significance, based on the experiences of the people she interviewed.

# Chapter 9

## Anthology: places

*Compiled by Sheila Peace and Dorothy Atkinson*

Caring takes place everywhere: in the domestic home, the hospital ward, the day centre or the care home, for example. These are all built environments that provide the context for the everyday lives of children, parents and grandparents, families and friends, service users and professional staff, such as nurses, care workers, doctors or occupational therapists. As buildings these environments will have been designed for particular purposes at particular points in time and their different histories may mean that they meet people's needs in different ways.

This anthology unpicks the theme of caring in place by offering a collection of excerpts from a range of publications, both contemporary and historical. At first sight they may seem quite disparate as we hear from older and disabled people about support and adaptations at home; about the importance of environment from a woman with dementia; about life on a long stay ward for people with learning disabilities; and nursing staff talking about how their place of work affects their performance. What these pieces have in common is how the way in which people and places come together affects their quality of life and well being.

## 9.1 Experiencing home care

This is an excerpt from an interview[1] with Reg Martin who was born in 1935. He was interviewed by Wendy Rickard in 1995 and the recording is deposited in the National Sound Archive at the British Library. For the 'home help' of the past or the 'home carer' today, being able to come into someone else's home and enable them to make decisions needs a particular type of social relationship, which Glenda managed with Reg.

---

**Excerpt form interview with Reg Martin (b. 1935)**

And I was put onto the Social Services. It was fine, except for the Home Helps. I could never understand a Home Help who was coming to clean who could come in and say, Now what do you want me to clean (laughs). I could never understand a Home Help asking

---

[1]Punctuated as transcribed.

such a question because if you have a home you do what's mostly, the bathroom, the living room, the bedroom. If it needs doing, you do it, you shouldn't need to ask. But they insisted and I couldn't cope with this. And it was all so different. So I had to keep on thinking of what did I say to the last one because there were things they could do and things they couldn't do. And I wasn't feeling well, to have to sort of argue. And then there was the food. I used to buy as I required but now I had to buy in advance of things. But I didn't know what I wanted. I didn't know whether I felt, you see (indistinct) it was very difficult to buy with the Home Helps. And after about six of them (laughs) I decided that this was a bad no go. It was definitely a no go time. And I was thinking, Oh I must be happy, just to let go, forget about it. But then they sent one around, Glenda. She never introduced herself as the Home Help, because we had an entry phone to come up, she just said, Glenda, Glenda from the Social Service Department. And she came up the stairs I opened the door and there was a great big smile. She said (indistinct) she said I'm Glenda, I'm the Home Help, I've come to do some shopping. I said. Oh, well I, you're a bit early, I haven't written out the list. Oh, it's all right she said you know. And we sat down and I was getting sort of tied up with this list. Eh, I wasn't sure and. And then she, Shall I have a look at it? And she had a look. And she said, Don't you need this. Don't you need that? And…And she was suggesting things. Well, god what a difference in a person. And she went off and she left her bag here, in the flat and she had an umbrella she didn't want to take with her so she left that there, you know. Off she, off she went and and end of half an hour she was back with a few things you know. And she sat and chatted, you know. And I spoke to her and asked her lots of questions and eh she laughed. And she was always having a laugh. She'd a great big grin. It was so nice. It really was. And, so she came again on the Monday, I was expecting somebody else. But she came back and this time she went and took the laundry down and while it was washing she came back and sat and chatted again and…I'm thinking I like this, I like this one. And I made up my mind when she finished, it was either this Glenda or nobody at all. So I rang Janine at the Home Care and I told her I said, The situation is this, I've got this girl called Glenda. I said, Well I want her. If I can't have her then I, just forget it. Oh, she says, I don't know whether, she said it's possible to immediately give you Glenda, because she's got other clients. But as it turned out Glenda had, a couple of clients, unfortunately, had died and it seems as though it was eh, shall I say, a partnership made in heaven really because it was at the right time. These people had died and she had the space for me to fit into. And that's, was fine. It was lovely. She came and we chatted and sometimes I wasn't feeling so good and so she wouldn't do, she would do very little. She would just sit, and chat, or if she thought you were really down, you just wanted to be quiet, she would just quietly go round and do things. You didn't have to tell her, you didn't have to tell her at all. You didn't have to tell her the bathroom needs cleaning, the kitchen needs cleaning you know, the bedroom, you know. She just did it as she would her own, her own home. That was nice. Shopping she got to know that I didn't know what I fancied or not, you know, because was losing, because I wasn't eating properly, I was losing, I was losing much more (coughs). And I hated the stuff they were still trying to give me, it was awful, it was like poison and Glenda, she used to find things, little pots of things, you know all sort of tasty and I used to have a fridge sort of full of little pots of things that she'd found. And it was just on the shopping day, which was so nice. She'd be shopping for somebody else, on another day, and see something and she'd buy it and she's bring it in, you know, on her way past. And, I saw this, I thought you might like this. And I'd pay her for it. And off she goes. Just a matter of seconds that she'd be in And it was so nice to think eh she was thinking about you. She obviously does it to others as well you know. I'm not saying I'm so special but it makes you feel eh happy and confident with, with her, and trusting. Which you, you have to trust people when they are coming into your home. You must feel happy, you must have a rapport, a compatibility, between you and I had it with her and I had it with Janina also and I had it with Jai. It all went very well indeed.

*Source*: C743/02/07 (F4935), tape 5, side b, National Sound Archive, 1995.

## 9.2   Adapting for disabled living

Bertie is one of 54 older people who took part in in-depth interviews for a study of the relationships between environment and identity in later life.

Born in Luton 84 years ago, Bertie had lived in Bedford for the last 50 years and was recently widowed. In the early 1990s his wife had suffered a number of strokes that left her disabled. As a retired architect, Bertie decided to use his own design skills to create an environment within their home that would better suit their needs and allow his wife to be cared for at home. These adaptations took place over a period of time and included structural alterations to the house and gardens; experiments with different kinds of off-the-shelf aids and devices; and small tailor-made adjustments to meet specific needs … Having both the financial ability and knowledge necessary to take this path, Bertie focused on the adaptation of the given environment rather than on other kinds of option such as moving house or looking for residential care.

The first time that his wife was ill, Bertie decided to create an extension and a downstairs toilet so that she could live in the more sociable space of the ground floor. He approached the local social services department for help:

I had a letter which said that if by any chance we were lucky enough to get a grant I would be expected to pay between £6–7000. Well, I was horrified, so I called the whole thing to a halt and said 'fair enough'. So I went it alone and I put a shower in myself, I had a lavatory basin put in, took a cupboard out and had the boiler put in the kitchen … . But, she was interested in her clothes and so of course when she wanted to get dressed in the morning, what did I have to do? Go upstairs and I would bring the wrong one down and she said what she wanted and I wouldn't have a clue [laughs] so I trundled up and downstairs and the first thing we did was bring down the wardrobe and stuck it here behind me here. She got all her clothes down here.

One of the things that I don't think is always appreciated is how important access and doors are. You came in this morning through the front wall where the first thing I did was widen it by three feet because if you've got the car in the drive you couldn't push a wheelchair right by it.

I got to the position in the end where the only way to get her out of here [front room] in a chair was to go out through here, through that porch where there was considerable congestion, down a ramp into the garden into a door at the back of the garage, back through the garage right around the front wall … it was a major issue. …

She couldn't negotiate the steps, so I did a ramp myself which went up one side so that you could get a wheelchair up and I adjusted the steps a bit so that you could also walk in and there was a rise between so that she had the option. She wasn't embarrassed by the fact that everything pointed to the fact that her being incapacitated.

You can see yourself if you're with a person and perhaps that's where I had the advantage on the OT, I was with her all the while so I could see whether a handle was needed and one of the vital ones is at the top of the stairs on the newel post as you get off the stair lift, at the top of the stairs, you have a handle to grasp … .

Upstairs we've got a toilet and the very same situation arose, I put handles both sides, but then you've got a 2'6" door swing in and you sterilize 2'6" of the floor space and so I put bi-fold doors up there and I did the same in the bathroom because there we wanted additional room. You see it wasn't only the patient, we wanted a carer alongside her and there wasn't room or if there was room the door swing was in the way, so I put bi-fold doors in there.

I would say that the authorities have been very helpful, but I do believe that a lot of things … if you do have the inclination to be a do it yourself, you can do it yourself and I have done a lot, I shouldn't say it really, but I have. I mean, even raising the height of a thing, I mean I have got a milk bottle carrier outside the back door, it is a nonsense really it has been up years, but instead of having to bend down to pick my milk up I put my hand out and it is at the right level.

*Source*: Sheila Peace, Caroline Holland and Leonie Kellaher (2006) *Environment and Identity in Later Life*. Maidenhead: Open University Press, pp. 138–140 (abridged).

# 9.3   A dementia-friendly environment

Christine Bryden was a top civil servant in Australia and single mother of three children when she was diagnosed with Alzheimer's disease at the age of 46.  She has written a book about her experience of living with dementia, the effects of memory problems, difficulties in communication and the exhaustion of coping with simple tasks. She has also given many talks on the topic which can be viewed on her website at www.christinebryden.com In this extract she describes what she means by a dementia-friendly environment.

Our environment is a critical part of our disease. How we exhibit symptoms will very much depend on our environment and how well we can cope with it. We need love, comfort, attachment, inclusion, identity and occupation as our world around us becomes strange and our ability scrambled.

The importantce of the person's environment in coping with the experience of dementia has been the focus of work by Kitwood who made a detailed study of the impact on the manifestation of dementia related to the institutional care environment. He suggested that dementia arises from a complex interaction between various factors unique to the person, which would explain the great variability of symptoms and progression of losses that accompany any particular type of dementia in different people.

First there is the personality, or resources for action, including a set of avoidances and blocks acquired through life's experiences of failure, fear or powerlessness, accompanied by various defences against anxiety. Next is the biography, or life story, including all losses and current social support. Then there is physical health, including sensory function, which may affect the degree of confusion and ability to communicate. These all affect the way the person copes with the actual brain damage.

The most important factor for improving care is the environment, as this can be changed quite easily to ensure that it enhances the person's sense of safety, value and well being. It needs to validate the person's experiences and emotions, facilitate the person's actions, celebrate the person's abilities, and provide sensory pleasures.

But sometimes the family home is where past conflicts, present tensions and well-worn patterns of behaviour may profoundly affect the expression of dementia. Please try to make sure you get help, to address any underlying emotional issues. As emotional beings, we are buffeted by our environment, with few cognitive resources to cope with stress. So we are very susceptible to our environment and to any family dysfunction. We cannot cope with stress, tension, arguments or unease around us.

As environment is so important to the expression of dementia, there is a great deal you can do to help. How we exhibit symptoms will very much depend on how well we can cope as the world around us becomes strange and our ability scrambled. Our behaviour is usually a perfectly reasonable response to our environment given the degree of brain damage we have.

Avoid background noise, which will make me tired and confused, anxious and even aggressive. A quiet environment helps avoid additional confusion. I wonder why so many day care centres and nursing homes have a TV, radio and talking all happening at once? No wonder the people sitting there look so blank! Maybe think about ear plugs for a visit to shopping centres or other noisy places.

If children are underfoot, remember we will get tired very easily and find it very hard to concentrate on talking or listening as well. Make sure we face away from any visual disturbances, and that we are in a quiet place.

Encourage routine so that we can feel safe and secure in a familiar environment, with a set of activities that we can recall. This will reduce the stress of trying to make sense of our surroundings.

Make our spaces uncluttered, particularly in areas like the kitchen and bathroom. Use a combined shampoo and conditioner so there are not too many bottles. Try to have a shower that is easy to get into, and a tap that only has one control, and no very hot or cold water.

We may have difficulty in vision and coordination which mean we might knock things over and feel clumsy. Decanting things into plastic containers might avoid breakages. If we do knock things over, and stare blankly at the mess we have made, please help us clear up, as we can't think through the steps needed, and get flustered and confused.

The entry and exit doors to toilets in public places, such as community centers, are a real challenge. They never seem to be painted a contrasting colour, so that we can find our way in and out of the toilet. There can be so many doors in there to confuse us, and our care-partner may not be able to go in there to help us. Whenever we have gone out with groups of people with dementia, this is always an issue. Someone is late coming out, and you hear doors banging as someone tries to work out which door is the right way out of the toilet. If only the entry and exit doors were a contrasting colour to all the other doors, we wouldn't get as confused and might be able to go out more often!

*Source*: Christine Bryden (2005) *Dancing with Dementia*. London: Jessica Kingsley, pp.144–146.

# 9.4   Life on a locked ward

This extract is taken from a research report written by Katherine Owen for the Judith Trust. It is a pen picture of 'Greenfield', a locked ward for women with learning disabilities as she – the researcher – experienced it. The ward subsequently closed (in 2000) and the women were moved into residential homes.

## Rules

### Rules for everything

The women's life on the ward was also greatly restricted by various rules. Some rules and regulations are crucial for the smooth and efficient running of any institution, but on Greenfield these rules permeated every area of the women's lives. There were rules about where they could go, both outside and inside the ward, rules about behaviour and even rules about the expression of emotion.

The rules which defined where the residents could and could not go were enforced by the locking of doors. It resulted in the women's lives being narrowed to the world of the ward. However, some of them made it known that they wanted to go out. Several of them waited by the front door, occasionally trying the door handle to see if it had been left unlocked, or waiting for an opportunistic opening of the door, which would allow for their escape.

### Vulnerable and dangerous

The ward was described as a 'locked' ward, which meant that none of the women, except one, were allowed to leave the ward unescorted. This rule was said to exist both for the protection of the women's 'vulnerability' and for the protection of others from the women's 'dangerousness'. It was linked to incidences of their past 'behaviours', for example, 'absconding', 'ingesting cigarette butts', and 'unpredictable violence'.

Locked doors were also a feature within Greenfield. The kitchen, the office, the laundry, the staff room, the staff toilet, the individual bedrooms, and the bathroom and shower room were locked at all times. Only the toilets and the main compartmentalised bedroom were left open. The staff justified locking the doors by describing how Elizabeth would go into rooms and throw objects out of the nearest window in her way of tidying up. Such rules had a significant impact on where the women spent their time during the day.

## Staff have keys. Patients don't

They were confined to the two main communal rooms, where they were surrounded by others. If they wanted time on their own they had to stand in the corridors. All the staff had keys to open the doors. None of the women who lived on the ward had keys.

If the women wanted something from their bedrooms, they had to ask permission from the staff. Even those who shared the compartmentalised room were dependent on staff to unlock their wardrobes, or 'lockers', so they could get items of clothing, or other desired possessions. However, individual women, who were thought to be capable and to some extent trustworthy, were given keys to do specific tasks. For example, Gillian was allowed to get her coat from her bedroom. Sally was given the most freedom with staff keys. She was allowed into her bedroom on request, and also allowed to go to the bathroom and start running herself a bath in the evening.

Many rules existed about the women's behaviour, an example of this being mealtimes. Whether it was lunch or supper, the women sat in their set places at four tables placed around the dining room. A member of staff wheeled in a trolley from the kitchen. One member of staff stood in the centre of the room with the trolley, took off the lids of the pre-packed, pre-heated food, and dished out the food onto plates. Another placed it in front of each woman. The women were required to stay sitting in their seats. In Greenfield ward the staff did not eat at the same time as the residents and they did not sit down at the same tables.

## Eat; sit up; sit down; no talking

During mealtimes staff walked about the room or sat on the radiators at the edge of the room, enabling them to be raised above the dining tables and direct the proceedings. The women would be told to eat their food, stop talking, use their knives and forks, sit up straight, or sit down.

Tensions were often high at mealtimes, as the woman attempted to get their needs met in the midst of these restrictions. The fact that they were given food and drink without the opportunity to choose it meant that if someone wanted something different, for example, a glass of water instead of squash, then they were dependent on the good will of the staff to go and get them their preferred drink. If they did not like the food that had been served, they were rarely offered an alternative and would go hungry. The women would push against the rules in different ways. Eva would get round being made to eat by either throwing up in the toilet after the meal, or by dropping her food onto the floor so that it would be too dirty to eat. Clare would push her food onto Samantha's plate. Francesca would avoid being moved back to her seat, if she had got up, by sitting down on the floor. Gillian would often ignore the staff's requests to be quiet and continue to talk.

## Smile. No whingeing or whining

The women were encouraged to 'smile', and 'be happy'. Eva was told not to 'whinge and whine' and was also asked not to talk about her particular conversational preoccupations. The women would cry often, usually for short periods. Sometimes it would be acknowledged, but in the main it was ignored. There was a sense that the staff did not want, perhaps could not bear, to dwell on negative emotions.

### Control

The staff ensured the women's adherence to the rules through various means: a system of rewards and penalties, medication, and observation. Rewards included cups of tea, biscuits, being allowed to take staffs keys and go to their bedroom, and trips out. In terms of penalties, it was not so much privileges that were withdrawn, but usually things of value to individuals: cigarettes for Eva, puzzles for Gillian, leaving the ward for Anita, and for all of them, access to bedrooms. Being allowed to go to the day service was also used as a bargaining tool in the control of people's behaviour. The women became distressed over the withdrawal or withholding of the things that were important to them, and some of them would begin to cry. Gillian followed staff around repeating, 'I'm good now, I'm good aren't I?', and try to do things to win the staff over. Eva smiled a false smile and once danced as a way to please the staff and get a cigarette. Anita tried to hug or cuddle the staff, as a way of saying she was sorry and that she wanted her punishment to be over.

The women's behaviour was also controlled through the use of medication. All the women were on regular medication, including a mixture of anticonvulsant, anti-muscarinic, anti-psychotic and sedative drugs. Many of the women were prescribed anti-psychotic drugs to stabilise their moods and several were also prescribed sedative drugs on a regular basis. However, if this was not thought to be having the desired effect, PRN ('when necessary') medication was also given. It was given if people were perceived to be 'high', or if there had been an incidence of violence or aggression on the ward. Sometimes the threat of medication was used as a means of controlling behaviour. For example, on one occasion when one woman refused to take her oral medication she was threatened with an injection.

Observation is a common controlling feature of institutional life. The women were watched both formally, through practices such as 1:1 staff supervision, observation checks every 15 minutes, or information sheets for periods, behaviour and bowel evacuation, and informally, through keeping the doors locked and the women in two main rooms. The women also disciplined themselves, regulating their own behaviour, for fear of 'getting into trouble' or 'doing something wrong'. As a result personal development and personal freedom were denied them.

*Source*: The Judith Trust (2003) *Going Home? A Study of Women with Severe Learning Disabilities Moving Out of a Locked Ward.*

# 9.5   The role of hospital design in the recruitment, retention and performance of NHS nurses

This research was commissioned by the Commission for Architecture and the Built Environment (CABE) and [carried out by Pricewaterhouse Coopers LLP (PwC) in association with the University of Sheffield and Queen Margaret University College, Edinburgh] undertaken between September 2003 and April 2004. The primary aim was to explore whether hospital design has an influence on the recruitment, retention and performance of NHS nurses in England, and to examine which aspects of design matter to nurses.

The Commission for Architecture and the Built Environment (CABE) … believes that improving the design of public buildings is fundamental to improving public services and that well-designed healthcare buildings can lead to better health outcomes. CABE's … report, … provides evidence that well-designed hospitals have a significant influence on the performance of nurses in their work and have a positive impact on their recruitment and retention. The research also shows that nurses are acutely aware of the role that hospital design plays in their everyday work and, consequently, want a greater say in shaping their working environment.

Whilst … a number of studies … examine the influence of the workplace on *office* staff, less research has been done on the effect that the healthcare environment has on the staff, particularly nurses, working within it. Much … information to date about design in hospitals is focused on patients.

## Methods

In carrying out the research … three major strands of work were undertaken:

- a review of existing literature…
- a series of qualitative focus groups with nursing staff were held in London, Leeds, Birmingham, Bury-St. Edmunds and Bristol
- a major quantitative survey of 479 Directors and Assistant Directors of Nursing throughout England.

## Nurses and their working environment – the evidence

'The outline and shape of a ward can influence how a group of nurses work – this has an effect on both management style and infection control issues' (Nurse, Leeds). Whilst findings of this study indicate that hospital design has the greatest impact on the performance of staff, followed by their recruitment and retention, it also recognizes the complex links between all three. Overall the research findings show that:

- well-designed healthcare buildings contribute to enhanced performance and motivation, leading to better health outcomes for patients
- good design is a factor in nurses' choice of hospitals
- a focus on internal design should be a priority – in particular the organisation of space on wards and units, storage and lighting (both natural and artificial)
- nurses want to be consulted about design, believe they can play a positive role in improving the design aspects of the areas in which they work and that consultation should begin early on the process.

[…]

## The impact of hospital design on performance of nurses

The relationship…between the organisation and layout of workplaces and levels of employee fatigue and stress is becoming increasingly clear. In this study, 86 per cent of Directors of Nursing say that hospital design is 'very important' or 'important' in nurses' performance, with the most crucial aspect being the design and organisation of the internal hospital environment … 'If you get exhausted in working in those sorts of conditions you get low, then depressed and morale goes' (Nurse, Birmingham).

Nurses view flexible working space as highly significant to their performance, that rooms and wards can be too functional, making them inflexible and only suitable for very specific purposes. Of particular importance is the layout and use of space – for example, so that nurses can observe patients as well as move around easily and perform procedures. The distance travelled between tasks can also contribute to performance and fatigue. 'A large proportion of our job is observation, and if we can't see a patient easily that's one of our senses that is rendered useless' (Nurse, London).

Constant exposure to artificial light, in particular fluorescent tube lights, is commonly mentioned by nurses as one of the most draining aspects of working on a ward. The capacity for nurses and patients to control the air temperature, rather than rely on hospital air conditioning systems, is seen as important, as is having the ability to open windows. 'It makes you happier to be working in a nice environment, pleasant view, sufficient daylight and the possibility of opening a window for fresh air' (Nurse, Bristol).

The particular stresses associated with nursing mean that dedicated areas for staff rest and relaxation during the working day are beneficial. Attractive outside spaces, gardens and landscaping are aspects of a hospital's design that both attract and retain nursing staff, especially relevant where the spaces allows staff to spend time away from their day to day work.

This might also extend to providing space for confidential discussions with patients and relatives, and between staff members. Often, if a staff room exists, it is the only place available to hand over between shifts and staff are trying to hand over to one another in the same space; rooms are frequently communal and used by doctors, ward and clerical staff and for meetings, leaving staff with nowhere to go. 'Ideally the staff rest area should be away from the ward area…so that staff actually get the chance to go away from the work area to relax' (Nurse, London).

Storage space is seen to have a particular impact on the ability of nurses to be able to work efficiently, with examples given of equipment having to be stored in inappropriate places such as patient bathrooms, with additional problems brought about by equipment being stored away from where it is needed. 'Equipment should have a place to live, not be stored in front of an exit or in a corridor' (Nurse, Birmingham).

Nurses feel that the location and quality of staff facilities – lockers, showers, on-site banks, canteen and crèche facilities – are very important elements … contributing to their ability to focus on their work by allowing them to carry out non work-related tasks easily.

The quality of fixtures and fittings is also seen as important with many nurses highlighting what they consider to be 'cost-cutting' measures that result in inferior quality fittings – door frames and locks, taps that do not encourage good infection control practices and sinks that are not big enough. 'You go into the staff toilets and turn the tap on by hand, but you have to turn it off by hand – you've just washed your hands because they were potentially going to contaminate a patient – how do you turn it off without recontaminating your hands?… There is no logic, no rational thought at all' (Nurse, London).

[…]

*Source*: Commission for Architecture and the Built Environment (CABE) (2004) *The Role of Hospital Design in the Recruitment, Retention and Performance of NHS Nurses in England.*

# Chapter 10

## Estates

*Lynsey Hanley*

We lived in Area 4. It was on the edge of the Wood – an estate on the periphery of Birmingham – in a row of terraced houses that led into a fistful of dead-ends. Between the house and my primary school there were no more than a few yards of road, the rest being a series of inter-connecting walks and avenues lined with more terraces and maisonettes. You could walk past the school and as far as the shopping centre, a mile away, and only have to cross the road once. […] Nearly 60,000 people lived there, on what was one of the biggest council estates in Europe.

The Wood. I was born there, and lived there between the ages of eighteen months and eighteen years. Even though I have lived away from home for over a third of my life now, it continues to shape the way I think about the world outside it. […]

It's not something you think about when you're growing up. *Wow, I'm really alienated. My school is suffering from its single-class intake. What this estate needs is a decent public-transport infrastructure*. It's more a sense you have. […]

Council estates are nothing to be scared of, unless you are frightened of inequality. They are a physical reminder that we live in a society that divides people up according to how much money they have to spend on shelter. My heart sags every time it senses the approach of those flat, numbing boxes that prickle the edges of every British town. […] I can't think about council estates without having a pronounced emotional reaction to those very words. … But there's something about them that makes me brim over with pain, and a sense of wrongness; even the bits that anyone else would think right. It's not even a feeling of having been hard done by (or is it?). It's more a feeling of having been consigned, contained, delivered to a place, to serve a sentence that may never end.

A more rounded view would take into account the degrading living conditions endured by working-class families in industrial cities, in slums and shanty towns, before council housing provided millions of them with warmth and space for the first time since their ancestors left the fields. Our grandparents – even our parents – do not forget how good it feels to have your own bath and an inside toilet, but then neither do they forget what it's like to live in a place that feels knitted into the fabric of the town or city it forms a part of.

From: Lynsey Hanley (2007) *Estates: An Intimate History*. London: Granta Books [Extracts].

[…]

Play word association with the term 'council estate'. Estates mean alcoholism, drug addiction, relentless petty stupidity, a kind of stir-craziness induced by chronic poverty and the human mind caged by the rigid bars of class and learned incuriosity. In London, there's an estate at the bottom of almost every gentrified road, a self-contained world signposted by lopsided bollards, DO NOT PLAY BALL signs and standardized double glazing. The privet hedges stop where the sound of shirtless men shouting begins.

[…]

Sometimes, estates feel as though they serve to wilfully deaden or disrupt lives, but they were never intended to. … When the Wood's local football club plays a team from elsewhere in the borough, they compete to the sound of a terrace chant that goes 'Go back! To your council estate!', sung to the tune of 'Go West' by the Village People. Recidivists are reported in newspapers to live on this or that estate as though it were a matter of course that they would. Any rich or famous person about whom it's discovered that they were brought up in a council house, no matter what else distinguishes them, is understood to have something of the Pygmalion about them.

[…]

Council homes were once the golden standard for a bright, uncynical working class who had every reason to feel entitled to the best the state had to offer them. To get a council house in the immediate post-war period was to have a full stake in society. Ownership didn't matter: what did matter was that you had succeeded in persuading those in power that you deserved better than to live in a slum, at the mercy of an exploitative landlord. The dream of holding a fair and equable stake in the collective wealth of the nation – of which good housing formed a part – barely had time to bear fruit before it was punctured, without ceremony, by the idea that the only way to feel fully anchored to society, and therefore to be fully a citizen, was to own the property you lived in. Council homes were never intended to be holding cages for the poor and disenfranchised, but somehow, that's how they ended up.

[…]

Between the two world wars, about a quarter of working-class people moved from the inner cities out into new outer-urban – the word 'suburban' sounds too middle-class – housing estates. […]

Families who moved from the cities on to new estates such as Cutteslowe, [in Oxford], Wythenshawe in Manchester and Speke in Liverpool could place themselves on a new class spectrum according to the poshness of the part of the estate they found themselves seconded to. In interviews similar to those conducted as part of the means test, they were asked by housing officers to reveal how they did their washing, whether they kept noisy or quiet pets, and how – if at all – they budgeted for essential items. If you spent your money as you got it, you would get a rented terrace without a bathroom (the bath in the kitchen would serve as a countertop when lidded with a slab of wood). If you planned and saved for the future, your reward would be an inside toilet. Poorer council-house dwellers suffered accordingly. They could not afford to keep up with the Joneses, and yet were required for the first time to buy or rent curtains, and to ensure that their children had shoes. Those who could not, or did not, became the ultimate pariahs, and the predecessors of those people we now revile for the degrading circumstances in which they find themselves.

[…]

In newspapers and on television, every reference to a council estate is prefixed with the word 'tough', as though bare-knuckle boxing is the leisure activity of choice for every British person who doesn't own their own home. It does its stigmatizing work as intended. Estates are dangerous, they imply: don't visit them, and whatever you do, work as hard as you can so you don't have to live on them. All the people who live on estates are failures, and failure is not only contagious but morally repugnant. Any connection between the physical, economic and social isolation of council estates and the sometimes desperate behaviour of their tenants is ignored, or dismissed, or laughed at, because that's what they're there for: to contain the undeserving, un-useful poor.

[...]

# The wall in the head

Since the fall of the Berlin Wall, a phrase has been used to describe the outlook of former residents of the communist GDR who can't quite get over the fact that their country has been subsumed into its larger, richer, democratic neighbour. They call it *der Mauer im Kopf*, or 'the wall in the head'. ...

To be working-class in Britain is also to have a wall in the head, and, since council housing has come to mean housing for the working class (and the non-working class), that wall exists unbroken throughout every estate in the land. The wall may be invisible, in that no one has built a fortress of bricks around every area of municipal housing ... but it's there, heavy and strong, and as thickly invisible as Pyrex. [...]

The wall in the head is built up slowly, brick by see-through brick, over the course of a lifetime. Your knowledge of what's out there, beyond the thick glass walls, is entirely reliant on what you can glean from the lives of the people you know, which usually means your own family members. If your family and friends all live on the same estate, that's a little wall built for you right there. If you have links outside it – friends who live in a different area or type of housing, activities that regularly and repeatedly expose you to new experiences – then you've one less wall to knock down. [...]

'He loves me to bits. I really wanna have a baby with him now. I've told me mom, she says it's fine if I can look after it.'

I remember these words, spoken by a classmate in a Home Economics lesson in our fifth year of secondary school. ... She wasn't speaking to me directly, but to the girls on either side of her, as they absently plaited their long dye-streaked hair without looking at it and fiddled with giant cans of Superdrug mousse under the desk. ... She had moved in with her boyfriend, after a row with her mum meant, evidently, that they could no longer live in the same house together.

[...]

Think of the pity of what she said: 'I've told me mom'. There is pity in the idea that no one found the statement particularly strange. ... There is a lot of pity in the thought that a girl's life had come to this at fifteen, and that she had little idea of what this could mean for the rest of it.

[...]

If you attend a school on a council estate, having come from a council estate, you get a council-estate education. It's not so much that you get told that kids like you can't ever hope to achieve their full potential; it's just that the very idea of having lots of potential to fulfil isn't presented. You don't know what your potential is, because no one has told you about it. Nobody tells you that there are universities, where you can learn about more things than you ever knew existed, because it's simply assumed that you'll never get that far. If you do what is hoped, but not expected, of you and find these things out for yourself, you have to *tell* your teachers precisely how far you are going to go in life, and even then they're not always going to believe you. Inculcated into every child at a council-estate school is the idea that you shouldn't hope for too much. ... Your best bet is get a place on a vocational course at the local technical college, where you'll get to hang out with lots of other kids whose educational attainment is scandalous in an affluent, highly technocratic society. [...]

Unless you show extraordinary levels of ability, initiative and maturity – in a school context where 'extraordinary' can mean anything from merely turning up, to showing an interest and then applying yourself – you are unlikely to be let in on the little secret that is the World Beyond the Wall. I am a child of the little secret, which is not to say I showed extraordinary levels of ability, initiative and maturity. Indeed, I showed the sort of qualities that most middle-class parents would regard in their children as deeply average, which is to say that I was quiet, conscientious, anxious to please, anxious full stop. My teachers – the only middle-class people I knew – let me in on the whole thing purely because I stuck out. ...

The wall is about *not* knowing what is out there, or believing that what is out there is either entirely irrelevant to your life, or so complicated that it would go right over your head if you made an attempt to understand it. It's hard to articulate. ... Here's an example that might better illustrate what I mean. The first time I saw a broadsheet newspaper, when I was about seventeen, sitting in the upstairs library of my sixth-form college, I thought it was an obscure subscription service for professors. It was the *Guardian*. I never for a moment imagined that I – armed with seven grade-A GCSEs and a shelf full of books at home – would ever be able to read it and understand it. *It wasn't for me*. It was completely unlike anything I'd ever seen.

[...]

That wall in the head springs up just when you most need a hammer to knock it down. It manifests itself in ways of speaking, ways of dressing, the ways in which opinions are exchanged and how entitled you feel to express an opinion at all. When I arrived at a sixth-form college in the southern part of Solihull, I was the only girl, along with a small handful of boys, from my school year to go there. ... The sixth-form college was a place full of nice people who didn't have a problem with the fact that I sometimes wore glasses ... I was all set, for the first time in my life, to fit in like that last satisfying counter in a game of Connect 4. But really, I had no idea. I mean, I had *no idea*.

[...]

I wanted to know about everything, but I felt a barrier stronger than I was capable of breaking down alone, a barrier that seemed to exist only in my mind but was no less solid for it. [...] If I was to fit in and make the friends I longed for, I had to learn how to become middle-class.

It was horrible. It felt like exchanging one wall for another. [...] For a year I stayed silent, absorbing as much as I could, scared of opening my mouth lest I got it wrong. Then, slowly, it began to make sense. I began to knit together the strands of this other world to make a rope that would carry me over the final wall.

In the second year, things were different. I'd saturated my brain with information and gradually found the confidence to say out loud what I'd learnt and what I thought of it.

[…]

So different were the lives lived at either end of my half-hour bus route to college that I could almost feel a physical change taking place on the way from one to the other. […]

A new and different gap was emerging between my life and that of the other kids on the bus. At school, I'd been seen as nothing more than an oddball, a boff, someone from the same area but who inhabited a different internal world. I began slowly to realize that my external world was now changing to go with it. For the first time, I was moving in completely different circles, ones in which I seemed to be accepted, even liked. … It appeared to me that the kind, sensible, thoughtful people I'd met at the sixth-form college – and who represented the vast majority of students there – were all middle-class. I seemed to be more on their wavelength than anyone's at school; therefore, I thought, I must be middle-class.

[…] I started getting the *Guardian* on weekdays and the *Observer* on Sundays; our politics teacher advised that it would help me with my A levels; the newsagent had to get them in especially. It felt as though everything was opening up to me: the richness of culture, the power of language, the usefulness of politics and, most importantly, the possibility of deep and lasting friendships rather than bully-acquaintances.

The first wall had fallen, but that didn't mean I was happy. The shock of realizing how much, and how rapidly, I was changing was almost too much to stand. There were many ways in which I was frail. The certainties that had bound together our small, isolated family-island began to come apart, as though the centre could only hold if we all remained exactly the same for ever. I stopped eating and got a part-time job in a cake shop so I could look at food all day without tasting it. My head felt like it was being crushed slowly in a vice (it really, physically felt like that: as though the walls were closing in and I would die if I didn't get out).

My parents waged civil war in the house, outbreaks of which I tried to duck but they wouldn't let me: they were scared. I told my dad I was depressed. 'But people like us don't get depressed!' he raged, depressed. For the first time in my life, I felt entitled to be treated for feelings that I knew were treatable, rather than an inescapable by-product of living a life in which you don't really feel entitled to anything. The GP in the flat brick clinic told me not to be silly, but – to his eternal credit – he didn't put me on My First Prozac as preparation for a lifelong trek along the vale of tears. Instead, he signed me up to a course of therapy in which, once a week, I'd reel off every one of my bizarre new discoveries about the world and its workings to a sympathetic psychologist. It worked amazingly well: a year later, I left home for London, never stronger, never to return to live. I knew then that everything was going to be all right. I had reached the other side of the wall.

[…]

# Homes fit for living in

In Britain, we face a future without council housing, if not without social housing. […] In the years since 1980 we have become a society of homeowners, which is how those people who do rent from councils and social landlords have come to be so marginalized.

[...] Why does mass state provision in health and education continue to thrive and attract ever greater public investment, whilst council housing becomes more fragmented and marginal every year?

The reasons for this disparity are historical: since the 1940s, with the exception of a few years at the advent of the welfare state, governments and councils have treated housing as a problem that needed to be fixed quickly, rather than as a fundamental part of a healthy, equal society. If public housing were to have the same status as the NHS or the education system, it would have had to have been wholly nationalized in the same way that they were. A second NHS – the National Housing Service – might today be as much a part of the national make-up as the NHS we have got, assuming it would have been treated with equal reverence by state and electorate, and would have received such massive investment. [...]

It would be dogmatic and silly to renationalize the 1.6 million council homes that have been bought under the Right to Buy, especially now that most of us accept or even crave the responsibility of having our own home. But ... [t]here will be a need for affordable social housing as long as property is bought and sold according to demand, and as long as low incomes and wide income disparities exist. Whether it is run by the local authority or by a housing association, it needs to be more thoughtfully placed and designed, more attuned to the needs and desires of the people who will live in it, and above all, more able to provide a liveable and enjoyable alternative to privately owned housing, rather than a miserable sign of failure.

I have a few ideas of my own as to how this might be achieved. [...]

The redevelopment of estates whose surface problems – remoteness, graffiti, loitering youths, ugly buildings – are caused by bad design and planning will only work ... if physical and cosmetic improvements are carried out along-side a serious and prolonged investment in tenants' potential to participate in managing their homes and estates so that they attain a sense of ownership and control. If tenants feel as though the estate is theirs, it doesn't matter whether or not they physically own their home: they will treat it with the same care as they would if their home was something they would one day sell to the highest bidder. [...]

The management of housing by and for tenants is crucial to the success of an estate, whether it is to remain in the charge of the council or be transferred to a social landlord. You need to be able to recognize the people who come and mow the grass verges every few weeks, or the voice of the person you call to ask to have your door repaired or rubbish chute declogged. [...] You need to know that the person who is dealing with your query or problem will not have forgotten who you are the next time you call. [...]

My vision – my hope – for the future of social housing is simple. I want it to come to be regarded as an integral part of the national housing stock, and not something that is seen as shameful. I want the desirability of home ownership not to come at the cost of denigrating council housing at every turn.

# Chapter 11

## Independent living: a social model account

*Colin Barnes*

Firmly rooted in the ideological and cultural traditions of western society, the notion of independent living, as used by the international disabled people's movement, represents a radical challenge to conventional thinking on disability. It encompasses both an ideological and practical solution to the everyday economic and social deprivations encountered by the overwhelming majority of disabled people and their families across the world. Also independent living has the potential not only to enhance the quality of life of people directly affected by disability, but also that of other structurally disadvantaged groups such as women, minority ethnic groups, lesbians and gay men, and older people.

To explain these claims further this paper will first examine orthodox thinking on disability and an alternative view emanating from disabled people and their organisations. Attention will then turn to the idea of independent living and its impact on policy development. The final part will address the ideological, cultural and practical implications of these developments.

## Orthodox views of disability and the challenge from disabled people and their organisations

There is a wealth of anthropological evidence that throughout history people with accredited impairments, who would today be considered disabled, have existed in relatively large numbers in all societies across the world. It is also evident that social responses to impairment and disability are historically, culturally and situationally variable (Hanks and Hanks, 1948; Scheer and Groce, 1988; Ingstad and Whyte, 1995).

Originally published in *Review of Disability Studies* (2005), 1(4): 5–13.

Notwithstanding variations within Western culture, there is a discernable cultural bias against people with any perceived biological abnormality or flaw that can be traced back to the ancient world of the Greeks and Romans (Garland, 1995). Although variable both in form and degree at different times and in different locations across Europe during the dark ages and the feudal period, perceptions of impairment and disability have been fairly consistent since the Enlightenment and the industrial revolution of the nineteenth century (Finkelstein, 1980; Oliver, 1990; Stiker, 1998; Gleeson, 1999).

This bias is due to the ideological, cultural and material changes that accompanied capitalist development. During the eighteenth century, Enlightenment thinkers produced a range of progressive ideas including a critique of established religions, an emphasis on the value of rational science, a commitment to social progress, and the generation of philosophies of secular, rational self-interest such as Liberal Utilitarianism. Later, these ideas were compounded by the evolutionary theories of Charles Darwin and their use by Social Darwinists and the Eugenics Movement.

In the nineteenth century, industrialisation, urbanisation and the spread of wage labour further enhanced the problems faced by anyone either unable or unwilling to compete for employment in the newly formed factory-based work systems (Ryan and Thomas, 1980; Oliver, 1990; Barnes, 1991; Gleeson, 1999). Such people were scrutinised and categorised in various ways by doctors and related professionals and segregated from the community into long stay hospitals and various institutions. These policies proliferated throughout much of the Western world during the first half of the twentieth century. The eugenic legacy was particularly influential in many developed countries including the USA and Sweden. The eugenic impulse came to its logical conclusion in the death camps of Nazi Germany in the 1930s and 40s, with the systematic murder of thousands of disabled people considered a burden to the state and, therefore, unworthy of life. A more so-called humanitarian response to the problem of the growing problem of disability did not emerge until the post 1945 period (Drake, 1999).

Before the eighteenth century, impairment and any subsequent disablement was usually explained with reference to religious teachings and/or traditional superstitions, myths and legends from earlier times. Notwithstanding that these miss-interpretations are still evident in some circles, today the prevalent view is that impairment causes disability and that disability is an individual medical problem or personal tragedy with overtly negative economic and social consequences for the individuals concerned, their families and society as a whole.

Moreover, since impairments are the cause of the problem logic dictates that they must be eradicated, minimised or cured. But where cures are ineffective, which is more often than not the case, people with impairments who are labelled disabled are viewed as not quite whole, not normal, and incapable of participating in and contributing to the everyday life of the community. They are, therefore, in need of care. In many countries this has resulted in the generation of a thriving and costly disability industry comprised of state institutions, private businesses, charities and voluntary organisations staffed by vast armies of professional helpers including doctors, nurses, therapists and social workers. The end result is that disabled people's assumed inadequacy and dependence is assured and reinforced. These perceptions were not seriously challenged until the 1960s and the emergence of the disabled people's movement (Campbell and Oliver, 1996).

Underpinning the political demands of disabled people and their organisations is a socio/political re-interpretation of disability widely referred to as the social model of disability. Originally devised by disabled activists in Britain, this approach derives from disabled people's direct experiences of living with impairment in Western society (UPIAS, 1975). Since its development in the 1970s, the social model has been increasingly accepted and adapted by disability groups throughout the world, and now underpins, either implicitly or explicitly, their thinking (WHO, 2001). It is also evident in disability related policies and initiatives in countries as diverse as Britain, the European Union and China (Stone, 1999; European Commission, 2003; Prime Minister's Strategy Unit, 2005) and the World Health Organization's recently devised 'International Classification of Functioning Disability and Health' (WHO, 1999).

The social model of disability is nothing more complicated than an emphasis on the economic, environmental and cultural barriers encountered by people viewed by others as having some form of impairment. These barriers include (a) inaccessible education, information and communication systems, and working environments, (b) inadequate disability benefits, (c) discriminatory health and social support services, (d) inaccessible transport, housing and public buildings and amenities, and (e) the devaluing of people labelled as disabled by negative imagery and representation in the media – films, television and newspapers. From this perspective, people with designated impairments are disabled by society's failure to accommodate their individual and collective needs within the mainstream of economic and cultural life (Barnes, 1991).

Although the social model has been linked to various theoretical approaches (Priestley, 1998) it is not, nor never was, conceptualised as a social theory of disability. The social model has provided the conceptual foundation for the development of a fully comprehensive materialist account of the social creation of disability, rooted in the work of Karl Marx and Antonio Gramsci and evidenced in the work of Vic Finkelstein (1980), Mike Oliver (1990), and Brendan Gleeson (1999). However, and in view of recent  misrepresentations by some writers (Shakespeare and Watson, 2001; Watson, 2002), there are three main points that need to be reiterated about the social model of disability:

1   In contrast to the conventional individual medical/deficit model of disability, the social model is a deliberate attempt to switch the focus away from the functional limitations of impaired individuals onto the problems caused by disabling environments, barriers and cultures.

2   The social model is a holistic approach that explains specific problems experienced by disabled people in terms of the totality of disabling environments and cultures.

3   A social model perspective does not deny the importance or value of appropriate individually based interventions in the lives of disabled people, whether they be medically, re/habilitative, educational or employment based, but draws attention to their limitations in terms of furthering their empowerment and inclusion in a society constructed by non-disabled people for non-disabled people.

In short, the social model of disability is a tool with which to gain an insight into the disabling tendencies of modern society in order to generate policies and practices to facilitate their eradication (Oliver, 2004). It is this train of thought that has influenced the concept of independent living as it is understood in the new millennium in the United Kingdom (UK) (Barnes, 2003).

# Independent living in the 21st century

The phrase 'independent living' first entered the English language in the 1970s, follow-ing its adoption by disability activists in the USA. What became known as the American Independent Living Movement (ILM) emerged partly from within the campus culture of American universities and partly from repeated efforts by American disability activists to influence US disability legislation. During the 1960s, some American universities had introduced various self-help programmes to enable students with 'severe' physical impairments to attend mainstream courses. But these schemes were rarely available outside university campuses. This unacceptable situation prompted some disabled students to develop their own services under the banner of 'Centres for Independent Living' (CILs).

Unlike other services *for* disabled people controlled by mainly non-disabled profession-als, these new CILs were self-help organisations exclusively run and controlled by disabled people. Further, in contrast to other professionally dominated provisions that focused almost exclusively on medical treatments and therapies within institutional settings, effec-tively removing disabled people from everyday life, CILs provided a new and innovative range of services and support systems designed to enable people with impairments to adopt a lifestyle of their own choosing within rather than apart from the local community.

Subsequently, the phrase 'independent living' has had a considerable impact on disabil-ity policy throughout the world. Disabled people and representative organisations are increasingly involved in the development of disability policy at both the national and international level. Also, there are now CILs or similar user controlled organisations pro-viding services and support for disabled people and their families throughout Britain (Barnes, Mercer and Morgan, 2000) and many countries across the globe (Charlton, 1998; Alonso, 2003).

Part of the reason for this apparent and unprecedented success is the almost universal appeal of the concept of independent living within Western culture. The term is apolitical in the sense that it appeals directly to advocates of the politics of the right and of the left, and it is political in that the environmental and cultural changes needed to facilitate mean-ingful independent living for disabled people will benefit everyone regardless of impairment or status.

Early exponents of independent living allied themselves with the radical consumerism of the 1960s and 70s. Consequently, the independent living movement has a particular appeal to proponents of the ideological cornerstones of capitalist development such as eco-nomic and political freedom, consumer sovereignty, and self-reliance. This realization prompted some critics to suggest that the philosophy and policies of the ILM favoured only a relatively small section of the disabled population; notably, young, intellectually-able, middle-class white males (Williams, 1984).

This is, however, a misrepresentation of what the term independent living has come to represent. Indeed, though they are often characterised as providing services for people with physical impairments only, historically, CILs have struggled to provide services for all sections of the disabled community. Where they have not, this is usually due to limited resources, material and human, and/or entrenched opposition from vested interests within traditional disability service providers.

Furthermore, in view of the dangers of misinterpretation, some disability activists, particularly in the UK where social model thinking is especially influential, have adopted the terms 'integrated' or 'inclusive' living rather than the original 'independent' living to characterise the philosophy on which their activities are based. Such terms have a far greater appeal to the left of centre elements within Britain's disabled people's movement. They recognise that humans are by definition 'social' beings, and that *all* humans, regardless of the degree and nature of impairment, are interdependent and, therefore, that a truly independent lifestyle is inconceivable (Barnes, 2003).

From this perspective, the ideologies and practices that justify the systematic oppression of people with impairments within capitalist society are similar to those that legitimise the oppression of other disadvantaged sections of the population such as women, minority ethnic groups, lesbians and gay men, and older people. Taken together, they represent an increasingly costly and complex barrier to the development of a truly meaningful inclusive and representative democracy.

Due largely to the intensifying politicisation of disability by disabled people and their organisations during the 1980s and 90s, both in the UK and elsewhere, the phrase 'independent living' has been increasingly evident in policy documents produced by health and social service professionals in the context of 'community care' services for disabled people. Usually focusing on professionally-led assessments of functional ability and inability, these initiatives bear little resemblance to the principles and practices of the international disabled people's movement. It is therefore important in the context of political and policy analysis to establish clearly the fundamental principles of independent living according to the writings of disabled activists, their organisations and supporters around the world.

Despite terminological differences there is general agreement amongst disabled activists and their allies that the philosophy of independent living is founded on four basic assumptions. These include:

1   That all human life, regardless of the nature, complexity and/or severity of impairment is of equal worth;

2   That anyone, whatever the nature, complexity and/or severity of their impairment, has the capacity to make choices and should be enabled to make those choices;

3   That people who are disabled by societal responses to any form of accredited impairment – physical, sensory or cognitive – have the right to exercise control over their lives; and

4   That people with perceived impairments who are labeled 'disabled' have the right to participate fully in all areas, economic, political and cultural, of mainstream community living on a par with non-disabled peers (Bracking, 1993; Morris, 1993; Charlton, 1998; Barnes, 2003).

# Discussion: a way forward?

Clearly the concept of independent living is a broad one that encompasses the full range of human experience and rights, including the right to be born with access to appropriate medical treatments as and when they are needed. Moreover, although independent living is commonly associated with disabled people with physical or sensory conditions in the younger or middle age groups, it applies to all sections of the disabled population. This includes people with complex and high support needs, people with cognitive conditions who are labelled in various ways ('learning difficulties', 'behavioural difficulties', 'mental illness', etc.). Equally important, disabled activists have long since pointed out that disabled women, disabled lesbians and disabled gay men, disabled people from minority ethnic groups, disabled children and older disabled people are particularly disadvantaged due to sexism, heterosexism, racism, ageism and other forms of structural oppression and prejudice.

Furthermore, people with designated impairments, however defined, will always experience varying degrees of economic, political and social disadvantage in societies organised around the core capitalist values of individual self help, economic rationally, and the profit motive. In the current socio/political context, in order for disabled people to secure an independent lifestyle, they are required to make a considerable effort. Hence, we need to re-configure the meaning of work for disabled people with complex and comprehensive support needs (Oliver and Barnes, 1998; Abberley, 2002; Barnes, 2003).

To pursue the goal of a 'society in which all disabled people are able to participate as equal citizens' (DRC, 2004), we must generate a cultural environment that places the needs of the many on a par with those of the few, and rejects the market led policies of the past. We must also celebrate rather than denigrate the meaning of social welfare, and the state's role in its provision (Oliver and Barnes, 1998). This is not to suggest that we need more of the traditional top-down approach to state welfare; quite the reverse. There is mounting evidence, from a variety of sources, that conventional professionally-led services are counter productive both in terms of the effective use of resources, financial and human, and the elimination of dependence.

What is needed is a significant shift away from government support for services controlled and run by professionals and non-disabled people, whether they be state-run or in the voluntary sector, and far greater investment in user-led initiatives at both the national and local levels.

Two notable examples in the UK include direct payments to disabled individuals, and the network of user controlled service providers and advocacy groups known variously as Centres for Independent, Integrated, or more recently, Inclusive Living: namely, CILs. The former allows the disabled individual to devise, pay for and, therefore, control their own support systems including the employment of personal assistance according to their own requirements. As in many countries across the world, Britain's CILs provide a range of services for disabled people, their families and related professionals. Examples include user-controlled information, advice and peer support systems, self-operated personal assistance schemes, personal assistant users' support groups, and advocacy and campaign groups. The general ethos of these organisations is to enable people with impairment/s, regardless of cause, to achieve an independent lifestyle of their own choosing and commensurate with that of non-disabled peers (Barnes, Mercer and Morgan, 2000).

Moreover, given that thousands of disabled people across the UK are denied the chance to achieve independent living due to the reluctance of many local authorities to implement a direct payment policy (Glasby and Littlechild, 2002; CSCI, 2004) (legalised under the 1996 'Community Care [Direct Payments] Act', following years of lobbying by disabled people's organisations [Hasler, Campbell & Zarb, 1999]), the distribution of direct payments should be centralised. This could be achieved by setting up a new national body accountable directly to the National Centre for Independent Living (NCIL), an organisation controlled and run by disabled people that emerged from within and is accountable to Britain's CIL movement.

Besides the distribution of direct payments, this new national body could have two further roles; first, to produce an appropriate and standardised assessment procedure for accessing direct payments and, second, to develop and support the nationwide network of locally-based user-controlled agencies and groups providing services for local direct payment users. To fulfil these roles, NCIL would naturally draw on the wealth of experience that already exists amongst its member organizations, many of whom have been providing these and similar services for more than twenty years (Barnes, 2004).

To achieve a lifestyle comparable to non-disabled peers, disabled people need far more than simply user-controlled services. To attain Independent living disabled people need equal access to mainstream schools, jobs, transport, houses, public buildings, leisure etc. or all the things that non-disabled people take for granted (Bracking, 1993: 14). It is a goal that is far from being achieved despite the introduction of the UK's 1995 Disability Discrimination Act and subsequent amendments. It will be necessary to strengthen and enforce the law and ensure that people with an awareness of disability and 'independent living' issues are integrated fully into *all* government departments at *all* levels, nationally, regionally and locally. The aim is to initiate and develop effective policies with which to eradicate the various barriers to inclusion in *all* areas of economic and social activity and, in so doing, usher in a further stage in the on going struggle for a truly equitable and inclusive society.

It is inevitable that this strategy will have significant implications for those charged with the responsibility for managing the economy, as effective barrier-removal will prove costly. But these short-term costs must be offset against the long-term gains of a barrier-free environment in which socially created dependence is considerably reduced if not eliminated altogether. Moreover, whilst such a policy may fly in the face of recent economic and political trends in Britain and elsewhere, it is important to remember that any notion of an inclusive and equitable capitalism is unrealistic and unachievable. And that over recent decades the gulf between the rich and poor has increased rather than decreased within and across nation states, environmental instability remains unchecked, and political and social uncertainly has intensified at both the national and international levels. If these tendencies are not to intensify further it is high time that politicians and policy makers, both in Britain and throughout the world, acknowledge this fact and take appropriate steps to develop a meaningful and just alternative.

For disabled people this alternative must be a society in which all human beings regardless of impairment, age, gender, sexual orientation, social class, minority ethnic status can coexist as equal members of the community, secure in the knowledge that their needs will be accommodated in full and that their views will be recognised, respected and valued. It will be a very different society from the one in which we now live. It will be a society that is truly democratic, characterised by genuine and meaningful equal opportunities and outcomes with far greater equity in terms of income and wealth, with enhanced choice and freedom, and with a proper regard for environmental and social interdependence and continuity.

The creation of such a world will be a difficult arduous process and progress toward its construction will be inhibited by cynics who will argue that such a world is unachievable, and little more than a utopian dream. However, as Oscar Wilde so cogently pointed out over a century ago in *The Soul of Man Under Socialism* (first published in 1891):

A map of the world that does not include Utopia is not even worth glancing at, for it leaves out the one country that Humanity is always landing. And when Humanity lands there, it looks out, and seeing a better country sets sail. Progress is the realisation of Utopias (Wilde, 1966[1891]: 1090).

# References

Abberley, P. (2002) 'Work, disability and European social theory', in C. Barnes, M. Oliver, and L. Barton (eds), *Disability Studies Today*. Cambridge: Polity, pp. 120–139.

Alonso, J. V. G. (ed.) (2003) *El movimiento de vida indepeniente*. Madrid: Foundacion Luis Vibes.

Barnes, C. (1991) *Disabled People in Britain and Discrimination: A Case for Anti-discrimination Legislation*. London: Hurst and Co.

Barnes, C. (2003, December 3) *'Work' is a Four Letter Word? Disability Work and Welfare Presentation*. Paper presented at the meeting of the Working Futures: Policy, Practice and Disabled People's Employment Conference, University of Sunderland, United Kingdom.

Barnes, C. (2004, December) 'Direct payments and their futures', *Independently*: 2–3.

Barnes, C., Mercer, G. and Morgan, H. (2000) *Creating Independent Futures: An Evaluation of Services Led by Disabled People. Stage One Report*. Leeds: The Disability Press.

Bracking, S. (1993) 'An introduction to independent living', in C. Barnes (ed.), *Making Our Own Choices*. Belper: The British Council of Disabled People, pp. 11–14.

Campbell, J. and Oliver, M. (1996) *Disability Politics: Understanding Our Past, Changing Our Future*. London: Routledge.

Charlton, J. I. (1998) *Nothing About Us Without Us: Disability Oppression and Empowerment*. Berkeley: University of California Press.

Commission for Social Care Inspection (2004) *Direct Payments: What are the Barriers?* London: CSCI.

Disability Rights Commission (2004) *Disability Rights Commission*. Available online at www.drc-gb.org/

Drake, R. (1999) *Understanding Disability Policy*. Basingstoke: Macmillan.

European Commission (2003, October 30) 'Communication of 30 October 2003 from the Commission to the Council, the European Parliament, the European Economic and Social Committee and the Committee of the Regions', *Equal Opportunities for People with Disabilities: A European Action Plan* (COM/2003/0650 final).

Finkelstein, V. (1980) *Attitudes and Disability*. Geneva: World Rehabilitation Fund.

Garland, R. (1995) *The Eye of the Beholder: Deformity and Disability in the Graeco-Roman World*. Ithaca: Cornell University Press.

Glasby, J. and Littlechild, R. (2002) *Social Work and Direct Payments*. Bristol: The Policy Press.

Gleeson, B. (1999) *Geographies of Disability*. London: Routledge.

Hanks, J. R. and Hanks, L. M. (1948) 'The physically handicapped in certain non-occidental societies', *Journal of Social Issues*, 4: 11–20.

Hasler, F., Campbell, J. and Zarb, G. (1999) *Direct Routes to Independence*. London: Policy Studies Institute.

Ingstad, B. and Reynolds Whytte, S. (1995) *Disability and Culture*. California: University of California Press.

Morris, J. (1993) *Independent Lives*. Tavistock: Macmillan.

Oliver, M. (1990) *The Politics of Disablement*. Basingstoke: Macmillan.

Oliver, M. (2004) 'The social model in action: If I had a hammer', in C. Barnes and G. Mercer (eds), *Implementing the Social Model of Disability: Theory and Research*. Leeds: The Disability Press, pp. 18–31.

Oliver, M. and Barnes, C. (1998) *Disabled People and Social Policy: From Exclusion to Inclusion*. London: Longman.

Priestley, M. (1998) 'Constructions and creations: Idealism, materialism and disability theory', *Disability and Society*, 13(1): 75–95.

Prime Minister's Strategy Unit (2005) *Improving the Life Chances of Disabled People*. London: Cabinet Office.

Ryan, J. and Thomas, F. (1980) *The Politics of Mental Handicap*. Harmondsworth: Penguin.

Scheer, J. and Groce, N. (1988) 'Impairment as a human constant: Cross-cultural and historical perspectives on variation', *Journal of Social Issues*, 44(1): 23–37.

Shakespeare, T. and Watson, N. (2001) 'The social model of disability: An outdated ideology', *Exploring Theories and Expanding Methodologies: Research in Social Science and Disability*, 2: 9–28.

Stiker, H. J. (1998) *A History of Disability*. Ann Arbor, MI: The University of Michigan Press.

Stone, E. (ed.) (1999) *Disability and Development: Learning from Action and Research in the Majority World*. Leeds: The Disability Press.

Union of the Physically Impaired Against Segregation (1975) *Fundamental Principles of Disability*. London: UPIAS.

Watson, N. (2002) 'Well I know this is going to sound very strange to you, but I don't see myself as a disabled person: Identity and disability', *Disability and Society*, 17(5): 509–528.

Wilde, O. (1966[1891]) 'The soul of man under socialism', in J. G. Foreman (ed.), *Complete Works of Oscar Wilde*. London: Collins, pp. 1079–1104.

Williams, G. (1984) 'The movement for independent living: An evaluation and critique', *Sociology of Health and Illness*, 6: 175–200.

World Health Organization (1999) *International Classification of Functioning Disability and Health*. Geneva: WHO.

World Health Organization (2001) *Rethinking Care from Disabled People's Perspectives*. Geneva: WHO.

(Other relevant literature can be down-loaded free from the Disability Archive UK at: www.leeds.ac.uk/disability-studies/archiveuk/index.html)

(An earlier version of this paper was presented at the 'Social Care Institute for Excellence' Conference on Independent Living: Copthorne Tara Hotel, London, 22nd November 2004).

# Chapter 12

## Losing your home

*Alison Norman*

It is not sufficiently realized that the loss of one's home – however good the reasons for leaving it – can be experienced as a form of bereavement and can produce the same grief reaction as the loss of a close relative. Peter Marris in his book *Loss and Change* (1974) quotes a study of the reactions of families moved from the West End of Boston under an urban renewal scheme in which it was concluded that:

> for the majority it seems quite precise to speak of their reactions as expressions of *grief*. These are manifest in the feelings of painful loss, the continued longing, the general depressive tone, frequent symptoms of psychological or social or somatic distress, the active work required in adapting to the altered situation, the sense of helplessness, the occasional expressions of both direct and displaced anger, and the tendencies to idealise the lost place. At their most extreme, these reactions of grief are intense, deeply felt and, at times, overwhelming.

> Altogether about half the 250 women and 316 men studied said they had been severely depressed or disturbed for a while, and another quarter had been more mildly upset. A quarter of the women were still very depressed two years after they had moved, while a fifth had taken over six months to recover their spirits. The unhappiest exiles described their loss in similar phrases to the bereaved: 'I felt as though I had lost everything.' 'It was like a piece being taken from me.' 'Something of me went with the West End.'

Similar reactions were described by Young and Wilmott (1957) when they studied families moved from the East End of London to a suburban housing estate and by Marris in a study of slum clearance in Lagos, where residents complained bitterly 'it seemed like being taken from happiness to misery', 'I fear it like death'. Marris suggests that, like bereavement, a change of home should be understood as a potential disruption of the meaning of life. Those for whom a move represents the realization of a social status and way of life with which they already identify will be able to work through the loss and re-create what they valued in their former neighbourhood. 'But,' he says:

From A. Norman (1980) *Rights and Risk*. London: Centre for Policy on Ageing, pp. 14–19.

for some, it may be a profound disturbance from which they never recover. And such tragedies are, I believe, more likely, the more slum clearance is used as an instrument of social change, not merely physical development; and the more it is directed against groups in society, whose non-conformity with the ruling values seems to stand in the way of progress. (Marris, 1974)

Old people who are moved into sheltered housing or residential care may or may not be moved from slum conditions, but the sense of loss must surely be equally great for them. Indeed it may be greater if, in the process, they have to sacrifice not only a home and neighbourhood but the greater part of the possessions of a lifetime. It must also be true that they are likely to work through the loss only if they make a positive identification with their new life. If they are being moved in conformity with ruling social values which are offended by letting them stay where they are, or are forced to go by the physical duress of having no viable alternative, they are still less likely to recover from the loss.

A good deal of research data, much of it American, supports such a conclusion, and it is clear that the loss of a home may be particularly serious for those who are mentally impaired, physically ill, or depressed and thus unable to make a positive effort to identify with the new life. Gutman and Herbert in 1976 quoted 13 studies which showed that the death rate of elderly persons was unusually high during the first year after 'relocation' and particularly during the first three months. This was so regardless of whether the movement was from the community into a mental institution, from one institution to another, from one ward to another within the same institution, or from old to new facilities. (The same researchers showed from their own study however, that this effect does not obtain when the community moves *en bloc* to a new building with improved facilities and every effort is made to prepare patients and relatives for the move well in advance, to keep friends together in their new quarters and to transfer staff as well as patients.)

M.A. Lieberman, in an important paper on relocation and social policy described four studies which he had made: 'one on healthy moving into affluent high-care, sophisticated institutions; others involving sick, highly debilitated human beings moving into circumstances that would delight a muckraker' (Lieberman, 1974). These 'have yielded roughly comparable findings. Namely, no matter what the condition of the individual, the nature of the environment or the degree of sophisticated preparation, relocation entails a higher than acceptable risk to the large majority of those being moved.' Given that relocation may sometimes be inevitable, Lieberman goes on to ask what steps can be taken to minimize the risk but cannot suggest a solution. He concludes that careful preparation and 'working through' of the transitional process and impending loss, important though it may be in relieving human misery, is not a powerful tool in minimizing relocation risk. 'The reason,' he says,

is not poor practice but rather incorrect strategy. Relocation is a risk to the individual not because of the symbolic meaning that such transitions imply, but because it entails radical changes in the life space of an individual that require new learning for adaptive purposes. Over and over again, studies on relocation report findings that physical status, cognitive ability and certain other characteristics of personality are powerful predictors to the outcome of relocation.

In other words, those who need institutional support the *least* are those who are most likely to survive the move into it, and 'it is often the very people who require supportive services that can be shown to entail the greatest risk'. (He adds that this is another illustration of how the results of empirical research often fail to help with the nitty-gritty of policy issues.)

A study of fatal home accidents made by the Tavistock Institute of Human Relations on behalf of the Department of Prices and Consumer Protection also suggests that old people are not necessarily safer when they are 'in care'. The authors found that out of 133 fatal accidents studied in the '65 and over' age group (75 per cent caused by falls) 35 per cent were in institutional care, although only 4.8 per cent of this age group live in institutions. They comment: 'Even considering that residential institutions contain a higher proportion of the infirm, the difference in accidental deaths is high' (Poyner and Hughes, 1978).

It would seem to follow from all this, that if avoidance of 'risk' is indeed a prime objective, moving people out of their homes may not be the best way of achieving it, and that the more they appear to be at risk where they are, the worse will be their prognosis if they are moved. Yet this is a factor which is seldom taken into consideration when considering transfer into residential care, and still less is it taken into consideration when deciding on hospital admission.

Elderly people, like members of any other age group, are of course often admitted to hospital for surgery or investigation which could not be provided in their own home; and they may benefit greatly from such treatment. (For example, a study of 248 patients over 80 admitted as emergencies to acute surgical wards of the Reading hospitals in 1976 showed that the overall mortality rate was 21.8 per cent and it fell to 12.5 per cent if terminal disease was excluded. All but seven patients were discharged home: Salem et al., 1978.) However, there is another large group of elderly people who become patients not so much because their condition demands full-scale hospital treatment as because there is a crisis in their system of social support. The social crisis then has a medical label attached to it in order to make the admission acceptable to the hospital. For example, if an elderly person develops pneumonia and the spouse finds the anxiety of nursing at home too much to bear, an admission will probably be arranged, but the diagnosis is pneumonia, not 'anxiety in spouse'. Very often the admission may be occasioned by some incident or accident which proves to be the last straw on an already overstrained support system, or because there is no time to arrange for the domiciliary services required by a change in circumstances (such as the caring relative becoming sick). Or, if an elderly person presents at an Accident and Emergency department of a hospital after, say, a fall in the street, a harassed houseman may 'play safe' and keep the person in for 'investigation' just to make sure no damage has been done.

The problem is that it is much easier for an elderly person to become a hospital patient than to cease to be one. There are a number of reasons for this. The 'social space' in which the person has been living may close behind him on admission, so that he cannot get back. A family may heave a sigh of relief, having realized, perhaps for the first time, what a burden it has been carrying and say, 'He's not coming back here.' A landlord may take the opportunity to repossess his house, or the warden of a sheltered housing complex say, 'He needs too much nursing now, I can't cope.' Ironically, it is often the person who would appear to be most at risk, who lives alone in his own home, who is in least danger of having his social space close up on him.

It is also often the case that if a person has only just been coping with independent life, hospital admission breaks a tenuous level of confidence which can only be restored with time, care and skill. Elderly people who are suffering from some degree of dementia are specially at risk because the experience of admission to a totally strange and unfamiliar environment is likely to increase confusion and generate problems such as falling and incontinence which may not have been present before.

Another possibility is that hospital 'investigation' may show up undiagnosed diseases which a person has been living with for years, but which, once diagnosed, the hospital may feel compelled to treat. Observation after a fall may then become treatment for something quite different, so that the person is confirmed in his patient status. Moreover, if the person is being treated in an acute ward, the nursing staff may not have the time, interest or training to help the patient to retain independence and mobility, and even a few days of inactivity may produce disuse atrophy which involves not only loss of muscle power but also loss of the range of movement normally possessed by a joint. Simple skills required for daily living such as combing one's hair, fastening a button or rising from a chair may then be lost. (It has been shown that even the muscle disuse occurring during normal sleep leads to significant weakness on waking: Browne, 1978.) A period of treatment in an acute ward may therefore mean that an elderly person requires a prolonged period of rehabilitation in a geriatric ward before he can recover his skills sufficiently to manage at home again – and the longer the period in hospital, the more likely it is that the 'social space' at home will have closed up.

For all these reasons, hospital admission – which can undoubtedly be 'life saving' – may also be dangerous to elderly people, and the dangers need to be weighed against the advantages when deciding whether or not to admit someone to hospital.

# References

Browne, B. (1978) 'Inactivity in the elderly', *Health and Social Service Journal*, 88(4575), 10 January.

Gutman, G. M. and Herbert, C. P. (1976) 'Mortality rates among relocated extended care patients', *Journal of Gerontology*, 31(3): 352–357.

Lieberman, M. A. (1974) 'Symposium – long term care: research, policy and practice', *The Gerontologist*, 4(6).

Marris, P. (1974) *Loss and Change*. London: Institute of Community Studies/Routledge & Kegan Paul.

Poyner, B. and Hughes, M. (1978) *A Classification of Fatal Home Accidents*. (Report to the Department of Prices and Consumer Protection, 2T140). London: Tavistock Institute of Human Relations.

Salem, R. et al. (1978) 'Emergency geriatric surgical admission', *British Medical Journal*, 2: 416–417.

Young, M. and Willmott, P. (1957) *Family and Kinship in East London*. London: Routledge & Kegan Paul.

Johnson, J  De Souza J (2010)
Understanding Health + Social
Care: OUP London

# Chapter 13

## Total institutions

*Kathleen Jones and A. J. Fowles*

[Erving] Goffman introduced the term 'total institution' and defined it more carefully than many of his imitators have done. A 'total institution' is 'a place of residence and work where a large number of like-situated individuals, cut off from the wider society for an appreciable period of time, together lead an enclosed, formally administered round of life' (Goffman, 1961: xiii).

Not all institutions are total institutions, though 'every institution has encompassing tendencies'; but some institutions, such as homes for the blind or the aged, mental hospitals, prisons, concentration camps, army barracks, boarding schools and monasteries or convents, are 'encompassing to a degree discontinuously greater than the ones next in line'.

Goffman's concept of the 'total institution' can be represented as follows: there is a continuum from open to closed institutions, but there is a break towards the closed end, separating off a group of closed, or nearly closed, institutions which can be described as 'total'.

In fact, both the completely open institution and the completely closed institution are abstractions. No institution is ever completely open: if it were, it would have no distinguishing characteristics at all. No institution is ever completely closed. If it were, it would die off. Open systems theory has taught us that all human systems are dependent to some extent on their immediate environment, and that they cannot survive without it. A mental hospital or prison imports staff, inmates, policy, material supplies and public reactions from the outside world; it exports staff on completion of contract, inmates on completion of stay or sentence, empirical material which may affect policy, the product of work programmes (mailbags, assembled electric switches, carpentry, scrubbing brushes, fancy paper hats, those curious toys which are made in occupational therapy, and so on), garbage, and stories of strike, threat and crisis which form the basis of public reactions. All sorts of people cross the boundary: inspectors, professional superiors, inmates' visitors, research workers, workmen, students, policemen, magistrates and others. But these considerations do not invalidate Goffman's argument about the relatively closed or 'total' institution. His contention is that this group of institutions has features in common: he qualifies it by

From K. Jones and A. J. Fowles (1984) 'Goffman: the radical', in *Ideas on Institutions*. London: Routledge & Kegan Paul, pp. 12–16.

adding that none of these features is specific to them, and that not all of the features may be found in any one of them. What he proposes is not a list of features to be identified in all cases, but a constellation of features which tend to occur in most cases, and which have some relation to each other. He is embarking on a sort of verbal cluster analysis. What he describes as a 'total institution' will probably not fit any real-life institution exactly. It is a Weberian ideal type against which the practices of real-life institutions may be measured.

It is important to clarify this definition, because the term 'total institution' has become something of a catch-phrase, and is often applied unthinkingly to particular prisons or mental hospitals. Goffman is much more scholarly than some of his imitators, and his frame of reference is precisely defined.

'Total institutions' have four main characteristics: batch living, binary management, the inmate role, and the institutional perspective.

'Batch living' describes a situation where 'each phase of the member's daily activity is carried on in the immediate company of a large batch of others, all of whom are treated alike, and required to do the same thing together'. It is the antithesis of individual living, where there are large areas of life which may be pursued on a basis of personal choice. It is characterized by a bureaucratic form of management, a system of formal rules and regulations, and a tight schedule which allows little or no free time. It allows the inmate no freedom of movement between different social groups, and no choice of companions: he lives with the same group of people, elected and defined by outside authority, 24 hours a day, without variety or respite. This is contrasted with 'a basic arrangement in modern society. … the individual tends to sleep, play and work in different places, with different co-participants, under different authorities, and without an overall rational plan' (Goffman, 1961: 5–6). In the institutional situation, individuals are not merely constrained by, but are violently attacked by, the system. They live under surveillance, and any infraction of the rules 'is likely to stand out in relief against the visible, constantly examined compliance of the others'.

Goffman is not clear which came first, the 'large blocks of managed people' or the staff who manage them; but 'each is made for the other'. 'Total institutions' typically consist of these two groups of people, the managers and the managed – staff and patients, prison officers and prisoners, teachers and pupils.

This is 'binary management': 'Two different social and cultural worlds develop, jogging alongside each other with points of official contact, but little mutual penetration' (ibid.: 9). The managers have power, and social distance is their weapon. They exercise this most tellingly in withholding information, so that the managed exist in 'blind dependency', unable to control their own destinies. The very fact of being an inmate is degrading: 'Staff tend to feel superior, and righteous. Inmates tend … to feel inferior, weak, unworthy and guilty' (ibid.: 7). Because the two groups do not and cannot know each other as individuals, they set up antagonistic stereotypes. Staff tend to see all patients or prisoners or pupils as being alike – 'bitter, secretive and untrustworthy'. The managed draw similar hostile pictures of the managers. The two groups may use a special tone of voice in talking to each other, and informal conversation and social mixing may be frowned upon by both sides.

How do ordinary people, with their own way of life and personal networks and round of activities, become inmates? Goffman thinks that this is not a process of 'acculturation', which involves moving from one culture to another, but of 'disculturation' or 'role-stripping' so powerful that the individual who is subjected to it may be rendered incapable of normal living when he returns to the community. He has been reduced from a person with many roles to a cipher with one: the 'inmate role'.

Much of this process is achieved through admission procedures, which Goffman sees as 'a series of abasements, degradations, humiliations and profanations of self' – a mortification process. Institutions are 'the forcing houses for changing persons'. To become an inmate involves a total break with the past, symbolized by the acquisition of a new name or number, uniform clothing, and the restriction or confiscation of personal possessions. All this may be done in a highly ritualised admission procedure in which the inmate may be forced to recite his life history, take a bath, possibly without privacy, and submit to weighing, fingerprinting, intrusive medical examination and head-shaving. The overt reason for these activities is administrative necessity: the real purpose is role dispossession. The bath, in particular, is a highly symbolic ritual, involving physical nakedness as the midpoint of a process of abandoning one life for another. 'The new arrival allows himself to be shaped and coded into an object that can be fed into the administrative machinery of the establishment, to be worked on smoothly by routine operation' (ibid.: 16). The new clothes are likely to be standard issue, the property of the establishment. Combined with a loss of 'personal maintenance equipment' such as combs, shaving sets or cosmetics, they create a new and humiliating appearance. The process is one of personal defacement.

As the stay is prolonged, so the loss of personal identity becomes more marked. There may be systematic violation of privacy through the practice of group or individual confession. The inmate's defences may be repeatedly collapsed by a process called 'looping' where the mere fact of defence is taken as proof of guilt (ibid.: 35–37). There may be 'indignities of speech or action' – inmates are forced to beg humbly for a glass of water or a light for a cigarette, to move or speak in a markedly deferential way indicating their lowly status. They may be beaten, or subjected to electric shock treatment, or physically contaminated – there are some particularly nasty examples drawn from concentration camps and political prisons.

Control may be kept by means of a system or rewards and punishments, petty by outside standards, but assuming Pavlovian dimensions in a situation of deprivation. Rules may not be made fully explicit. The inmate cannot appeal to them for protection, and may break them unwittingly, and be punished for it. Like Kafka's K., he exists in a half-world of guilt and apprehension. He has no privacy, no rights, and no dignity.

How does the inmate survive these attacks on his personality? Goffman suggests four types of 'secondary adjustment' (ibid.: 61–64):

1   The inmate may withdraw, cutting himself off from contact.
2   He may become intransigent, and fight the system.
3   He may, in a vivid phrase, become 'colonised', paying lip-service to the system like the inhabitant of some African or Asian country awaiting the day of independence.
4   He may become converted, genuinely accepting the institution's view of himself, and what is acceptable behaviour.

The last of these is not really survival, but a kind of personal extinction. Curiously, and on the face of it illogically, it is the only adjustment acceptable to the authorities of the institution. Any attempt by the inmate to immunize himself against the destructive forces focused on him will be seen as non-co-operation, and may be used as an excuse to detain him longer.

He may develop a 'line', a sort of edited account of how he came to be an inmate, repeated to his fellows and to anyone else who will listen with increasing self-pity. He may have a sense of 'dead and heavy-hanging time' – of life wasted, and the months or years ticking away without gain or satisfaction. Against these reactions, the authorities offer 'the institutional perspective': a view of life which denies his individual perspective and validates the institution's existence. It is promoted by such means as the house magazine, the annual party, the institutional theatrical, the open day and the sports day, which create an artificial sense of community. These formal events offer certain minor possibilities of role release for the inmate – recognized and routinized liberties, forbidden in normal circumstances, may be allowable; but the total effect is to reinforce the power of the institution, and the 'assault on the self': 'These ceremonial practices are well suited to a Durkheimian analysis: a society dangerously split into inmates and staff can through these ceremonies hold itself together' (ibid.: 109).

# Reference

Goffman, E. (1961) *Asylums*. New York: Doubleday/Anchor.

# Chapter 14

## Bedroom abuse: the hidden work in a nursing home

*Geraldine Lee-Treweek*

In Western society the bedroom has been constructed as a place of privacy. It has a unique symbolism for the individual in terms of personal choice. Even if other parts of the domestic home are open to public view the bedroom usually is not. (See Willcocks et al., 1987: 4–6; Goffman, 1959: 124.) Yet in forms of institutionalized care this is problematic, as these rooms are also workplaces for staff. The way that homes are organized leaves those with the least training to undertake the physical care work. This work is often bedroom-based work. It is physically hard and dirty. Also it is hidden.

The physical work behind the scenes is not seen, yet it is essential if the patient is to be presentable to others. In Goffman's (1959: 126) terms the preparatory work of the bedroom is backstage 'technical work' and is often undertaken by low-status workers whose product is then presented by higher-status workers. In the case of the nursing home the patient that the auxiliary washes, dresses and organizes is placed in the lounge where nursing staff then present the sanitized patient to visitors. [...]

This paper argues that in many homes the bedroom world is ordered and arranged by the nursing auxiliary [...] the aim of their work being the creation of the acceptable patient for public view. In this world mistreatment and punishing behaviours become acceptable, mistreatment being part of the daily grind of getting through the work – of organizing people in conveyor-belt fashion to time and chore constraints. Punishment, apart from being a more deliberate and personal form of cruelty, involved getting back at the job and taking it out on the objects of care. Both also appeared to create a subdued patient who was then easier to order. Lastly, I discuss how mistreatment and being hard towards patients had become part of the auxiliaries' subculture and had been elevated beyond simple necessity to being an essential attribute of the good worker. [...]

## The home and bedrooms

Cedar Court was one such home, sited on the outskirts of a major town in the south west of England (the name has been changed to preserve anonymity). On arrival I was immediately

Originally published in *Generations Review* (March 1994), 4(1): 2–4 (abridged).

struck by the isolation from the general community by a large garden surrounded by trees and a long gravel drive. The exterior of the building was modern and anonymous, unlike a domestic home. [...] Heavy glass swing doors at the front of the building gave the appearance of a hospital entrance. Inside, the home was carpeted from bedrooms to lounge with a 'seconds flawed' carpet and the walls and ceilings were all painted magnolia. To the visitor the buzzers, smells of disinfectant, uniforms, trolleys and wheelchairs gave an impression of hospitalization and a medical order. Yet, although trained staff dominated public areas, the majority of staff were untrained auxiliary workers who worked mainly in the more private area of the home. [...]

## The bedroom job

The bedroom was the main site of work for the auxiliaries and most of the patients' time in the home was spent there. Morning work was virtually all bedroom work and was officially begun by the auxiliaries entering patients' rooms on the tea round. This was a point of the day at which cups of tea were served and bottoms were washed. It was customary to present the patients to the new shift intact, clean and quiet in their rooms for 8 a.m. Presenting well-ordered bodies seemed to symbolize the job properly done. The next shift spent all the morning in the bedrooms, washing and dressing patients. The workers spent most of the morning getting patients ready, then taking them down to the lounge. By lunchtime they were all down, but straight after lunch it was time to put them back to bed for a nap and later get them up again.

  In the evenings work again revolved around the bedrooms as staff got patients ready for bed. By the time the night shift came on, all patients were in bed. In this way the auxiliaries' work could be said to revolve around the bedroom. And it was in this private world that they were able to decide the rules and had total hidden control.

## The aim and nature of the work

The aim of work in the bedrooms was generally the creation of patients who could be presented into the lounge area: 'the lounge standard patient'. Those who were 'displayed' in the lounge were those who fitted the home's construction of the ordered patient – the physically and mentally ordered patients, dressed tidily, unsmelly and clean. The patients with whom the auxiliary worked in the bedroom was, by comparison, highly disorderly. Some states only existed in the bedroom areas: violent outbursts, confusion outbursts involving noise; shouting, spitting and other anti-social behaviour, such as continual rapping on tables or banging sticks on floors, and also very persistent and distressing crying and sobbing. Acute sickness was also visible only in the bedroom; but in these cases the trained staff took charge. All patient who exhibited these behaviours in the lounge were immediately physically confined to the bedrooms by the auxiliaries.

# Depersonalization and mistreatment – part of the job

Mistreatment appeared a fairly everyday strategy to get through the work. It involved deper- sonalization – ignoring the individual's spatial rights, ignoring the patient's words, or even their presence – to save time. Workers' felt resistance to the individual's emotional needs was central to time-saving. Emotional work had to be repressed and physical labour prioritized. Patients who demanded too much emotional time and refused the role of 'object' were neg- atively labelled as 'whiners' and were avoided. The more that patients demanded, the more resistance was employed to prevent their emotional needs from being fulfilled.

Auxiliaries often ignored the presence of patients, preferring to talk about them in the third person, and saying insensitive things. [...]

At night treating patients as objects was virtually the sole form of interaction observed. But for workers this was a time-saving device, as illustrated by the rituals of rounds.

> The same ritual is observed in each room entered: the auxiliaries go alone or in pairs, the toilet light is switched on, a jug is collected from the toilet, the patients' bed sheets are pulled back exposing them to the air, their night clothes are pulled up to allow the leg bag to be emptied. They might need to be rolled over to allow access. The urine is then thrown down the toilet which is flushed, the jug is washed, the sheets are pulled back over each patient and the auxiliary exists. If two auxiliaries are in the same room on the round they very often chat over the patients while they deal with them. Should a patient stir or open their eyes during this ritual they are told to go back to sleep. Any patient awake at night is considered an inconvenience to this two-hourly ritual. Many patients lie motionless with their eyes open and staring blankly as this ritual is performed. (fieldwork notes: nights)

Personal space and presence was also disregarded in the format of entrances and exits into rooms. Auxiliaries would often enter a room with little regard for the convention of traditional greetings. Brief introductions were often followed by invasive procedures to find out whether the patient was soiled, such as pulling sheets back, rolling patients over to look at their bottoms, and then giving some brief explanation of what the auxiliaries were doing.

The exit out of the room also tended to be unmarked by the usual rituals. Once a work chore was done the shutting of the door seemed to suffice as the end of the interaction. [...]

These acts of mistreatment involved the staff ignoring patients and not involving them in care. But other forms did involve the patient. Making jokes at the patient's expense was seen as 'having some fun with the patients' and workers argued that it involved patients in some way with the work. For example, patients who could not walk properly were told to 'race' down the corridor, and jokes would be made about Nigel Mansell, etc. Patients who were crying in pain would be told to buck up and smile. Mimicry was also common, with staff copying the words of confused residents. Most patients either could not hear, see or understand jokes that the workers made at their expense, while others became distressed at them. But 'joking' appeared to help auxiliaries get through the work; it broke up the stress and gave them some sort of control.

Mistreatment involved a wide range of behaviours all of which served to create compliancy in patients. Mistreatment served to give workers more control over the objects they had to process, within strict temporal constraints around the space of the home. They were partially a product of constraints on the job and also appeared to stem from ignorance about how to work with confused people and elevation within the subculture of the role of restraint and containment as part of the job.

## Punishment

Auxiliary staff believed that physical abuse towards patients was unacceptable, and many gave accounts of whistle-blowing on violent colleagues in the past. However, there was no notion of mental or emotional cruelty. Telling people off, ignoring them and 'teaching them a lesson' in ways other than physical violence were seen as acceptable. When working with nursing staff the auxiliary took the role of the verbally punitive partner. It was her role also to deal with the patient who behaved badly in the lounge, to make it clear that certain behaviours were not acceptable. [...]

Use of call buzzers was particularly disliked and one of the ways a patient could be punished was for their buzzing to be ignored. Due to immobility of patients, ignoring buzzing induced a powerlessness they could do little about. [...] Active stratagems were used to deal with other less capable 'buzzers'. [...]

Others 'harsh' night remedies included pulling the bed out from the wall, thus leaving the patient unable to reach the buzzer. Some 'naughty', persistent buzzers had begun to confound this punishment by calling to other patients to get them to use their buzzers for them. On one occasion a patient who was talking to another in the four-bedder was put in a chair, taken downstairs to the lounge and sat in a corner on her own until she 'seemed quiet'. Communication and group resistance from patients were not tolerated.

Day punishments went on mainly in the form of telling people off, teasing them or even denying their realities. More lucid patients were punished mainly through avoidance; their buzzers would be ignored and they would be left until last. 'Confused' patients were generally treated with a much more confrontational form of punishment. For example, they were called names: 'dying duck', 'moaning Minnie' or told they were 'pathetic', 'stupid' or 'being childish'. With these patients fear tactics, such as using a threatening tone of voice or physically being noisy in the surrounding environment, ramming the metal sides of hospital beds down violently, were observed daily. Punishment and control strategies such as these seemed a way to get back at the job.

## The hard culture

Auxiliary work in nursing homes is hard work: low paid, low status, dirty, physically backbreaking and tiring. However, far from complaining about the conditions of their work the nursing auxiliaries appeared to have elevated the notion of personal hardship within their subculture. Personal hardship and hard behaviour towards patients seemed central to auxiliaries' understanding of what they were supposed to do. They spoke about others, such as residential home workers, and trained staff, as too 'soft'. A strong emphasis was placed upon coping and getting on with the work, even avoiding the use of hoist and aids, despite the frequency of serious back problems.

Violence from patients was experienced on a daily basis. Verbal and physical violence were common: swearing, biting, kicking, hitting (with the hand, stick or frame) usually occurred when patients were having personal care chores done. The physical violence was usually exhibited by those considered to be suffering from forms of confusion. Physical abuse was seen as funny – the basis for staffroom stories and myth-making; part of the job. Auxiliaries often invited me to watch certain chores that illustrated this type of violence. For example, one auxiliary invited me to observe a patient who was always aggressive in the evenings, referring to the chore as 'fun'.

The violent behaviour of patients was discussed at the end of shifts. The auxiliaries would recount patients' aggressive acts and compare bruises with pride. In situations where a trained staff member was present and a patient exhibited violent behaviour it was the auxiliary who physically positioned herself to take the brunt of it, restraining the individual and ticking them off for their behaviour. Taking and containing aggression was being 'hard', which itself was part of the role of being an auxiliary.

Within this subculture of personal hardship and the elevation of containment and ordering aspects of the job, it is unsurprising that acts of mistreatment and punishment were pervasive and unquestioned. […]

# Conclusions

[…] In Cedar Court, bedroom work was auxiliaries' work and in some ways they had colonized the space as a workplace, with the patients having little control over these areas. The physical state of the patient was the only indicator of the job being done. Physical care was attained at Cedar Court through practices of daily mistreatment. Through these the individual could be ordered around the routine quicker, and they did appear to effect a state of compliance in most patients. Both punishment and mistreatment rapidly helped to create 'the lounge standard patient', which indicated that care was being carried out. Within this hidden bedroom world non-physical abuse was very difficult for trained staff, visitors or others to perceive. For example, it appeared that the trained staff who worked in fairly close proximity, but rarely in the bedrooms, were not aware of the existence of such abuse. The hard culture which had developed amongst auxiliaries positively sanctioned non-physical abuse as part of the work. Thus abuses could be carried out in front of other auxiliaries without being commented upon.

In Cedar Court the principal aim of the auxiliary was the ordering of the patient in the private world of the bedroom, and care was judged by the state of the patient's body. In this context non-physical mistreatment of the patient becomes routinized and difficult to detect. Research on institutional abuse needs to uncover both the hidden nature of care tasks and the meanings of such work to staff, to understand abuse more fully.

# References

Goffman, E. (1959) *The Presentation of Self in Everyday Life*. Harmondsworth: Penguin.
Willcocks, D., Peace, S. and Kellaher, L. (1987) *Private Lives in Public Places*. London: Tavistock.

# Chapter 15

## Virtual togetherness

*Maria Bakardjieva*

## Infosumption: the rationalistic ideal of internet use

Accounts of participation in virtual groups cropped up in the stories of some of the people I interviewed, without specific questioning. Invited to explain how they used the Internet, they started with their online groups. With others, no mention of any social life online was ever made. My pointed question about whether they took part in virtual groups or forums received sometimes very sceptical and even derogatory responses:

> I am reading a few groups, not much. But again, nothing intrigues me to participate. So I don't know how widespread that communal thing is. I have no idea. I haven't participated. Chats, I find, are a horrible waste of time! I tried it once or twice and said, forget it! [What is so disappointing about it?] Oh, the subjects, the way they talked about it ... (Reiner)

> I am aware, like you say, of newsgroups or usegroups, whatever they are called, I tried, two or three years ago, some and I just didn't care. The crap that came back and the depth of the level of knowledge didn't really strike me, it wasn't worth going through these hundreds of notes – somebody asking this or that to find ... But I couldn't find any substantive issues and I did not care, I did not want to use it to advertise my own knowledge, so I just left them alone. (Don)

Garry, the naval radio-operator, summed up this particular position regarding Internet group discussions in a useful model. According to him, a good radio-operator sends as little as possible, but receives the maximum:

> Because the radio-operator is there just to get all the information he can about the weather, the time signal, about what's happening in different countries and orders from different places.

From: Maria Bakardjieva (2005) *Internet Society: The Internet in Everyday Life*. London: SAGE, pp. 169–180 (abridged).

And if he can get that efficiently without going on the air too much, then it is to the benefit of everybody. If everybody is on the air asking questions, then you cannot hear really anything but miles and miles of questions being asked. That's why the etiquette of the professional radio-operator was to say as little as possible. Like telegrams used to be ... To me, it is a matter of getting information across. (Garry)

Coming from this perspective, Garry, like the other respondents quoted previously, scorned the 'noisy people out there on the Internet', 'the empty heads' who were out there first: 'There are always people out there who just have their mouth hanging out and they are just talking, and talking, and talking, and just creating a lot of babble' (Garry).

These empty heads produced 'garbage upon garbage' on the Internet, a low level content with which Garry did not want to engage. He believed that his contributions, had he made any, would not have been appreciated. To post in newsgroups, for him, would have been like 'casting pearls before swine – that means it is pretty pointless to be intellectual when you are dealing with people who just want to talk about garbage'.

A closer look at the 'radio-operator' perspective reveals the underlying communicative values to be 'substantive issues', 'information', 'efficiency'. The respondents in this category upheld a rationalistic ideal of information production and exchange and judged the content of the discussions they found on the Internet by it. The high expectations they had to the quality of communication prevented them from contributing any content themselves because of an 'expert knowledge or nothing' attitude. From the perspective of this rationalistic ideal, these respondents repudiated sociability understood as the pursuit of human contact, acquaintance, friendship, solidarity and intimacy, as legitimate motives for using the Internet. The users in this category were going to the Internet for timely, accurate, reliable information and, quite naturally, were finding it in the online offerings of traditional information institutions such as news agencies, radio stations, newspapers, and government sites.

# Instrumental interaction: rational and yet social

My son has an Attention Deficit Disorder ... and it was really interesting to get online and to talk to people from all over the world about this issue. It was called the ADD forum – a really good way for providing information. (Martha)

In Martha's narrative, one noticed the persistent authority of the rationalistic ideal with information as its central value. Recognition of other users on the Internet, not necessarily experts or expert organizations, as sources of information and ideas was also apparent. Information remained the leading motive stated for going on the Internet, however 'talking to people online' was not perceived as its antithesis:

At one turn of the conversation when Martha admitted that she missed the ADD forum that was available only through CompuServe, she took care to emphasize: 'It wasn't chatting to meet people and get to know people. It was chatting about ideas and exchanging information', thus paying tribute to the rationalistic ideal.

Similarly, John perceived his participation in the SkyTraveler's Digest, a mailing list for motor glider hobbyists, as a valuable resource in problematic situations when decisions regarding new equipment had to be made or technical problems to be solved. He had approached news-groups in the same way: in cases when he needed a question answered, a problem solved, a new experience illuminated: his wife's diabetes, a new type of apple tree he wanted to plant, his new communication software, etc. He enjoyed the helpfulness and solidarity demonstrated by people who took the time to answer his queries in their specifically human and social aspects, but admitted that once the problem was solved, the interpersonal communication would fade away:

> We don't normally communicate socially – how are you, what's the weather … It's usually when a technical question comes up. After that question is solved, we may talk a little bit about how old we are, what we did. But once the problem is solved this fades away. But yet, those people are still in the background. And when I am looking at postings and see their name, a bell rings. (John)

Thus people with expertise and experience in different matters of interest were coming into 'attainable reach' through the medium. John himself would only respond to questions others had asked on the mailing list when he had 'something positive', meaning well-established, proven, to say and believed that this reserved culture of 'positive', substantive exchange made his mailing list work well.

Merlin, too, was quite scrupulous as far as the quality of the contributions in his virtual group was concerned. He insisted he was on this mailing list in order 'to learn', 'to expand my understanding of the electrical components used in the electric car'. He saw the list as a 'semi-professional community' and only felt the right to contribute when he had hard evidence to show for it: 'somebody says something wrong or asks a question, especially connected to hybrids, because I have thought about it, I haven't done any real calculations, [only] very simple calculations which answered some questions that were asked'. Despite the preponderance of strictly technical content on the list, the personalities of participants had come through and Merlin had developed some curiosity as to what kind of people they were. When he had happened to be in the locations of some of the men on the list, he had driven by their houses or shops and had met some of them. Putting a face to an e-mail address or alias, a living image and context to stories told on the list, seemed to have been a transforming experience in terms of how Merlin felt about his list:

> Now, I have met these people, so it actually means a lot more to me, now that I have met [emphasizes] … I thought Jerry was a wealthy guy, in fact, you have to categorize him as poor, he is a postman and he hasn't worked for over a year, he is obviously not rich. And I have seen him, and I have seen his wife Shauna, I actually saw his two daughters in passing. I have seen the truck, the car, that had this plasma fireball incinerated inside of the car, I saw the battery – there were three batteries welded together in a T-junction, I mean really, to do that damage, it really had to have a lot of energy … (Merlin).

Thus, unexpectedly, the rationalistic model of Internet use (Merlin insisted on his loyalty to it) was showing cracks where it would have seemed most unlikely – on a technical discussion list.

[…]

# Chatting: sociability unbound

The cases discussed so far derived in a significant way from the rationalistic model of Internet communication, albeit implanting in it interpersonal interaction and sociability in different degrees and variations. However, when I listened to Sandy I realized that a qualitative break with the rationalistic model was taking place. Sandy spoke for a markedly different model of Internet communication, one that had sociability as its central value. Ironically, as I explained [earlier], Sandy was first introduced to the Internet through a university course she was taking. That means finding information had been the foremost rationale for using the medium presented to her by authoritative sources. However, it did not take long before Sandy discovered the chat lines and got fascinated by what they had to offer. In her open and emotional statement Sandy showed no signs of guilt or remorse for abandoning the rationalistic model of Internet use. In fact, she did not seem to notice the major subversion to which she was subjecting the medium as perceived from the 'radio-operator' perspective. She was happy to be one of those noisy people who were out there 'talking, and talking, and talking' (see Garry's quote earlier in this chapter). Her main reason for being on the Net was 'meeting people in there and having a great time talking to them' (see Martha's statement in the opposite sense above).

> I was drawn to the rooms that were like the parent zone, health zone and things like that, just general interest ... I would talk to people in there and then I met this guy who lives in Ontario and his wife and they had a room called the Fun Factory. It was about 10 of us. We just hung out there, we went in there and just chatted about life. All kind of fun things – we goofed around, told jokes, stories, whatever. The same ten people. Oh, I still talk to them all. In fact we've flown and we have met each other and some of us ... Lots of times other people came in, but this was the core. (Sandy)

Paradoxically, what started as 'goofing around' ended up having dramatic consequences for Sandy's 'real' life. In Sandy's own reflections, as a direct result of her hanging out in chat lines, her marriage fell apart completely. That was because online she met 'really good people' who helped her to regain her self-confidence: 'then, all of a sudden, I was reminded that I was a real person [emotional tone] with real emotions, and real feelings and I was likeable by people'. One of her new online friends was the first person to whom she revealed that her husband was beating her:

> And he just said – get out! You have to get out, Sandy, you cannot stay there! And he and I became really close good friends and he convinced me that life could go on and even that I would lose a lot of materialism, I would gain so much more, if I could fight this fight and get out. And I did. I left. (Sandy)

Another person Sandy met on the chat line also became a close friend and shared a lot in Sandy's marital problems. He was also instrumental in helping her with the technological challenges of the Internet. He was a computer professional and taught Sandy skills that she needed to move and act freely online. Thus, one can notice how, starting from a close personal relationship established online, Sandy had occasionally gone the full circle back to hard information and proficiency in one particular area:

And he made it easy. I would say 'I don't think I can do that', and he would say – 'I remember you saying that about such and such, but if you just think about how it works'. And he would explain to me how it worked. And then I would go and do it myself. (Sandy)

The chat room Sandy was describing could hardly meet the high standards of community raised by the critics of the idea of virtual community. The interactions in that room had been vibrant, and yet superficial, intense, and fleeting at the same time:

In the room it was mostly goofing around, telling cracking jokes. And also there was always stuff going on in the background in private conversations and then you'd have the public room. And often you would have three or four private conversations going at the same time as the room. (Sandy)

What was actually happening in this environment was that people were meeting previously anonymous strangers and treating them as someone 'like myself', someone who could laugh at the same jokes, talk about the same topics of interest and then walk away and go on with his or her own life. That is, what the room was providing for its visitors was an environment for 'fluid sociability among strangers and near-strangers'. [...]

## Community as in commitment

With Ellen, the concept of community dominated the conversation from the first question. Ellen had hooked up to the Internet from home after she became housebound and diagnosed with a rare, crippling chronic illness. Her explicit motivation for becoming an Internet user was to be able to connect to a support group. She simply felt 'very desperate for information and help'. 'Getting information' and 'getting support' were two inseparable reasons for her to go online. Thus, Ellen joined an invisible, dispersed group of people who were logging on everyday to get the 'gift of making this connection' with each other:

to discover that thousands of people are going through exactly the same incredible experience and nobody in their family understands, their husbands and wives don't understand, the doctor doesn't believe them and they have this terrible difficulty of functioning. And yet, there is this tremendously strong community of people who have never met and probably will never meet but who are so loyal to each other and have such a strong support because it is a lifeline for all of us. (Ellen)

The list was experienced as a safe environment by these people, a place where they felt comfortable saying:

I've had a really bad day, I had to go see a specialist and I had such a difficulty and couldn't breathe and it was such a challenge to get there and then the doctor was awful to me. And then I got home and my husband was complaining because the house wasn't clean ... (Ellen)

And immediately after a complaint like that would pop up in members' mail boxes, there would be a 'flurry' or supportive responses. Loyalty, high tolerance for 'dumping', safety, family-like atmosphere, compassion – these were all attributes Ellen used to describe the quality of interaction in her 'wonderful group'.

The real-life effects consisted of 'a lot of confidence', 'getting my life in proportion again', 'getting a sense of myself' (compare with an almost identical formulation by Sandy) 'feeling much less a failure'. Learning a lot about the disease was among the benefits of list membership, however Ellen took care to distinguish the particular kind of learning that was taking place there:

> I learnt so much from these people who had had the disease for years. I had tried to get hold of some medical information. But getting online is different because there, for the first time, you get information from people who have trodden this path already! (Ellen)

For good or ill as the case may be, the victims of the disease Ellen had were short-circuiting the medical establishment and the expert knowledge produced by it and were learning from each other. More accurately, they were collectively appropriating and using expert knowledge in ways they had found relevant and productive in their own unique situations as sufferers and victims. On the list they were creating this culture of appropriation and a stock of knowledge stemming from their individual and yet intertwined lifeworlds.

A similar sense of gain from online support group discussions came through clearly in Matthew's comment. According to him, people with similar medical problems learnt from each other about the existence of a variety of treatment options, which, consequently, empowered them when dealing with the medical profession. Matthew challenged the very notion of a patient. In his understanding, people with health problems were clients, customers and in the best case, collaborators with doctors, nurses and prosthetists. To be able to act in this capacity however, they needed to be informed and acculturated in their disability. This is, Matthew believed, what online support groups, such as the mailing list for amputees he himself had initiated, were instrumental in doing. 'I learnt more about being an amputee in the one year on the mailing list than throughout the twenty years I had lived with my disability', Matthew insisted passionately.

What distinguished Ellen's experience from other, more detached, forms of learning like those described by previous respondents was the fact that the people she was interacting with online had come to constitute a collective entity with its own distinctive culture. Her virtual group had a relatively stable membership communicating on a daily basis and feeling responsible for each other's well-being. Both commonality of interest and diversity could be found in that group. Most of its participants were people seeking alternative approaches for dealing with the chronic devastating disease they had. In Ellen's estimate, most of them were highly educated and articulate. Women were in the majority. At the same time, members of the group came from different religious backgrounds and life experiences in terms of profession, family, nationality and other factors. Yet, characteristically, they were entering their shared space ready and eager to listen to interpretations coming from viewpoints different from their own:

> Like this woman in Israel, a Hebrew scholar, a convert to Judaism, she has the most fascinating perspective on things. There are amazing things coming from her ... But nobody has ever tried to push one point of view above another. There has been very much a sense of sharing. (Ellen)

Ellen's account describes a 'warmly persuasive' version of a robust online community distinguished by interpersonal commitment and a sense of common identity that could meet the highest standards. Ellen's Internet was thus markedly different from the rationalist model of Internet communication defended by the 'infosumers'. Yet, as we have seen from the cases cited earlier, not all home users of the Internet recognized or were eager to grasp this opportunity offered by the technology. It took a particular configuration of situational factors: a rare disease, physical and social isolation, a vital need to come to terms with a radically new experience, and mastery of language and expression (recall that Ellen was a philologist, editor and writer) for this rather extreme form of online community involvement to materialize. And it should be noted that even in this case online community was not displacing face-to-face community where the latter did or could have existed. It was rather filling the gap left by the impossibility of face-to-face community or the inability of existing face-to-face communities to satisfy important needs of the subject. Furthermore, online community was, helping the individual member, at least in the evidence presented by Ellen's case, in her struggle to regain confidence and motivation for rebuilding face-to-face relationships.

I would now like to go back and revise the theoretical debate about virtual community in the context of the various experiences of my respondents. Let me start the interpretation of the emergent continuum between what I called 'the rationalistic model of Internet communication' and the 'community as in commitment' experience with the observation that in all of the cases discussed above, the respondents had access to principally the same technology with some variations in computing power, speed and access time which, I found, were not related to the prevalent type of use.

The users who denied the communal aspects of the Internet (most of them men) came from a strictly utilitarian value orientation. They were using the Internet to find positive, reliable, scientific, professionally presented information and were more often finding it in the virtual projections of institutions such as online magazines and newspapers (Reiner), radio and television stations' sites, government sites (Garry), news agencies (Norris) and scientific publications online (Sophie). To most of these users, newsgroups and mailing lists had little to offer and respectively, communal forms were questionable in principle. The everyday practice of such users, I suggest, is organized by the consumption model of the Internet. The everyday practice of the infosumer, for its part, continuously reproduces the consumption model of the Internet as a social institution.

On the other hand, representatives of disenfranchised groups – in my study these were clearly Ellen and Matthew, both disabled, but also in some sense Sandy (a victim of spousal abuse) and Merlin (unemployed long term) – were using the technology as a tool to carve spaces of sociability, solidarity, mutual support and situated, appropriative learning in communion with others. As I tried to show, these two forms of Internet use were not separated by empty space but by a whole range of intermediate modalities. Martha and John appreciated the empowerment stemming from the opportunity to draw on the knowledge, experience and practical help of otherwise anonymous people in the areas of their specific interests and concerns. [...]

# Section 3
## Approaches

## Introduction

How care is provided is the focus of this section. Most of the chapters are about approaches to health care although they have wider applicability to social care practice. Chapter 17 by Jocelyn Lawler about body care, for example, looks at ways in which nurses can be helped to acknowledge rather than deny the complexities of body work, which involves the contravention of social norms about touching and intimacy, and its emotional content. This clearly has resonance for home care workers and care home workers who, as Lee-Treeweek's chapter in the last section demonstrates, often repressed the emotional side of their work and gave priority to the physical aspects. It is of course the case that those engaged in day to day body work, which is so highly challenging, are likely to be the least qualified and the lowest paid. Chapter 18 examines the role of health care assistants and raises issues about patient safety and the quality of care provided by these unqualified support workers. The authors argue that with the shortage of qualified nurses and the increasing amount of paperwork associated with audit and care planning, health care assistants have moved beyond the support role to more direct work with patients involving, for example, giving injections, dressing wounds and setting up infusion feeds. Such developments they suggest may be putting patients at risk.

Chapter 19 focuses specifically on the issue of risk. With the move towards consumerism in the NHS, issues related to risk and possible litigation have come to the fore. This chapter reports on how nurses and midwives perceive this climate of risk and examines the impact it has on relationships between patients and front line workers. One strategy for managing risk and possible litigation has been the introduction of protocols to guide health care practice in Britain. Chapter 20 looks critically at the use of protocols or guidelines in the NHS. It concludes that successful implementation requires the right balance to be struck between the standardisation of practice and allowing professionals to exercise their clinical judgement.

In the following two chapters the focus turns to patients and, in particular, the impact of the internet and of electronic records on their experience of illness. The internet is changing the way people learn about health and illness and health sites are one of the most popular resources on the web. Chapter 21 reports on research which has explored the impact of this new source of knowledge on people's experience of cancer and concludes that it enables people to acquire expertise in how to manage serious illness that might otherwise not have been available to them. Chapter 22 is a fascinating account of people's reactions when given the opportunity to access their online patient records.

The final chapter in this section describes a collaborative project between health and social care to support children who are affected by HIV/AIDS. The project, run by Barnardo's, used groupwork with these children to overcome the secrecy and stigma surrounding the illness and the consequent isolation.

It would be impossible to cover every aspect of health and social care practice in a section such as this. However, these chapters offer an interesting insight into some of the issues facing service providers and service users in the 21st century. The contrast with the anthology pieces which begin this section is quite stark. For example, Barbara Prynn's description of what happened to children who were 'boarded out' with foster parents in the early 1950s or Ian Vokins' account of how his diabetes was treated around that time, when set alongside the following chapters in the section demonstrate just how much things have changed over the last 50 years or so.

# Chapter 16

## Anthology: approaches

*Compiled by Joanna Bornat*

We become involved in health and social care in different ways. The five items included in this anthology draw on research into the history of fostering by a social worker, the memory of someone growing up with diabetes in the 1950s, a debate between two philosophers about visual impairment, hospice doctors and nurses developing ways to deal with patients' pain, and family history for children orphaned by AIDS in South Africa.

All very different, and an eclectic choice perhaps, but with a common theme: perspectives of need. Approaches made towards providing for people perceived as being in need of care and support vary according to contexts of time and geography. Some of the accounts here describe very different forms of provision, because time has moved on and more is now known about particular conditions. In their different ways, however, they illustrate how uneven the experience of health and social care has been, and continues to be, and how practitioners have, at times, adopted approaches which have had long term implications for the lives of the people they work with. All evoke empathy in their different ways, a reminder of the importance of acknowledging similarities in human experience, as much as difference.

## 16.1 Growing up alone

Barbara Prynn, a retired social worker with a professional background in fostering, interviewed people who had been in the care of Dr Barnardo's Homes and the Foundling Hospital. Both these organisations fostered or 'boarded out' children until they were thought old enough to learn a trade. In this extract, adults born in the 1920s and 1930s recall the pain of separation from their foster parents.

---

The children who were placed with their foster families in infancy assumed that they were their biological children. While some of the foster parents explained the nature of their relationship, others did not. This meant that when the children came to leave, it was unexplained and unexpected.

Geraldine describes how her foster mother explained her situation when she was eleven,

…we sat down and she said er 'I've got to tell you now because you're getting older you know' and she said that 'You're not really my little girl'. So I said …'Yes, I am'. So she said 'No, and nor's Bridie [another Barnardo girl in the foster home]. 'Cos she was littler than me. So she said 'You come from Dr Barnardo's'. And erm …well it was a sad time and we was all crying and er I didn't want to know (*long pause*) but then of course I – I knew, and that was that. So it sunk in afterwards,

Rosalind was the same age as Geraldine when she had to 'go back.' She describes learning about this three weeks before it was to happen and its long-term effects,

…how they told me I'll always remember, I used to change um 'Schoolgirls' Friends', we used to have a book, you know magazines, and we used to change swap them with other people, and I was going to do it this afternoon and my Dad said 'I shouldn't bother to get too many, because you've got to go back to the Home'. He was abrupt, but um …I don't think they knew how to tell me, and that was you know they just got it over sort of thing.
…as a child, I never showed a lot of emotion, I still don't, I think (*sigh*) …you know, I keep everything sort of inside; so I never showed a lot of emotion about it, but that day on the train when I got on the train, and I vowed then that nobody else would hurt me and that, you know … it takes a lot now to make me cry, but um, I think it hardens you.

Henry who was a foundling, describes the situation in his foster home. His foster parents were farmers:

My foster parents whom I only knew as Mum and Dad …they had had their own family …of about six children, and subsequently from 1896 until about …1920 I suppose …they had …eight foundling children …we were there from the age of a few months until …about …five earlier and then it became six, it meant that there was one young child, one getting to the time of leaving, and so …erm …my foster mother had a continuous flow of children from the Foundling Hospital as did numbers of the other, foster mothers.

When he was six years old he went with his foster mother and a number of other children with their foster mothers in 'a special horse bus' to the Foundling Hospital. He and the other children were left there. He now knows that the arrangement probably was that his foster mother would have taken another baby home with her. These exchanges took place on quarter days. Henry was fortunate in that his foster mother always made a point of coming to see him on later quarter days when she brought back or collected other children. She also sent him food parcels from the farm. He paid one visit there when he was older.
[…]
Henry and the other interviewees who entered the care of the child care institution as infants did so because they were illegitimate. Their experience differed radically from those who did so at a later stage in their childhood. Their entry came about because of parental death or misfortune. One important area of difference was that children in the second group

were not alone. They usually had one or more siblings who shared their early life experience.

Walter and Ronald both lived with their parents during their early years. Walter's mother had had a son before her marriage to his father and Walter was one of four children of the marriage. Ronald was the eighth child of a family of twelve children. Walter was seven when he and his three younger siblings were removed from home by a court order. Ronald and his four younger siblings left home when he was five after their mother's death in childbirth.

[...]

Ronald and his five siblings were also taken to Stepney Causcway [Barnados]. His description of this event and its long-term effects is very vivid:

> Ah, I don't know how long we were there, but that place has a, it is really a dreadful memory it's something that I've struggled with for years. It inculcated a kind of fear in me which I think I, I kept right up until adulthood. Erm, we had not been there very long ...when erm one morning part of the routine I remember it was that after the – the two girls being mere babies were separate from us [Ronald and his brother] – but the routine was that after breakfast they would bring the babies down to play with the younger children in the Nurseries. And on this particular occasion Irene and Joan didn't turn up, and I asked the Matron where my two baby sisters were. And I can remember almost her exact words 'Ooh you won't see them again. They've gone to Babies' Castle'. You can imagine the effect on a five-year-old who only a few months before had been told Mummy won't be coming home with the baby; they've gone to Heaven. It's a memory which er (sighs) used to cause me tremendous ...I didn't realise how deeply it had gone till recently quite frankly.

> ...I'll give you an example of the effect it had on me. When I was in my early thirties and had been, at teacher training, we did the usual course on child development in the course of that looking at children in care – the institutionalised child. And somebody who knew me said 'Well, you were a Barnardo boy weren't you'? And I said 'Yes'. 'Were you at Stepney' So I said 'Yes'. 'Don't you think you could arrange for us to go to Stepney, you know and look around' So why not? Good idea. So I did.

> And when it came to going. I got as far as Stepney Causeway and I couldn't go – I couldn't go near the place. I just made an excuse and went home. I've never been there since.

*Source*: B. Prynn (2001) 'Growing up alone', *Oral History,* 29(2): 62–72.

# 16.2    A diabetes story

Ian Vokins' story appears on the website 'Diabetes Stories: personal tales of diabetes through the decades' (www.diabetes-stories.com). He was interviewed by Helen Lloyd for a project funded by the Wellcome Foundation and run by Dr David Matthews at the Oxford Centre for Diabetes, Endocrinology & Metabolism (OCDEM). Ian Vokins is one of 50 people diagnosed with diabetes whose life stories contribute to the history of medicine. Copies of the recordings are archived at the British Library and on the project's website (address below). An excerpt from the beginning of his interview has been included here.

Well, I was born in 1942...when I was five, we moved to the next village across, called Milton, and … I spent my early years there, until I started work when I was fifteen. My father, originally, was a gardener, before I was born, and then he became a chauffeur and a driver for the RAF, as a civilian, through the war, actually, then. And my mother was in service before I was born, and then she worked for a petroleum company – Esso. And I have a brother, who's six years younger than me. Had a similar upbringing, and he developed diabetes when he was in his late twenties … I had a fairly normal upbringing. We didn't have much money – it was just after the war… I hated school with a vengeance … I was a – what they call – a late starter; I started learning after I left school … we always ate very well. My mother was an exceptionally good cook, and we always managed to get, you know, good food, because that was the most important thing.

… But my childhood, I can… mostly I can remember spending most of my childhood over the local fields, and fishing in streams and things. It sounds a bit Huckleberry Finn, but really, that's what it was like. It was… I knew, you know, at the age of nine, I knew all the names of all the birds, all the trees, all the… I could tell you what tree a leaf came off and things like that, because it was just passed on from…

*And how did your diagnosis with diabetes come about?*

Well, it happened in July 1954. I can distinctly remember an aunt of mine coming to tea and noting that I was drinking excessive amounts of anything I could get hold of. And my mother took me to the doctor's on… at the first opportunity, and I was diagnosed within an hour or two, and in hospital the next day.

… I wasn't feeling very good, but I wasn't really ill either, but I was sent into the Radcliffe Infirmary, as I said, the next day…and I was in there for three or four weeks. I think the insulin that I was put on was called Insulin Zinc Suspension, and I was on approximately eighty units; that was just one injection a day. A few weeks or months later, I was admitted to the children's ward in the Churchill Hospital. I guess I was having problems with control, and I remember having to eat large quantities of potatoes, and nothing – not even a trace – of sugar.

… And I wasn't making any progress at all with the control, and they were upping my insulin dose every two or three days. And then my doctor was changed, and I can remember a Dr Smallpiece coming on the scene, who was a lady doctor, and she took over and allowed me to have a slightly more liberal diet. Remembering that this was 1954, and I was only twelve years old, it was quite a strain for me to have to eat all these potatoes and, you know, bread with hardly any butter on, and stuff like that. And she allowed me to have a scrape of marmalade, I remember, or jam on bread, and stuff like that; but only small amounts. But there was a definite response to my control, and after being in there for actually eleven weeks, on a hundred plus units a day, they allowed me to go home.

*Can you remember, back in the Radcliffe, being taught to inject yourself?*

Yes, I can – yeah. That was using an orange. I remember them giving me an orange and a syringe, and saying "pinch it up". And if ever you've tried to pinch an orange up, it's not that easy, but that was how we were taught to do it. And I think they also used a pillowcase as well… a pillow as well to do it, but I can distinctly remember the orange!

*Did you find it difficult?*

No, not at all, no. I accepted, after the initial shock – you know, at that age, and I'd never heard of diabetes before, and I don't think my parents knew that much about it either, so it was quite a shock to everybody, so… – but once we'd accepted it, after, you know, quite a short time, everything seemed to slot into place with the managing the diet and the insulin.

*How did you test for sugar levels?*

Well, we didn't actually… 'cause, in those days, blood testing could only be done in hospitals and laboratories. It was done… I can remember in the hospital, we used to use various… it was a urine test, but we didn't even have tablets in the hospital. We used to mix some ammonia and something else in a test-tube with urine, and boil it over a Bunsen burner. And mine used to go orange nearly every time, I remember, which means plus two per cent. And then they brought in a thing called Clinitest, which was a tablet you dropped in so many drops of water, and that gave you a similar result.

*And what did they teach you about diet?*

Well, first of all it was fairly strict – you know, don't eat… I could eat as much meat, fish, eggs or cheese – I can remember that being on the diet sheet. Meat, fish, eggs or cheese were free, but the carbohydrate intake was extremely strict. And I remember being given a set of scales by the almoner, and they only went up to eight ounces. And I used to have to weigh the bread and my cereal and just about everything on these scales.

*Source*: www.diabetes-stories.co.uk/transcript.asp?UID=44 (accessed 15 May 2007).

# 16.3   Sight unseen

Martin Milligan was a philosopher who was blind from the age of 18 months. Brian Magee is also a philosopher who has an interest in exploring how people experience the world differently. He and Martin Milligan discussed this question in letters, starting from the point that if someone is visually impaired then it might be assumed that their understanding of things will not be the same as that of someone who is sighted. In this excerpt, Martin Milligan writes about his experience of awareness of difference.

You may ask what right I have to opinions on such matters, being someone wholly without visual experience of my own. Part of the answer to that question must be that an advantage which most born-blind people have over most sighted people in considering the importance of sight, and the relations between blind and sighted people, is that they are likely to have had more relevant experience. For whereas most sighted people will have known few if any blind people, and (if any) will often not have known them very well, born-blind people will usually have known a lot of other blind people, including blind people who have had sight, *and also* a lot of sighted people, and will have known some of both groups very well. They are also likely to have had more experience of interaction between blind and sighted people. For that reason – and also because an enormous preponderance of what is written and said in literature and the media deals with sighted people, and not with the blind – blind people are apt to know a good deal more *about* sight and sighted people than the latter can know about blindness and blind people.

To take my own case. In the close-knit family in which I grew up, both of my parents and my brother were sighted. All my early playmates were sighted. I had the privilege (admittedly rare at that time in this country) of being educated in ordinary primary and secondary schools predominantly for sighted children, schools in which there were some additional staff, together with special books and equipment, for the support of a relatively small number of blind pupils, but where, like most of the other blind pupils, I spent most of my time as a member of sighted classes: so I had close friends among the sighted as well as among the blind pupils. During most of my student days, and throughout the greater part of my working life, the overwhelming majority of my friends and acquaintances, including almost all my close friends, have been sighted. Of the women whom I have loved and lived with intimately one was totally blind, one fully sighted, and the third has had a significant amount of sight, although she has little left. My son, with whom I have shared much, has a lot of sight, although he is visually impaired. In short, I have had a great deal of experience of what I have regarded, and what I know *they* have regarded, as 'everyday moment-to-moment human interaction' with people whose visual experience I could not directly share – as well as some experience of living only with other blind people. This latter experience, of course, differed in some respects from the other. Blind people living together need more help from outside. At the same time, because they face some problems not encountered by others, they can form special bonds. But it is my experience that these are not necessarily stronger than bonds that can be formed between blind and sighted friends.

My whole life therefore seems to me to stand in contradiction to the views expressed in those passages of your letter. When I was young and did not get the sighted girl-friends I wanted I was sometimes tempted to think that this was because they were put off by my being blind. But when I saw the success some of my blind friends had with women I realised that my blindness had very little to do with this. Although most sighted people are naturally a bit nervous and tentative when they first meet a blind person, and although some have initially a tendency to treat a blind person as if blindness were associated with mental inferiority, or at least with insuperable problems of communication, I have found that all this usually wears off pretty quickly on closer acquaintance. Sighted people in fact often say to me, as I know they do to many blind people, 'Most of the time I'm with you I forget that you're blind.' This isn't the compliment it's sometimes supposed to be, since I see nothing to be ashamed of or embarrassed about in being blind, but I think it's very often quite simply a statement of the truth. When a friend and I are working together, or listening to music, or attending a meeting, or talking about politics or economics or history or science, or even about sport or holidays or people we know, my blindness usually doesn't come up, because it isn't relevant. Even if my friend tells me about the goal [...] scored for Leeds United last Saturday, his description won't usually differ in any way from one he would give to a sighted friend who hadn't seen the match.

More important: when my blindness does come up, as of course it sometimes must and should, it's very rare for me to experience it as a barrier between me and a sighted friend – and also, I think, rare for my friends to do so. True, it *is* sometimes an occasion for problems between me and *some* sighted people. In the first place, I can believe that there may be a small minority of sighted people who are so strongly repelled by blindness that they fiercely resist forming relations with a blind person. I think I may have had one or two experiences of this; but of course it's difficult to be sure whether it is one's blindness or something else in one which is putting someone else off. Even where I have suspected that revulsion at my blindness may have been the distancing factor, I haven't thought that what repelled was simply or chiefly my inability directly to share visual experience, for my impression has been that people who care specially about their sight and who get a special amount of pleasure from seeing want to try to share that with blind people, and that their descriptions of what they see – although no doubt, as I have conceded, often seeming to them to fall short of their actual experience – are not only of real help and interest to me but serve to draw us closer. In any case, if blindness repels people, that isn't primarily our problem, but theirs. More troublesome, sometimes, than people who are repelled by blindness are people who are attracted by it because they see in it an opportunity to 'take over', to manage, or at least to patronise. If that were all that was present, the relationship with such a person would be relatively simple: it would be one of battle. The complication often is, however, that mixed in with these more doubtful motives there is quite often a strong element of straightforward kindness and good-heartedness. But in any case, what is at issue is, again, not the inability to share visual experience but the problems involved in the giving and receiving of help. That blind people often do make *friends* with sighted people shows that where there are compatibilities of disposition, common interests or just the right 'chemistry', such problems are not insuperable, or even often very serious. The differences in experience between blind and sighted people who are friends often serve, in fact, like other differences in experience between people, to enrich their relationships.

What I am saying therefore is, first, that although there are significant differences between blind and sighted people they need not be divisive, and are often not so. I also want to say, second, that not all the differences between blind and sighted people are to the advantage of the sighted, as the part of your letter under discussion seems to suggest. Many born-blind people learn to use their ears, their fingers, and even their noses to explore their environments to a much greater degree than most sighted people do. It's possible, at least, that on average blind people *think* a bit more than sighted people. There is also another difference, which I would like to approach through another bit of autobiography.

For the dozen years or so after I left school I had almost no occasion to meet any other blind people. And I had no special wish to do so – apart from one or two old school friends, and a splendid blind teacher I had had – as I was inclined to think of blind people as just ordinary people minus sight. But when it seemed that I wasn't going to get an academic job, and that if I was to earn my living I had better learn to do something that employers were already willing to pay blind people to do, I went to a blind training centre to learn to be a shorthand-typist. There, for the first time in my life, I spent several months living and working with a number of adult blind people, most of whom had lost their sight recently, though some of them had been born blind. To my surprise I found this a rather inspiring experience. What inspired me was the exceptional spirit and courage of the people around me. Perhaps it shouldn't have surprised me. These were all people still recovering from the trauma of loss of sight, or emerging from gross over-protection and sheltering, who were now faced with the necessity of learning to get about by themselves, and to enter or re-enter the ordinary sighted world. They just *had* to show a bit of extra spirit and courage. I think these qualities are probably present in slightly above-average doses in most blind people 'out in the world'. I didn't think of myself as brave at the time, because I had grown up as blind in the ordinary world; but looking back on that time from my present less active condition I'm inclined to think that I was quite brave too then. But I don't want to make too much of these differences either way. Just as there are certainly some blind people who are more perceptive than many sighted people, there are certainly some sighted people who have shown more grit and determination than most blind people.

So, although I don't want to under-play the differences there are in experience between the sighted and the blind, I can't see reason for saying that they 'can only be described as "vast" or "huge"'. At any rate I am sure that the difference in experience between a sighted civil servant in London and a sighted peasant in Tibet, or even a sighted miner in Kent, is likely to be a great deal 'vaster' than that between him or her and a fellow civil servant in the same office of the same sex and rank who is blind. And I'd be surprised if the differences in outlook and experience between you and me were as 'huge' as the differences between either of us and a Japanese, or American or even British millionaire, blind or sighted, who had made his or her money in cement, coffee, or the money markets. What matters anyway 'on the human scale' is not the 'vastness' of differences between human beings – the experience of every one of us differs a good deal from that of every other – but the extent to which we can unite in a community within which we can gain from and be strengthened by the differences between us. From that point of view the difference between those who have sight and those who do not is easily bridged compared with other differences between human beings such as differences of class, nationality, race, religion, sex and even age.

*Source*: B. Magee and M. Milligan (1995) *Sight Unseen: Letters between Brian Magee and Martin Milligan*. London: Phoenix.

# 16.4    An oral history of the modern hospice movement

By interviewing people who helped to pioneer the modern hospice movement in the UK, the authors of *A Bit of Heaven for the Few? An oral history of the modern hospice movement in the United Kingdom* wanted people to talk about how they felt about their careers and their work so that they could build up a feeling for how and why certain things worked and happened. In this excerpt, doctors and nurses who worked in hospices in Sheffield and Belfast describe changing understandings about pain management.

Well there was one patient who, when I said to her, 'Well, Mrs Hinson, tell me about your pain' – this was the day after she was admitted – and she said, 'Well, Doctor, it began in my back; but now it seems that *all of me is wrong*,' and she talked about one or two more symptoms, and she said, 'I could have cried for the pills and the injections but I knew that I mustn't. Nobody seemed to understand how I felt and it seemed as if all the world was against me. My husband and son were marvellous but they would have to stay off work and lose their money, but it's wonderful to begin to feel safe again.' So she's really encapsulated the whole thing in the answer to one question. And I quoted her many times and that's the start of what has gone through hospice literature: *total pain*.

*Continuing with this theme, Tony Crowther provides a detailed case illustration from his own experience in the hospice setting of St Luke's, Sheffield in the 1990s:*

...the patient who came in ... she'd been home for a week, from the oncology hospital, came in because they couldn't manage at home because of the pain. So we knew she'd had active treatment recently, and yet her pain was totally uncontrolled, in spite of being on ...something like 1,200 milligrams of diamorphine in a syringe driver in 24 hours, which isn't a massive dose, but it's big enough. And in two or three days it all unravelled ... that ... well first of all she'd seen the consultant who had said, 'Oh well, I can't do any more, you'd better go to a pain clinic.' When she came into us, we found that her husband had hardly been seen while she'd been in the oncology hospital; he hardly ever visited ... so we needed to unravel why. She was only a youngish woman, 41 or 42. Was he too poor to travel? I mean, in fact that was what he'd said when we tackled him about it. He lived in Rotherham which was costing him, I think it was about £3.50 return and he said, 'I can't afford to come every day.' So that was easily sorted. We then found that he, while his wife was at home, had had a blazing row with her father over the care he was giving to his wife, to his daughter. We then found that [their] daughter, who lived in Birmingham with two young children and a husband in the army, had rung one evening, say the Tuesday, asked how Mum was and he had said, 'Well, I haven't visited today,' so they'd had a row; that he was neglecting mother.

So there were so many family turmoils going on, and this had rubbed off on the patient. And I'm not saying that we got her pain controlled completely, it took us a fortnight to unravel all that little lot, but we managed to get the daughter and grandchildren up from Birmingham, we managed to get enough money for the husband to travel every day, and we persuaded him to come in at lunchtime and have lunch in the unit and stay with his wife, and explained why ... there's no reason why lay people should understand why; the effect that has on patients. So there is a lot more to this now and, and I'm getting more and more interested in the power of ... where the patient is in their family, or in their own ... I don't know, in their, their capsule of society. The influence that has on the patient I find fascinating, and on how it influences them.

*Sam Ahmedzai, also working in Sheffield, but in the acute hospital rather than the hospice, draws on the concept of total pain in the following example from the late 1990s, showing how a variety of interventions and forms of support may have to be marshalled to tackle a particular problem:*

What we're saying is that of course the severity determines what you offer, but really it's a case of looking at each patient's symptom now with all faces in mind. So that if you have a patient comes in with a mild cancer pain from a bone metastasis you'll say, what can we do from the anti-cancer point of view? – a shot of radiotherapy. But that's not going to work for a month so we also go to the analgesics, let's give you some paracetamol and a non-steroidal. By the way, you know this, the reason they're having the pain is because there's a fracture in their femur, well, maybe an orthopaedic surgeon can fix that and you get over night pain relief and then we can give radiotherapy to give you long-term relief. And this patient is living alone or with a very, very distressed family, we need a nurse to come in here or a social worker to come and support. Really looking at the sort of the 'total pain' concept.

*Ivy McCreery, a nurse working in the Marie Curie Centre in Belfast, makes the point about pain relief quite strongly, as something absolutely fundamental to the hospice and palliative care approach:*

...when people come here, you can do nothing till you've sorted out somebody's pain – so once you get their pain managed then there are other outstanding symptoms that are causing them distress that you have to try and manage, and once you get those managed then they begin to get comfortable, they begin to get their personality back and be able to cope with, with life other than just being a sick person. And from then on you have to move on into communication, because who are you communicating with, you have to be able to communicate with the patient to get them, to let them know what pain relief they're on, why they're on it, to let them know what pills you're giving them for whatever symptoms – not only them, but the relatives, you have to let, you know, keep the relatives up to date of why you're doing things. Because there's less problems then. If you have open, honest, appropriate communication, hopefully there's less barriers.

*John Hunt, a nurse with experience of working in hospice and palliative care units in different parts of the country, both in the independent sector and the NHS, draws together some of the fundamental principles of pain management that by the end of the twentieth century had become orthodoxy within the field:*

...one of the things I do think is that the, if you like, the underlying philosophies of the use of the medications probably haven't changed. And what I mean by that is that the, the old hard and fast ideas of looking at oral medicines, looking at trying to work from a simple base of starting with one medicine, looking at the effects of that, adding in others slowly, but also looking at – for example with pain – looking at managing pain in a very careful step-by-step way, the old idea of *by the mouth and by the clock*, and also the ideas of the goals of pain management, the old goals that we used to recite about enabling people to have no pain at night and be able to sleep, enabling people to have no pain at rest, and then enabling people to have no pain as they were able to be more active. I don't think those things have changed. I think the use of combination medications – again there may well be a much broader range of medications now – but again I think the same, the same theories apply – again if we take pain because it's probably the best one to do, looking at the type of pain, looking at the level of analgesic effect that your initial drug will get, and then thinking about co-analgesics which may not necessarily be analgesics: steroids, non-steroidals etc, etc and in particular thinking about neuropathic pain and not only being able to relieve the pain but being able to give people back some sort of function. So thinking about that in terms of the analgesic plan. So whether I am right or not, I don't know because I only have, if you like, the past to reflect on, but I don't think those theories have necessarily changed: I think some careful theories of looking at the problem and thinking about the management by using medications in a step-by-step way are still there.

*Source*: D. Clark, N. Small, M. Wright, M. Winslow and N. Hughes (2005) *A Bit of Heaven for the Few? An Oral History of the Modern Hospice Movement in the United Kingdom*. Lancaster: Observatory Publications.

# 16.5    Memory work and resilience in times of AIDS

This excerpt is from a manual for people working with AIDS orphans in KwaZulu-Natal in South Africa. The participants mentioned were support group workers who were HIV-positive and who had been trained in memory box work. Memory boxes were at the heart of the Simanlondo project which emphasised the importance of family history in developing resilience amongst orphaned children.

## Family conversations

Eight of ten of the participants talked about the history of their family. All the participants who had started making a memory box had written down elements of their family history. They felt that it was important for themselves and for their children to document that history. Here is an example:

> I wanted to know about what made my family unique, so I spoke to my father and my aunt. I also wanted to know more about my mother who died when I was thirty-two. I have written down their place of birth, where they lived before coming to Durban and the reason for their move. I have written down the names of all my relatives on my mother's and my father's side. I have also written down the date of birth of all the members of my family, the names of their children and the dates of their marriages. Finally I have written down the date of death of the deceased members of my family and how these persons have died.

The interviews show that the creation of memory boxes prompted families to talk about health issues and the history of the family. Nine of the participants had started to speak to their families about their history. They also told their children about their place of birth, their ancestors and their origins. Undoubtedly, the memory box has initiated an open dialogue between parents and children, especially between mothers and daughters. One of the participants told her child that she had been sexually abused and she offered her words of advice for the future. Another one spoke to her daughter about the Zulu culture and the role the ancestors played in her life. She explained how the family history had affected her and expressed the sadness she felt when her father deserted her family. She also said that it was important to talk to her daughter about death:

> I told her all the funny things that we have done, our religion and our culture. I explained why people wear skins and snakes. I also told her about the bad things that happened; when people died and how they died. My parents broke up and I told her now frustrating it was growing up without a father. So she knows.

One of the participants described her difficulty in persuading her mother to talk about her father, because of the painful memories this brought back to her.

> When I ask my mum, she cries. I want her to try and find him so I could meet him. I think about it a lot. I think she gave me another surname, because when I look at

the phone book there is nobody with the same surname. If they are painful memories for her, I must leave them hidden, I will never know what kind of family I had. What hurts the most is my mum denying my father.

The same interviewee said that it was very difficult for her to discuss her family history with her children, because her mother would not expand on her relationship with her father. She did not know much about her family history and wanted to explore it with her mother before she spoke to her children.

For one of the participants the training was a time of self-reflection. She came to a deeper understanding of her family history. She became aware of the fact that her mother had not told her the full truth about her father's death. The training prompted her to trace one of her relatives who told her more about her ancestry:

I realised that when you are a child, many people die and you do not know why. You do not understand what happened. It is difficult to know the full story. It is important to let your children know. It happened to me when I was younger. When my father died, my mother did not tell me what had happened to him. She said that perhaps my brother had poisoned him, but she did not tell me the full story. I used to say my last name without knowing where it was coming from. Thanks to the Memory Box Programme I found out that my name comes from my uncle in Kranskop. I found my father's brother and his family in the South Coast. I asked someone in town and they showed him to me. This is how I found members of my family. I think the Memory Box Programme is a very good project.

## Memory boxes

Nine interviewees had encouraged their children to create a memory box. The only reason why the tenth interviewee did not do so was that he did not live with his child. Discussing the memory boxes gave the children the opportunity to ask questions about their family, their origins and their culture. Often this led to a discussion about death. All questions were answered in a caring, supportive environment. The parents made a point of being truthful with their children.

I always used to communicate with my child, but now it has become more serious. I have to make sure she is alright. I can't just leave her to cry when she is angry. I have to find out why because otherwise I lose out. I want her to see me as a supportive mother. For example, if she has done something wrong I used to shout and scream at her, but I realise now that I have to find out why. If she has done something wrong and she explains it to me, then I must tell her the correct way to do it. She won't learn if I scream. I must advise her.

The dialogue between parents and children helps build resilience in the child. The daughter of one of the interviewees, for instance, felt confident enough to talk to her mother about her father's absence. This conversation raised her self-esteem and strengthened her sense of identify.

At school the children were told to make a family tree. We put the family trees in their memory box. My daughter did not know her father. So she wrote a letter entitled

'If I knew my father'. She wrote: 'I do not know if he was handsome, I do not have a photograph. If my father was here, I would be in a fancy Indian or white school. If he was here, I would have lots of nice dresses.' She kept saying: 'I love my mum. She is taking care of me. She raises me alone without the help of anyone'.

Seven of the ten participants, two of whom were men, had started creating a memory box. The other three were collecting items for a memory box. One of the participants had regular contact with his nieces and nephews and they had begun to make a memory box.

*Source*: P. Denis (2005) *Never Too Small to Remember. Memory Work and Resilience in Times of AIDS*. Pietormaritzburg: Cluster Publications.

# Chapter 17

## Body care and learning to do for others

*Jocelyn Lawler*

Nursing care requires access to every part of the body which is potentially touchable. However, in Western cultural traditions, certain parts of the body are more (socially) accessible and more readily touched than other parts. We are culturally 'non-touching' and this is especially so for the British. As nurses learn how to perform their work, therefore, they must overcome their own sociocultural backgrounds and adjust to a particular professional subculture and its established methods that permits handling other people's bodies. They must also confront the symbolism of certain parts of the body, in particular parts which have sexual significance, and they must find ways to manage social interaction during those times when they break taken-for-granted rules about the body.

The people whose experiences are discussed in this study [...] found some of their first experiences of working with other people's bodies to be socially awkward. Coming as they did from a non-touching cultural background, many of the nurses I talked with found that they were, among other things, acutely embarrassed in having to perform body care for others.

Those who had the least difficulty touching and handling the bodies of patients came from backgrounds with a relatively relaxed attitude to the body and exposure (but they were few in number) or had friends or family who were nurses. Most of the interviewees described a style of family life and upbringing where body functions were dealt with in a 'civilized' manner (see Elias, 1978). The sensitive bodily functions were carried out in private and they were not discussed. The body was almost always kept covered, consistent with the established cultural patterns of their families, and this socialization was acknowledged as a difficulty for a beginning nurse, as one nurse explained.

> *I:* I can remember the first man I had to wash. That was traumatic.... I was timid. I was embarrassed, I guess. The women weren't quite so bad, I mean that was a shock but a different sort of shock to the men.

From Jocelyn Lawler (1991) *Behind the Screens: Nursing, Somology and the Pattern of the Body*. Melbourne: Churchill, pp. 117–133 (abridged).

*R*:   Why are the men worse?

*I*:   I had never seen men naked and – even though I had brothers – three brothers. I mean you were just very modest, I guess, when you were at home.

*R*:   So you came from a family who kept things covered up?

*I*:   Oh yes.

*R*:   Did they talk about bodily functions?

*I*:   No, see they were very English in that respect. They were something that you didn't talk about. Nothing like that was.

*R*:   So when people went to the loo?

*I*:   It was behind a closed door and that was it.

*R*:   Did that make it very difficult for you as a nurse to then have to do for others what was [taboo], in your family life?

*I*:   Taboo. Yes, I guess so, yes.

[...] There are other factors, however, that influence these experiences, and they have their origins in the way the body is constructed in our culture. In particular the relationship of maleness and male power to genitalia and sexuality had a powerful effect on some of the female interviewees. The power invested in the male body is a theme which recurs throughout this study. [...]

## First experience of body care for others

While much has been written to educate nurses, [...] nurses are poorly prepared, educationally, for the breaking of social norms which many nursing acts necessarily involve. What they learn of these things they learn through experience.

> We are taught the proper way to carry out a bed bath, but not how to deal with the breaking of the social taboos when we wash a patient's body. Most nurses remember the fear they felt when doing their first bed bath. As a young female you work with a patient (who might well be male), behind drawn curtains and are expected to strip and wash his whole body. I remember feeling shamed and confused; my hands felt stiff, cold, awkward and useless. A bed bath can be embarrassing for the patient at the best of times – but far worse when the nurse herself [*sic*] is embarrassed. (Berry, 1986: 56)

Berry's experience is mirrored by that of the people interviewed for this study. They talked of feeling terror, embarrassment and timidity when they first had to confront other people's nakedness, and at having to undress people, particularly men.

Normal male–female relationships in society are disrupted in nursing, especially when a beginning female nurse encounters her first male patient. She has yet learned the interpersonal skills that will later make her work manageable. While male nurses experience some feelings of embarrassment when they encounter female patients for the first time, the data reported here suggest their discomfort is not as acute. It is possible, however, that my data reflect what men were willing to tell a woman about their sense of discomfort and also what women are prepared to discuss with another woman (see Warren, 1988).

For many, sponging a patient for the first time was highly significant, and they have retained vivid memories of that occasion. They acknowledge it as a major milestone – a time when the reality of nursing confronts them. After the first sponge, however, doing body care for others seems to become much easier. [...]

I asked each of the interviewees if they could remember the first time they had to 'do for someone else what that person would normally do for themselves'. Almost without exception they related stories of the first time they had to sponge a patient. [...]

## The naked male body

In many of the accounts I heard from female nurses there was an early sense of profound embarrassment, lack of social competence and sometimes fear associated with men and having to deal with male bodies, particularly when the genitalia are exposed. It is an aspect of nursing practice which is often surrounded by social awkwardness and uncertainty. The following accounts indicate the early discomfort and fear of having to deal with the naked male:

> Yes. I can [remember my first experience with body care]. We went to ... this *long* pavilion ward, a *men's*, ward. [I] begged not to go to a men's ward first. [...] Anyway, went there, and was terrified through the whole procedure. ... Just was terrified. ... I remember it really clearly. ... Women did not worry me. Men worried me a lot.

> I copped Male Ward. And I had to go to the corner [bed] – a boy about 18 he was. And he had a plaster on his leg, and so I gave him the dish and told him to wash himself, and he wasn't going to take his underpants off, and I wasn't about to take them off either! [*Laughter*] I can remember that as plain as day! [...] And I think that he was embarrassed and so was I. ... I had seen men before, but we'd been reared, you know, you don't look at men. And that to me was just a problem. I was too embarrassed. ... I still remember it as clear as day.

> I can remember the very first day on the ward ... *begging* that they let me do a female one [sponge] first because I couldn't bear the thought of pulling down a pair of man's trousers. At that stage I don't think it ever occurred to me that my father had genitals. I was that protected from the male anatomy.

The first sponge is often the very first clinical act which beginning nurses perform where the body is completely exposed, and where they touch socially proscribed parts of the body. As the accounts illustrate, the male genitalia are especially problematic and many were very reluctant to touch those areas, as one would expect in a society where the male sex organs are invested with such meaning and kept covered, and where body contact in the genital areas is almost exclusively reserved for sexual contexts. In the absence of learned skills to manage these situations, the beginning nurse feels socially awkward and embarrassed.

Some interviewees remember their first experiences as occasions where they first saw suffering, disfigurement and death. And like the naked body, one does not normally encounter these things extensively in one's daily life, nor are they necessarily discussed in detail, and even within hospitals there is a limit to what the public sees, or is allowed to see or know. [...]

> In the very early stages … they took us over to the hospital – it was one of those old Nightingale wards. … It was a male medical ward and there was a guy in a bed near the office and he was obviously on his last legs. Now I had had nothing to do with death except seeing my grandmother who was … very unwell but she wasn't unconscious, she was a bit delirious. This guy in the bed was, you know, vomiting blood, and the whole ward was like a zoo, and I walked in with one of my mates and I thought 'my God, what have I got myself in for?' … and we had this guy who was in a single room, you know, he was Cheyne-Stocking and he died [Cheyne-Stokes Breathing is a type of breathing seen in some serious nervous conditions]. When he died we looked at each other and said 'God what are we gonna do now? He's dead'. … We thought he was dead. We weren't real sure. We weren't real sure. We kept saying to each other 'Is he [dead]? Is he?' Well, we were sort of hysterical with laughter for a while because we thought 'yeah, well he is dead 'cause that dreadful noise had stopped', but then we got sort of sad because we hadn't witnessed anything like this before. …

Other nurses remembered their first experiences because, as beginners, they were disorganized, they lacked skill and they encountered scenes for which they were completely unprepared. As a consequence they felt inadequate. It is important for nursing students to feel a sense of competence in their actions (Davis, 1968) and without it they feel unable to adequately convey a sense of being in control – a sense that is needed in order to promote a particular context in which to perform highly intimate care for patients. The following two accounts, given by nurses who are now very experienced and skilled at their practice, illustrate their felt lack of competence – a lack which meant they had not yet developed the occupationally specific methods that they could later use to manage such situations. Speed is often used by nurses as a method by which difficult things are managed, particularly those things which are potentially embarrassing. The first account was given by a male registered nurse, now in his thirties and skilled at care for acutely ill and intensive care patients.

> I can remember we went to the ward, and … I can remember lining up with all the bits and pieces, the bowl and stuff and thinking to myself 'I haven't got a bloody clue what I'm doing here'. We'd done it on models and dummies and that in the school but never actually done it on a person and I looked at the man I was about to sponge. I can remember him, he was a big man, fat man, and he'd a cholecystectomy. He had an I.G. tube and he had a drain in and a drip and I thought 'where will I start with all this – how will I get the pyjamas off?' – that sort of stuff. I was slow. I know it took me 55 minutes … and even then I forgot to do things like clean his teeth and do all that sort of thing. I was so intent on getting him washed. It was awful. … I knew to wash him, and I knew what I had to do as far as washing and drying and all that sort of thing, but not having any idea of the organization – and being slow. And it was hard because he knew that we were new.

> I have often had that woman's situation in my mind since. You know, it's something I have not lost through the years, was going into a bathroom and seeing this elderly lady in a bath and seeing her arm and leg floating on top and she was weeping and couldn't express anything, and I later discovered she'd had a stroke and she was aphasic. She had been a doctor, and you know how stroke people cry, and she just cried and cried, and couldn't express herself and it was sort of a trauma to me that I have never really lost. I can remember her, ,and I think that's a terrible thing – for a woman like that to come to that state and – I mean she couldn't move

anything, her leg and arm were floating on top and the nurses were trying to bath her in a bath, and she was just crying and drooling and couldn't speak. ... It was 'Whatever do I do, whatever do I say?'

# Learning 'basic' nursing

When these nurses were taught how to do body care for others, it was in a particular manner – a manner that incorporated an emphasis on routine and procedure which involved no unnecessary exposure of the patient's body and which followed the recipe book approach characteristic of the texts. Additionally, the patient's embarrassment was to be considered, and nurses were also taught to maintain 'privacy' – a term which has a particular meaning where body care in nursing a concerned. Privacy has to do not only with avoiding unnecessary exposure, but it is also a notion about the vulnerability of patients. Instructions on clinical procedures emphasize privacy as a central consideration, along with the adherence to routine. [...]

## The emphasis on procedure

The accounts I heard in this study confirmed that nursing procedures, as they are described in texts, as step-wise and relatively stereotyped affairs, are indeed what nurses are taught as students. I asked those I interviewed how they had been taught to perform body care, especially sponging, which is the most central and comprehensive act of body care.

I: They [the teachers] were very strict, very 'thorough' – the word is.
R: But what did they teach you about how you might socially manage things like other people's nakedness, and embarrassment, and modesty?
I: I don't think they ever prepared you for that.
R: So they taught you how to do the procedure....
I: Physically do it, yeah. By the book! It was a procedure.

Yes, I can remember exactly what they [the nurse teachers] told us. Things they were more worried about were putting the sheets and the blankets in the right place and the towel in the right place and they never mentioned anything about how you should cope with the person, or the person coped with you. That was never, ever mentioned.

Others remembered being taught about a procedure which incorporated the notion of privacy, and how one might achieve this during the procedure. Privacy in this sense means not over-exposing the patient, and it also means ensuring a visual privacy such that others cannot see the patient's nakedness. In effect, it is dealing with the body in a privatised and 'civilized' way, but it is also somological – the nurse must 'do for' the body while simultaneously recognizing personhood. The procedure, though, was dominant in their early formal education.

We were always taught to screen the patient and we were always taught about privacy – privacy as in 'from the rest of the ward' – to screen the patient and make sure we were in this little closed-off area. We were taught nothing about embarrassment as far as the patient was concerned with the nurse. We were always taught to keep the patient warm which presumably meant you kept them covered, but then in the middle of summer you didn't need to be covered to be warm. We were always taught to keep them covered and taught to sponge by moving the sheet up and down various parts of the body – that sort of thing. ... Exposing one bit at a time, but then at the same time we had to expose other bits, but nothing was ever talked about as far as patients' embarrassment or nurses' embarrassment. We were taught about privacy but it was privacy as in screening the patient from everyone else in the ward. ... There was nothing about privacy between the nurse and the patient. It was always just there. ...

[...]

# Learning to control emotions

Much of what nurses' (women's) work entails, represents what Hochschild (1983) has termed 'emotional labour' – a commodification of feelings to suit the public (paid) arena. [...] Nurses are heavily involved in emotional labour because, as well as learning physically and procedurally how to wash another person in bed, there is an expectation that students will learn to control their emotions. Such emotional control is part of the nurse's 'professional' approach, that is learning how to do body care and perform other nursing functions in a manner typical of the occupation.

Many aspects of nursing have changed since it embraced the concept of individualized patient care. One such change is the recognition that some emotions are normal, if not desirable, and that it is probably not healthy for nurses (or anyone else for that matter) to suppress them. Historically, however, one characteristic of a 'good' nurse, was the ability to hide emotional reactions and to cultivate an air of detachment – a sort of professional distance from one's work. Many of the nurses I interviewed remember being expected to learn such emotional control and to learn it as they developed their nursing skills, and as they coped with a daily working life that was often difficult and disturbing.

One British nurse, who is now in her fifties, described what she had been taught as a student nurse.

I don't think we had very much at all on relating to people as individuals. ... You have to remember I'm British and the British stiff upper lip. ... I think it was just that it was not done. It was not done for the nurse to show emotion. ... it was to do with being professional and it upset the relatives. ... I think it had to do with being a professional person ... [and] we learnt it because I think if you showed any emotion you couldn't cope as a nurse you weren't made of the right stuff [*laughter*]. You weren't suitable if you showed emotion. ... We certainly didn't look sad, I mean, you were not allowed to look sad or grieve, but neither were you allowed to giggle around the place. You had to comport yourself – with dignity. ... No frivolity, not at all.

With experience and more generalized social change, many nurses re-evaluate those early influences, particularly as they affect the ways in which they help patients come to terms with illness experience and the lived body. The ability to control emotion is often used by experienced and expert nurses as one method to help patients through illness experience. [...]

Other nurses, who are much younger than the British nurse whose experience is related above and who trained in Australia, relate similar experiences to those of their British colleague. The occupational ethos of emotional control remains relatively pervasive.

> You were never allowed to [show emotion] – and you were never allowed to cry. You were only allowed to cry if the Charge Sister let you cry [*laughter*]. You weren't allowed to cry if someone died or was really sick, you just felt that you had to give a little bit more to the patient – and you weren't allowed to laugh either if you could see the funny side of things. ... You had to appear what they termed 'professional', which was very cold and caught up.

> We weren't taught about ... emotions ... and you weren't taught ... that it's normal to feel disgust or things like that, which it is, isn't it. You know, you have a job to do and you do it, but no, not enough emotion or feeling was put into it.

> [I was] always told not to get involved and become attached to the patient or – it's hard not to get involved, I mean you do get involved. ... I think it gets passed down, you know when you're looking after a really sick patient [other nurses say to you] 'you shouldn't get involved, you know' and so it goes on.

[...]

Emotional control, as an ideal aspect of professional practice, is now being seriously evaluated in the research literature. Benner and Wrubel (1988), for example, claim that it is impossible for nurses to care about what happens to patients and to help them during illness experience unless some degree of involvement occurs. Many of the nurses in my study would agree because they have recognized that emotional detachment does not work and that in some cases they have had to unlearn what had previously been taught to them. [...]

> I think probably we were taught that [emotional control] to start, but I think I've learnt over the years that that isn't always appropriate to the occasion, that there are times when I think ... that as a person I have the right to let that other person know that they are embarrassing me ... or that I feel uncomfortable in a situation. ... I think that's improved. I think once upon a time you weren't expected to be emotional about anything. We weren't expected to feel emotion if a patient we cared about or cared for died. ... Now I think it's quite acceptable for the staff to be just as emotional about the situation as the family is. I think that's good. I think it's important that we let the people we're caring about know – that we really do care ... you can't do that if you remain detached. Looking back I think that in our early training – that we were sort of expected to be a bit remote, you know [we were told] 'don't be silly, Nurse. Pull yourself together'.

[...]

## Lack of affect as a clinical strategy

Nurses were expected to be controlled – to show no emotion. Many of them interpreted this to mean that they were to be emotionless, but lack of affect is in itself a response – a way of dealing with what would otherwise be a social mistake, a deviant act, an affront, an insult, a source of embarrassment. To show no affective change, for example, at another person's naked body is a way of conferring a very different meaning on nakedness from the usual effect of running naked across the field at a sports event. [...]

Lack of affect is a means by which nurses construct context, so in that sense it serves to assist in the management of otherwise potentially embarrassing situations. The problem for nurses, however, is that lack of affect can become *the* standardized and expected emotional response, in which case it excludes the possibility of sharing difficult moments for patients in a way which allows the nurse to 'make contact' with the patient existentially (see Benner and Wrubel, 1988: Chapter 1).

In many ways nurses operate in a social vacuum because they are often naïve or ill-informed (at best) about the work they are expected to do and how they can behave, and little, if anything, in their lives prepares them for what they are required to do for others as basic nursing (body) care. Much of what nurses do is not public to protect patients' 'privacy', and it takes time and experience to feel comfortable in the role of nurse, doing things for other people. Talking with patients about some things is also difficult because there is a problem with language. Not only is it not always socially appropriate, or acceptable, to discuss what nurses do, there is a real difficulty in choosing appropriate words or simply having conversation about various things to do with the body. This [...] is richly indicative of 'the problem of the body' and privatized body functions and it highlights the silence of the body in discourse generally.

# The problem of language

I asked the interviewees what they found most difficult to do when they first began nursing, and while many found the physical and procedural aspects of caring for other people's bodies awkward, there was a very real problem with language and conversation. Nurses were taught always to explain what they were going to do to patients, because patients are often unaware of what could happen during a certain procedure. [...]

Explanation, however, is not straightforward because some people are not relaxed about discussing some body functions or body parts; and the choice of words is far from straightforward. The two accounts below illustrate some of the general aspects of this problem. I had asked the interviewees if they found it difficult to know what to say to people when they were doing nursing care.

> Embarrassing. Didn't know what to look at, what to say, because at those times I was quite shy and I can remember it was an old lady ... with a fracture and ... we had to ... sponge and we had to do the whole works not knowing what to say or what to touch when you got to those bits ... because it's something you don't ask. ... We didn't know if that person would be offended by what we said. If you said 'your boobs' would she be offended by that. Being older she would probably be a bit strict.

> We were never taught how to deal with that [the language difficulty]. I mean, to ask a patient if they wanted to wash, for example, 'would you like to wash between your legs?' or if you were being jovial you'd hear people say 'I'll wash down as far as possible and you wash "possible"'. And all this sort of thing – how do you ask someone if they'd like to wash between their legs. ... The language is *always* a problem.

One of the major problems of language in nursing care is that there are no widely accepted standards for the names of body parts and functions. If, for instance, nurses call various body parts by their anatomical names, there is a fair chance the patient will not understand, and if they use language that is in common usage, the choice is by no means simple; furthermore, there are some things which people do not readily discuss. [...]

> I think ... [some] patients, when we ask them if they've had their bowels open, they tend to say 'yes' routinely because they don't know what we're talking about. That happens on a regular basis because they're not real sure what we're talking about.... People tend to call having your bowels open a lot of stupid things.... I think it's classed as dirty. Whereas it shouldn't be. It's only your own body, but I think they're taught from a young age [that it's dirty].

With the civilizing process (Elias,1978), body functions concerned with excretion have become highly privatized, at least by some social groups, particularly those of higher social status. [...]

> Oh yes. I think it's definitely class related. Joe Bloggs off the river bank is easy to talk to. They shit, they fart, they piss. You can communicate. It's the people with a middle-class presentation who don't have the vocabulary to match.

In summary, learning to be a nurse involves facing the reality of the place of the body in our society. [...] Becoming socialized as a nurse, however, means taking on a new way of looking at the body and learning to 'do for'. It requires unlearning ways of viewing the body. Such unlearning is necessitated by 'the problem of the body' and by the extent to which nursing and illness are disruptive of social order and normal rules do not always apply. [...] There is also no professional jargon that can be used to describe body functions which would make it possible to sanitize things people regard as dirty. [...] In the absence of discourse and socially acceptable language, some nursing functions are located outside socially condoned and accepted practices – they are dealt with by their absence and the silence which surrounds them.

# References

Benner, P. and Wrubel, J. (1988) *The Primacy of Caring*. Menlo Park, CA: Addison Wesley.

Berry, A (1986) 'Knowledge at one's fingertips', *Nursing Times*, 3 December: 56–57.

Davis, F. (1968) 'Professional socialization as subjective experience: the process of doctrinal conversion among student nurses', in H. S. Becker, B. Geer, D. Riesman and R. S. Weiss (eds), *Institutions and the Person*. Chicago: Aldine.

Elias, N. (1978) *The Civilizing Process: the History of Manners*. Translated by E. Jephcott. New York: Urizen Books.

Hochschild, A. R. (1983) *The Managed Heart: Commercialization of Human Feeling*. Berkeley, CA: University of California Press.

Warren, C. A. B. (1988) *Gender Issues in Field Research, Qualitative Research Methods*, Vol. 9. Newbury Park, CA: Sage.

# Chapter 18

## Patient safety and quality of care: the role of the health care assistant

*Hugh P. McKenna, Felicity Hasson and Sinead Keeney*

The concept of the unqualified support worker in health care is not new. Indeed, from the beginning of formal health care, there have always been unqualified or untrained assistants working within the hospital and community settings (Abel-Smith, 1960). Over the years they have had a plethora of designations. For example, … 'generic support worker', 'health care assistant (HCA)', 'clinical support worker', 'ward assistant', 'care worker', 'home care assistant' and even 'bed maker' (Thornley, 2000) which reflect their varied roles. … Although this has not been enforced in any legal sense, HCA is now the most commonly accepted title.

There is currently no reliable or accurate official data on the number of HCAs employed in the National Health Service (NHS). One estimate (Andalo, 2003) is that there are about half a million in the UK. Although this role has been established for some time, there is no clear understanding of who makes up this workforce, what they actually do and what competencies they possess (Thornley, 2000). This means that the role often varies depending upon the country and the clinical area in which the person is employed.

[…]

In 2004, the Royal College of Nursing (RCN) document 'The Future Nurse' (RCN, 2004) incorporated the HCA within the 'nursing family' echoing the Royal College of Midwives (1999) who welcomed HCAs as members of the maternity team. The following year, the RCN (2000) balloted its members and found that 78.1% voted in favour of accepting HCAs into the College. While such recognition is laudable, it is still the case that HCAs are not regulated (Anonymous, 2004). This raises serious concerns, especially with regard to patient safety and quality of care.

Originally published in the *Journal of Nursing Management* (2004) 12: 452–459 (abridged).

# Growth of HCAs

[...]

In the late 1980s, before the introduction of Project 2000, students often undertook 'basic care' duties (Chapman, 2000). Post this reform, student nurses no longer made up an informal part of the workforce and the void was filled by qualified nurses who often found themselves carrying out 'non-nursing' domestic, portering and clerical duties. [...] Therefore, one of the main arguments for the increase in the number of HCAs was that they were necessary to undertake the lower level duties so that registered nurses would have time to meet higher level patient needs.

Initially, it was believed that this would lead to nurses spending enhanced time with patients with concomitant improvements in care quality and safety (Wakefield, 2000). However, nurses found that they had to spend growing amounts of time inducting, training and supervising the increasing number of HCAs (McKenna, 1995). It was ironic that the role that had been introduced to free up nursing time was actually eating up nursing time.

# HCA role evolution

[In 1988], the United Kingdom Central Council for Nursing, Midwifery and Health Visiting issued a position paper on HCA (UKCC, 1988). This paper stated that the role of the HCA should be developed in the areas of housekeeping, clerical tasks and other work related to the maintenance of the environment in which direct care is given. Therefore, there was official recognition that the HCA was to support the qualified nurse by under-taking ancillary work, such as domestic duties, answering telephones, maintenance of supplies, maintenance of hygienic environment, transport of patients, specimens, equipment, processing of documents, admission, transfers and discharges (O'Malley and Llorente, 1990). However, this role description is no longer viewed as being credible. With the short-age of qualified nurses and the increase in paperwork that audit and care planning bring, HCAs are undertaking more direct patient care activities. One UK study reported that HCAs believed that housekeeping duties should be assigned to another worker and complained that they had to leave patients' bedsides to do such routine housekeeping work (Philips, 1997).

[...]

Findings from Carr-Hill and Jenkins-Clarke (2003), who reviewed staff activities over a 7-day period in 19 hospitals in England and Scotland, reinforced the widely held view that a sizeable proportion of what many people would regard as nursing care is being under-taken by HCAs. They found that HCAs and nurses were interchangeable in many hospitals. The consequence of this has been that the role of the nurse in delivering bedside nursing care has gradually lessened, with many of the core skills of nursing being handed over to HCAs (Anonymous, 2004; Illey, 2004). [...]

Studies in the UK have shown how the role of the HCA is exceeding its original scope, not always to the benefit of the patient (Snell, 1998). One of the largest surveys in this field, sponsored by the union UNISON in 1997, revealed that HCAs undertake a vast number of nursing duties, including catheter care, dressing and wound care (Thornley, 1997). The survey identified that one in five HCAs carried out invasive procedures and one in 10 undertook venepuncture. The findings also noted that HCAs received little supervision while carrying out these tasks.

More recently, Duffin (2001) reported that more than half of all HCAs are dressing wounds and helping to formulate patient care plans. The survey also found that one in three HCAs set up or monitored diagnostic machines and helped train students or newly qualified nurses. It also revealed that some set up infusion feeds, give injections, liase with doctors, supervise staff, take charge of shifts and undertake sole care of patients who are at home. In midwifery, assistants undertake the monitoring of women using cardiotocograph machines or provide advice on parenting skills and breast feeding (Charlton, 2001). In UK operating theatres, consideration is being given to HCAs undertaking scrub duties presently performed by qualified nurses (Smith, 2003). According to Snell's (1998) study many were left in-charge of a shift and 53% reported that little or none of their work was supervised. To compound this, because of their increasing numbers and visibility at the patients' bedside, HCA are involved more in student learning. This idea is reinforced by Wakefield's (2000) work who reported that HCA are increasingly being used as advisors who feel free to pass judgement about the competence of students and their ability to implement nursing interventions.

The evolution of the HCA role can be attributed to a number of reasons, for example, as the role of the qualified nurse has changed, so has that of unqualified staff (Withers, 2001). Such a change is reflected in the Wanless (2002) report that illustrates how workload might be shifted from doctors to nurse practitioners, and from nurse practitioners to HCAs. Indeed since that the demand for nurses will increase by around a further 10% the report indicates that the gap could be filled if 12.5% of nurse workload could shift to HCAs. However, the increasing reliance on HCAs raises serious quality and safety questions.

Modern health care is complex and patients in hospital are often in the acute stage of their illness. Patient throughput has increased and new treatments and technologies have bought with them their own hazards. This is also true within the community where nurses are undertaking home-based interventions which were recently only practised in the safety of a hi-tech clinical setting. For the reasons identified above HCAs are spending more time in non-supervised direct patient care. As a result, many nurses have voiced concerns over patient quality and safety (Workman, 1996; Daykin and Clarke, 2000; Hind et al., 2000).

# HCA training

It is apparent that training and appropriate delegation is instrumental to quality and safety of care (McKenna, 1995; Micheli and Smith, 1997; Warr et al., 1998; Hogan and Playle, 2000; Thornley, 2000; Hind, 2001). Nonetheless, despite the fact that HCAs are at the front line in providing care, there is no statutory duty for them to have any training. Invariably, HCA training is considered to be the responsibility of the health care Trust or private hospital leading to informal or makeshift training programmes (see Chang and Lam, 1997; Ashwill, 1998; Davies, 1999; Steele and Wright, 2001; Field and Smith, 2003; Joy and Wade, 2003; McKenna et al., 2003a). This has led not only to wide variations in standards of training but also care (Kenward et al., 2001).

In the UK, National Vocational Qualifications (NVQs) were introduced in an attempt to standardize HCA training. The NVQs focus on the attainment of competencies gained in the workplace and the underlying theory (Francis, 1998). The NVQs are flexible; available at levels 1–5, there are no entry requirements and no examinations and they can be undertaken over a period of several years with virtually no time limit. The acquisition of an NVQ is not a permit to practice but identifies the holder as competent to undertake a range of duties in a care environment (BACCN, 2003).

[...]

HCAs who have qualified to NVQ level 3 are able to join the RCN as an associate member (RCN, 2000). Furthermore, NVQ prepared HCAs can often enter nursing diploma programmes (Coombes et al., 2003). [...]

Apart from NVQs there are no national mandatory educational programmes for HCAs in the UK. Their absence threatens public safety and therefore a nationally recognized standard for HCAs, linked to educational programmes, is long overdue (Barczak and Spunt, 1999; DoH, 1999; DoH, 2000a and b; Ramprogus and O'Brien, 2002; Field and Smith, 2003). Such training programmes have been implemented elsewhere, for example, the Irish Government, recently piloted a national training programme for HCAs. Its evaluation has shown it to be effective in producing skills and knowledge relevant to the workplace, enabling HCAs to practice safely and to a high standard (McKenna et al., 2003b).

# Nursing accountability for the HCA

The Nursing and Midwifery Council (NMC) Code of Professional Conduct (2002) is explicit on the issue of delegation and accountability:

> You may be expected to delegate care delivery to others who are not registered nurses or midwives. Such delegation must not compromise existing care but must be directed to meeting the needs and serving the interests of patients and clients. You remain accountable for the appropriateness of the delegation, for ensuring that the person who does the work is able to do it and that adequate supervision or support is provided. (NMC, 2002, para. 4.6)

This means that nurses should not delegate duties to HCAs if they are concerned that the care undertaken will not be safe or up to the quality standard expected by a nurse who would normally undertake the task (Dimond, 1995). Delegating to HCAs seems, at first glance, to be uncontroversial. However, it is impossible to ensure delegation is appropriate if roles are not clearly defined and training is ad hoc. Furthermore, for qualified staff to delegate appropriately and safely they need to have a firm understanding of their role and the role of the HCA. Reports indicate this is not the case (Hartig, 1998). [...] Scoullar (1991) warned that this can result in HCAs being left with unrelated tasks such as administration, cleaning and collecting X-rays, in between they are expected to assist with nursing care. This could lead to a task-oriented patient care approach. Furthermore, the HCA role not only varies from setting to setting but also within settings according to the pressures at any given time. As Nazarko (1999) suggested, if nurses are under pressure they may allow HCAs to carry out unsupervised tasks they would not otherwise consider, which could result in patients being put at risk. ... Therefore, delegating care processes to

HCAs is fraught with moral and legal difficulties ... and hard-pressed clinical nurses may sometimes forget that they have accountability for the safe and effective care of patients (Fell, 2000; Hind, 2001).

# Regulation and patient safety

The need to regulate HCAs was first raised in the NHS Plan (DoH, 2000c). While research findings recommended that HCAs should be regulated, Ministers could not win agreement from all four countries in the UK about how this should happen (Andalo, 2003). Therefore, HCAs are not currently subject to professional regulation and as a result are not professionally accountable.

The RCN and the UKCC fear that patient safety is being compromised by lack of HCA regulation (Caulfield, 2000). Currently, there is no system in place whereby a HCA's criminal record or level of competence can be checked. There have been some well-publicized cases where patients have been subjected to abuse at the hands of HCAs in nursing and residential homes (Caulfield, 2000; Faugier, 2004). In some instances, HCAs were dismissed from their work, yet commenced employment in another similar setting shortly afterwards. Unlike nurses, there are no regulatory mechanisms in place to alert the new employer to past offences. There have been reports that some nurses were removed from the nursing register and began working as HCAs, particularly in the private nursing home sector (Thomas, 1996). Not surprisingly, the regulation of HCAs has been an increasing matter of concern for patients, professionals and employers. Unregulated HCAs are undertaking increasingly complex and intimate activities – often in people's own homes and with the most vulnerable sections of our community.

In March 2004, the DoH (2004) issued a consultation document entitled 'Regulation of health care staff in England and Wales'. The document sets out the DoH proposals for extending regulation to those staff that have a direct impact on patients and have the potential to compromise public safety if their work or behaviour falls short of acceptable standards. However, the DoH has proposed that a new regulator be created with little mention of a role for the NMC. As HCAs undertake more nursing type roles, it is widely felt that regulation would be best handled by the NMC (O'Dowd, 2003; Anonymous, 2004). Meanwhile within this climate of regulation uncertainty, many nurses depend vicariously on HCAs to deliver unsupervised direct patient care without being totally certain of the safety or quality of such care.

# Conclusion

... This paper has attempted to outline some of the quality and safety concerns in relation to the HCA role. In a climate of a global shortage of registered nurses and a 'role creep' to accept medical duties, there is an increasing reliance on HCAs to fill the gaps in care. Because they are answerable to managers and not to nurses, HCAs are often pressured to go beyond their level of competencies to perform duties for which they are not qualified – potentially endangering patients. This includes administering medication, undertaking venepuncture, recording ECGs, siting intravenous cannulae, removing venflons, leading counselling sessions, making decisions about wound dressings and when patients will be seen in A & E departments.

The debate about the role of support staff undoubtedly disguises the debate about the future of nursing itself, as the distinction between a nurse and a HCA is becoming blurred. The challenge for nurses may be to define and control their working practices before they completely lose their claim to the core skills associated with nursing. The HCAs themselves are powerless, waiting on policy-makers to sort out the mess while they do their best to be part of the nursing family. In the meantime, the lack of a recognized training programme, regulation and their undefined role put patient quality and safety at risk.

# References

Abel-Smith, B. (1960) *A History of the Nursing Profession*. London: Heinemann.

Andalo, D. (2003) 'Slipping through the net', *Nursing Standard*, 17(31): 18–19.

Anonymous (2004) 'Nursing should seize the initiative to have its say on HCA regulation', *Nursing Times,* 100(9): 13.

Ashwill, J. (1998) 'The patient care assistant program: the nursing profession's response to educating unlicensed assistive personnel', *Journal of Continuing Education in Nursing*, 29(3): 126–129.

Barczak, N. and Spunt, D. (1999) 'Competency-based education: maximise the performance of unlicensed assistive personnel', *Journal of Continuing Education in Nursing*, 30(6): 254–259.

British Association of Critical Care Nurses (BACCN) (2003) 'Position statement on the role of health care assistants who are involved in direct patient care activities within critical care areas', *Nursing in Critical Care*, 8(1): 3–12.

Carr-Hill, R. and Jenkins-Clarke, S. (2003) *Improving the Effectiveness of the Nursing Workforce. Short Report of Analysis of NISCM Data Set*. York: The University of York, Centre for Health Economics.

Caulfield, H. (2000) 'Support act', *Nursing Standard*, 15(3): 18.

Chang, A. and Lam, L. (1997) 'Evaluation of health care assistant pilot programme', *Journal of Nursing Management*, 5: 229–236.

Chapman, P. (2000) 'Unknown factor', *Nursing Times*, 96(6): 28–29.

Charlton, D. (2001) 'Support workers in maternity care', *MIDRIS Midwifery Digest*, 11(3): 405–406.

Coombes, C., Arnold, J., Loan-Clarke, J., Wilkinson, A., Park, J. and Preston, D. (2003) 'Perceptions of nursing in the NHS', *Nursing Standard*, 18(5): 33–38.

Davies, J. (1999) 'Cinderella no more', *Health Service Journal*, 109(5681): 4–5.

Daykin, N. and Clarke, B. (2000) 'They still get the bodily care: discourses of care and relationships between nurses and healthcare assistants in the NHS', *Sociology of Health and Illness*, 22(3): 349–363.

Department of Health (DoH) (1999) *Making a Difference: Strengthening the Nursing, Midwifery and Health Visiting Contribution to Health and Health Care*. London: HMSO.

Department of Health (DoH) (2000a) *A Health Service of all Talents: Developing the NHS Workforce*. London: DoH.

Department of Health (DoH) (2000b) *Recruiting and Retaining Nurses, Midwives and Health Visitors in the NHS. A Progress Report*. London: DoH.

Department of Health (DoH) (2000c) *Meeting the Challenge*. London: The Stationary Office.

Department of Health (DoH) (2004) *Improvement, Expansion and Reform: The Next 3 Years. Priorities and Planning Framework 2003–2006*. Available at: www.dh.gov.uk/assetRoot/ 04/07/02/02/0407 0202.pdf (accessed 21 September 2004).

Dimond, B. (1995) *Legal Aspects of Nursing*, 2nd edn. New York: Prentice Hall.

Duffin, C. (2001) 'HCA take on more nursing tasks', *Nursing Standard*, 16(5): 9.

Faugier, J. (2004) 'Blurring boundaries is not progress', *Nursing Times*, 100(1): 16.

Fell, C. (2000) 'Letter', *British Journal of Perioperative Nursing*, 10(4): 180.

Field, L. and Smith, B. (2003) 'An essential care course for health-care assistants', *Nursing Standard*, 17(44): 33–35.

Francis, B. (1998) 'Regulating non-nursing healthcare workers', *Nursing Standard*, 12: 35–37.

Hartig, M. J. (1998) 'Expert nursing assistant care activities', *Western Journal of Nursing Research*, 20(5): 584–601.

Hind, M. (2001) 'Health care support workers and the scrubbed role', *British Journal of Perioperative Nursing*, 11(6): 262–268.

Hind, M., Jackson, D., Andrews, C., Fullbrook, P., Glavin, K. and Frost, S. (2000) 'Healthcare support workers in the critical care setting', *Nursing in Critical Care*, 5(1): 31–39.

Hogan, J. and Playle, J. (2000) 'The utilisation of the healthcare assistant in intensive care', *British Journal of Nursing*, 9(12): 794–801.

Illey, K. (2004) 'Nursing and healthcare management and policy. Occupational changes in nursing: the situation of enrolled nurses', *Journal of Advanced Nursing*, 45(4): 360.

Joy, P. and Wade, S. (2003) 'Opening the door to healthcare assistants and support workers', *Nursing Older People*, 15(6): 1820.

Kenward, G., Hodgetts, T. and Castle, N. (2001) 'Time to put the R back in TPR', *Nursing Times*, 97(40): 32–33.

McKenna, H. (1995) 'Nursing skill mix substitutions and quality of care: an exploration of assumptions from the research literature', *Journal of Advanced Nursing*, 21: 452–459.

McKenna, H. P., Hasson, F. and Smith, M. A. (2003a) 'Training needs of midwifery assistants', *Journal of Advanced Nursing*, 44(3): 308–317.

McKenna, H. P., Keeney, S. and Hasson, F. (2003b) *Evaluation of the Irish Pilot Programme for the Education of Health Care Assistants*. Dublin: Department of Health and Children.

Micheli, J. A. and Smith, C. E. (1997) 'Unlicensed assistive personnel in the perioperative setting', *Nursing Clinics of North America*, 32(1): 201–213.

Nazarko, L. (1999) 'Delegation dilemmas', *Nursing Standard*, 14(13–15): 59.

Nursing and Midwifery Council (NMC) (2002) *Code of Professional Conduct*. London: NMC.

O'Dowd, A. (2003) 'Next regulation wrangle on the way', *Nursing Times*, 99(3): 10–11.

O'Malley, J. and Llorente, B. (1990) 'Back to the future: redesigning the workplace', *Nursing Management*, 21(10): 46–48.

Philips, L. (1997) 'Support services. Domestic bliss', *Health Service Journal*, 107(55–75): 32.

Ramprogus, V. and O'Brien, D. (2002) 'The case for the formal education of HCAs', *Nursing Times*, 98(27): 37–38.

Royal College of Midwives (RCM) (1999) *Support Workers in the Maternity Services Position Paper 5a*. London: RCM.

Royal College of Nursing (RCN) (2000) *Royal College of Nursing to Admit Non-registered Nurses following Landmark Vote*. Press Release, 18 October. London: RCN.

Royal College of Nursing (RCN) (2004) *The Future Nurse: The RCN Vision*. London: RCN.

Scoullar, K. (1991) 'Health care assistants: a constant source of support', *Nursing Times*, 87(25): 29–31.

Smith, H. (2003) 'Assistants to scrub or not to scrub', *British Journal of Perioperative Nursing*, 13(10): 420–426.

Snell, J. (1998) 'A force to reckon with', *Health Service Journal*, April: 24–27.

Steele, V. and Wright, R. (2001) 'Cutting it fine', *Health Service Journal*, April(12): 28.

Thomas, L. (1996) 'Editorial', *Nursing Standard*, 10(48): 21.

Thornley, C. (1997) *Invisible Workers: An Investigation into the Pay and Employment of Health Care Assistants*. UNISON.

Thornley, C. (2000) 'A question of competence? Re-evaluating the roles of the nursing auxiliary and health care assistant in the NHS', *Journal of Clinical Nursing*, 9(3): 451–458.

UKCC (1988) *Position Paper on the Development of the Support Worker Role*. London: United Kingdom Central Council for Nursing, Midwifery and Health Visiting.

Wakefield, A. (2000) 'Tensions experienced by student nurses in a changed NHS culture', *Nurse Education Today*, 20: 571–578.

Wanless, D. (2002) *Securing our Future Health: Taking a Long-term View*. London: The Public Enquiry Unit.

Warr, J., Gobbi, M. and Johnson, S. (1998) 'Expanding the nursing profession', *Nursing Standard*, 12(31): 44–47.

Withers, R. (2001) 'No wannabes', *Nursing Standard*, 16(8): 25.

Workman, B. (1996) 'An investigation into how the healthcare support workers perceive their role as 'support workers' to qualified staff', *Journal of Advanced Nursing*, 23: 612–619.

# Chapter 19

## Working on the front line: risk culture and nursing

*Ellen Annandale*

This chapter begins with a discussion of nurses' and midwives' perceptions of the risk climate in which they work and its associations with culture of consumerism and the new NHS. This is followed by an analysis of the effects that this climate has upon relations with colleagues and with patients. [...]

## The data

The data come from a study of legal accountability in nursing and midwifery that was conducted in 1994. They are drawn from two sources: a questionnaire survey of all trained nurses and midwives who were employed in one hospital trust in late 1994, and in-depth interviews with nurses working on the neurology services of a different hospital trust. [...]

The data extracts are presented verbatim except where the notation (...) is used. Where the staff designation is in parentheses (i.e. staff nurse) this indicates that the data come from the survey sample. Where interview data are used, the designation precedes the dialogue (i.e. staff nurse: ...).

## A climate of risk

> You can't really put your finger on it, what it is. And it's like at the moment you feel you've got to watch your back all the time. That's the sort of atmosphere it is. That you can't ... if you're talking to somebody you've got to be careful. That's the feeling: the openness has gone. (sister)

Originally published in *Sociological Review* (1996), 94(3): 416–451 (abridged).

> I think nursing *is* stressful, but as far as accountability is concerned ... you see it's something you think about *all* the time. It's not here in front of your head, it's in the *background* and I think until something comes up, a mistake has been made, then you're made aware of it; that's when you start thinking about it. (staff nurse)

As these comments reveal, risk surrounds practice, it is in the *background*, there is an *atmosphere*: it is always there. As one staff nurse explained, it is 'always on your mind that you may be held responsible in a legal dispute for actions or words'. Or, as one sister more graphically put it, 'litigation is the "bogey man" that stands behind my shoulder as I practise as a midwife'. This atmosphere engenders a feeling of vulnerability, a fear that you may do the 'wrong thing' or, more worryingly, that whatever you do may not be 'right'.

> You hear of others 'being held accountable' and begin to fear that whatever you say or do may not be right. And you begin to feel more alone. (staff nurse)

Feeling vulnerable or under suspicion means working under 'a constant awareness that you may be subject to criticism, quite often in an unrealistic way' (sister).

The recognition that 'since we are all human, we can all make mistakes' only adds to this vulnerability, particularly when, as one nurse put it, 'I am constantly being made aware that every little thing that is done could in the future be used against me' (staff nurse).

Feelings of vulnerability, the sense that the future haunts actions in the present, can create a fair degree of stress. Indeed, only 23 per cent of the survey sample reported that concerns with legal accountability did not cause them 'any stress at all', while 60 per cent said it caused them a 'little' and 17 per cent a 'great deal' of stress. General fears of either making a mistake, experiencing a complaint or being sued, and a general fear of the nurses or midwives' actions being used against them, were identified as the source of this stress by just over 40 per cent (others referred to more specific aspects of practice which will be discussed, below).

It could be argued that these concerns are intrinsic and long-standing to medical and nursing work. Signs and symptoms do not order themselves into neat diagnostic categories, nor do they unequivocally signal the 'correct' treatment regimen. Rather, the process of acquiring, interpreting, managing and reporting 'the disorders of human illness' is an error-ridden process (Paget, 1988: 34). Yet the nurses in the survey and interview samples felt almost without exception that the concerns that they identified were of *recent* origin. Over 55 per cent of the survey sample felt that legal accountability had become a concern over the last three years, and 37 per cent over the last five years. The sample was asked to indicate (yes/no) whether *each* of the factors listed in Table 19.1 was a reason for increased concern about legal accountability.

Clearly, the awareness of patients and their relatives, the concern of professional bodies (like the Royal College of Nursing, Unison and the UKCC), and to a lesser extent, the professionalization of nursing, and increased concern expressed by hospital trusts, all heighten concern. However, a much clearer hierarchy emerges from the sample when they are asked to indicate the *main* reason for increased concern. Here the increased awareness of patients/relatives was the predominant factor by far, mentioned by 65 per cent. The concern of professional bodies (12 per cent), the professionalization of nursing (11 per cent) and the concern of trusts/management (6 per cent) were seen as far less significant. [...]

Table 19.1   Reasons for increased concern about legal accountability (those answering 'yes')

|  | Number | % |
|---|---|---|
| Patients/relatives more aware of their rights | 298 | 98 |
| Increased concern from professional bodies | 235 | 76 |
| Professionalization of nursing | 156 | 50 |
| Hospital trusts/management more concerned | 185 | 60 |
| Other | 38 | 12 |

The fact that some respondents referred to *both* patient awareness *and* the changing organization of hospitals (particularly managerial changes) suggests that they may have a combined, perhaps even mutually reinforcing effect, upon the climate in which nurses and midwives work:

> As the public becomes increasingly more aware, particularly with the Patient's Charter in force, and with the advent of trusts, it seems that nurses are more responsible for themselves and have less support from employers. (staff nurse)

## Consumers as risk generators

The phrase 'patients are more aware of their rights' was a constant refrain in both the nurse interviews and survey data. This *awareness* seemed to be an omnipresent cloud hanging over daily practice. Although consumerism need not be viewed negatively, it was often taken to be a new and rather malevolent presence which was resented by staff:

> *Staff nurse*: The introduction of the Patient's Charter gets Joe Public to go to bat. It's quoted considerably in the hospital, people quote it to you. So there's an emphasis on 'my granny needs to see a surgeon', you get quite a bit of that. You got it even *before* the Patient's Charter came out, when it was a White Paper.
>
> *Int.*: You mentioned talk about the White Paper around the hospital?
>
> *Staff nurse*: By patients and relatives. And in the community. People are more aware of what they're entitled to and expect standards to be higher than they used to be. Whether it's through the media, I don't know. But I've found that; they're very articulate.
>
> *Int.*: What about?
>
> *Staff nurse*: Nursing care, waiting lists: 'My mother's not been seen.'

The notion of 'patient awareness', which is really a summary term for an assemblage of concerns, is perceived as something that is imported into the hospital from without. Thus, as illustrated in the preceding dialogue, it is seen as motivated by the Patient's Charter. Broader social changes are also seen as culpable.

> People are becoming more aware of their rights, and appear to be more concerned with mistakes and unreliability in all aspects of life unfortunately. (staff nurse)

They know more, want and expect more information:

> Before, I think people used to sit back and say Oh, they're in hospital and, you know, 'let the doctors and nurses get on with it, they know what they're doing.' But with erm, there's so much hype, so much information from the media, they tend to question things because they're more aware of the things that *could* go wrong. (staff nurse)

The consumerist attitudes that are expressed in a desire for information can become particularly hard to take when they also involve a desire to blame someone for a 'bad outcome'. This is something that was particularly to the forefront of midwives' concerns:

> People generally have high, unrealistic expectations and think pregnancy, birth and newborns should be planned and perfect in line with their ideals. When it doesn't, they sue the pants off professionals. (sister)

The sense that patients and relatives are 'looking over the nurse's shoulder' undoubtedly generates personal vigilance over the nurse or midwife's actions and the actions of others:

> I think with the press, people are more aware of their rights and things like that ... Whereas before people, if they weren't happy with something, say they had a complaint to make, they perhaps wouldn't make it. Whereas now, I think they're more eager to because they're more aware of their rights from that point of view and you need to be *aware* of what you're doing more and more. I suppose you've always *been* accountable, *even more* so now because you need to document things more and be more aware of ... it's always in the back of your head, you know, that you've got to be careful what you do because patients, you know patients are more likely to complain. (staff nurse)

But since patients' awareness is an awareness of nurses' and midwives' practice, it can also be experienced as a form of threat and a lack of trust:

> Although at the time you feel you have done the right thing, often people, mainly relatives, interfere and question if you have given the right treatment in an attempt to intimidate you by suggesting they will take further action. (staff midwife)

[...]

Patient-consumers are expected, incited even, to secure their rights under a contractual model of social relations in the NHS, something which is made quite clear in the Citizen's and Patient's Charters (Walsh, 1994). If they feel that their rights and expectations are not being met patients are encouraged to complain to the relevant authority, which is reflected in the notable rise in NHS complaints over recent years. The 1994 Health Service Commissioner's report revealed a record 1,384 complaints for 1993–4, a 13 per cent increase over the previous year. Most strikingly, hospital complaints in England took a massive leap from 32,996 in 1990/1 to 44,680 for 1991/2 (DoH, 1994). Medical malpractice litigation has also increased markedly over the last decade, contributing to fears that a trust could find itself unable to pay if faced with a series of major damages over a short period. Indeed, Health Authority spending on awards for clinical negligence rose from £53 million in 1990/1 to an estimated £125 million in 1993/4 (Harris, 1994). In response to these concerns a Special Health Authority has been set up to manage a pooled Central Fund for Clinical Negligence.

Evidently a sense of moral panic has been created by a fear of complaints and litigation (Dingwall, 1994). As we have seen, some nurses and midwives see the Patient's Charter as a catalyst for the assertion of patients' 'rights'. Yet surveys suggest that up to 40 per cent of the population may not even have *heard of* the Charter (Cohen, 1994; Mahon et al., 1994). Similarly, while informal complaints may be increasing, there are as yet few examples of litigation against nurses in Britain. Very few of the respondents in the current research actually said that they had been involved in a formal complaint. Moreover, only a minority of those who were asked in interview were aware of what would happen in the hospital if a complaint was made against them, nor were they aware of the legal definition of malpractice. In their minds informal complaints, formal complaints and litigation seemed to merge to form an undifferentiated whole. There is, then, a sense in which the new consumerism may be more apparent than real. Perhaps, in line with findings for physicians in the US (Ennis and Vincent, 1994), nurses and midwives of overestimate the *true* risk of experiencing a complaint or a malpractice suit. [...]

A good part of nurses' and midwives' concern seems to derive from the perception of *individual* responsibility and accountability to patients. As Hugman (1994: 215) remarks, 'market consumerism in health and welfare can be seen as the attempt to promote the patronage model of professionalism' and to extend the power of service users over professionals. This is part and parcel of what Dingwall (1994: 47) has called a new mode of governmentality which 'segments individuals into bundles of discrete interests pursued through specific and limited agreements'. Sanctified by the individualistic model of the law, this new mode of governmentality has the effect of directing health care providers away from the holistic care of the individual towards 'the servicing of human bodies under a series of specific agreements between purchaser, provider and consumer, an auto-mechanic's model of medicine' (Dingwall, 1994: 60). Clearly, the 'accountability' that the health care provider now owes to her or his client is individualized. This was clearly recognized by respondents who stressed that 'errors and inaccuracies come back on the individual more' and consequently, 'at the end of the day, it's your neck on the line'. Nurses' individual responsibility is enshrined in the UKCC code of Conduct (1992). Indeed, the UKCC's assistant registrar for standards and ethics explains that while previously, the Code only said that *each* nurse was accountable, 'the 1992 document explicitly says that "you are personally accountable"'. This was changed, he states, to emphasize that nurses have a 'direct-personal accountability' for their practice (Pyne, 1994). Codes of professional conduct, then, are couched in the language of professionalism with duties and obligations described as 'individual ownership and responsibility for nursing actions' (Kendrick, 1995: 267).

But it is precisely this sense of ownership of one's own work that seems to be missing in the accounts that we have looked at so far. [...]

# Working in the new NHS

The radical changes set in train by the NHS and Community Care Act of 1990 (DoH, 1989) have gained so much momentum that the formal structure of health care now bears little resemblance to that which existed even a decade before. These changes were premised on the vision of a costly and inefficient service marked by stultifying bureaucracy and driven more by the needs of professionals than the provision of quality care to patients. The internal market has sought to introduce accountability into the system at every level, making clinical and financial decision-making more visible through contracting, standard setting and audit mechanisms. In line with broader changes in the economy, this shift has been accompanied by new '"leaner and flatter" managerial structures, decentralised cost centres, devolved budgets, the use of performance indicators and output measurement, localised bargaining, performance-related pay, and customer-oriented quality service' (Pinch, 1994: 207). On the face of it, this new organizational context would seem to cohere well with nursing's professionalizing strategy. Yet devolved authority 'does not in itself guarantee that the staff who are "close to the customer" will gain greater control over decision-making' (Walby et al., 1994: 16). As the following discussion will demonstrate, nurses feel that they have responsibility, but sometimes little control. In this context individual accountability can be experienced more as downward pressure than personal autonomy:

> I feel there is less support from management. More putting the blame on individuals. (staff nurse)

> I'm concerned because management won't back you up, and someone is always singled out to take the blame. What if someone sues me? (staff nurse)

> We feel that our numbers are more at risk than ever before and authorities use personal accountability to free themselves of responsibility. (staff nurse)

Apparently, in the nurses' and midwives' opinions it is '*individuals* who are blamed', 'someone is always *singled* out', authorities use '*personal* accountability'. The fact that many nurses and midwives may conceive of individual accountability as a management tool does little to lessen its impact on their day-to-day experience. [...]

Some nurses made a direct link between what they saw as the hospital trust's fear of the costs of litigation and downward pressure on them as individuals. For example,

> Trusts will shift blame on to individuals so as not to incur heavy claims for damages. (sister)

This may be bound up with the fear of actually losing one's job or professional registration:

> *Staff nurse*:    In the present climate, I think everyone wants to keep their job. And everyone is so aware that jobs that were once secure now aren't. And I think that's the one thing that frightens most nurses more than anything.
> *Int.*:    Why has that changed?
> *Staff Nurse*:    Because of the economic climate of the Health Service and because ... you know, *no one* in my group who I qualified with has got a permanent contract. So it's a matter of keeping your nose clean, otherwise you don't get your contract extended. And it's the same with a lot of other staff as well; they *can* be replaced. There are so many nurses out there.

The problem for many of the respondents was that in their opinion management expected them to assume responsibility as individuals, but consequently failed to provide a safe environment in which they could work. Ironically, in the minds of a number of nurses, this only served to increase the likelihood that mistakes would occur. This is made clear in the following remarks:

[...]

Lack of resources; equipment, manpower, time and finance, are taking their toll on the sort of service we can provide. People are given wonderful choices and they are disappointed when they are let down – they complain, quite rightly so. But we don't have the resources to back up the choices they are told they are entitled to. (sister)

# References

Cohen, P. (1994) 'Passing the buck?' *Nursing Times*, 90(13): 28–29.

DoH (Department of Health) (1989) *Working for Patients*. London: HMSO.

DoH (1994) *Being Heard, The Report of a Review Committee on NHS Complaints Procedures* (The Wilson Report). London: DoH.

Dingwall, R. (1994) 'Litigation and the threat to medicine', in J. Gabe, D. Kelleher and G. Williams (eds), *Challenging Medicine*. London: Routledge, pp. 46–64.

Ennis, M. and Vincent, C. (1994) 'The effects of medical accidents and litigation on doctors and patients', *Law and Social Policy*, 16(2): 97–121.

Harris, J. (1994) 'The price of failure', *Health Service Journal*, 14 April: 6–10.

Hugman, R. (1994) 'Consuming health and welfare', in R. Kent, N. Whitley and N. Abercrombie (eds), *The Authority of the Consumer*. London: Routledge, pp. 207–222.

Kendrick, K. (1995) 'Nurses and doctors: a problem of partnership', in K. Soothill, L. Mackay and C. Webb (eds), *Interprofessional Relations in Health Care*. London: Edward Arnold, pp. 239–252.

Mahon, A., Wilkin, D. and Whitehouse, C. (1994) 'Choice of hospitals for elective surgery referrals: GPs' and patients' views', in R. Robinson and J. Le Grand (eds), *Evaluating the NHS Reforms*. London: Kings' Fund, pp. 108–129.

Paget, M. A. (1988) *The Unity of Mistakes. A Phenomenological Interpretation of Medical Work*. Philadelphia: Temple University press.

Pinch, S. (1994) 'Labour flexibility and the changing welfare state: is there a post-Fordist model?', in R. Burrows and B. Loader (eds), *Towards a Post-Fordist Welfare State?* London: Routledge, pp. 203–222.

Pyne, R. (1994) 'Accountability'. Presentation to West Midlands Regional Health Authority, Advanced Nurse Practitioner Working Groups. 9 August.

Walby, S. and Greenwell, J. with Mackay, L. and Soothill, K. (1994) *Medicine and Nursing*. London: SAGE.

Walsh, K. (1994) 'Citizens, charters and contracts', in R. Keat, N. Whitley and N. Abercrombie (eds), *The Authority of the Consumer*. London: Routledge, pp. 189–206.

# Chapter 20

## Procedures and the professional

*Rebecca Lawton and Dianne Parker*

In recent years a range of risk management strategies have been introduced in the British National Health Service (NHS) in response to growing litigation and a transfer of the associated costs to the NHS Trust. One such strategy involves the increasing use of written procedures to control or guide practice. A further impetus to the drive to gain some control of medical practice came from the Griffiths report (Griffiths, 1983) which introduced the notion of business management into the NHS and gave managers the overall responsibility for delivering health care. In order to manage the budgets of healthcare organisations it was necessary for managers 'to establish some control over the activities of doctors and their use of resources' (Kelleher et al., 1994). In Britain, the White Paper for Health advocated the use of guidelines as a means of improving quality of care and cost effectiveness (Kleijnen and Bonsel, 1998). The development and implementation of clinical protocols and guidelines would also serve to reduce the traditional variation in the practice styles of physicians noted by Hunter (1994).

Internationally the development and use of clinical protocols has attracted a substantial research literature which suggests that there are three main reasons for the increasing drive to develop clinical protocols: risk management, the speedier integration of research into practice (Robertson et al., 1996) and the standardisation of practice to provide a more cost effective and efficient health care system (Chassin, 1990). UK research (see Grimshaw et al., 1995 for a review) has tended to focus on the characteristics of the guidelines themselves, e.g. the way in which they were developed and the process by which they are implemented as well as the outcome of their application.

[...]

It is clear that the mere introduction of a clinical protocol is not sufficient to ensure that it will be accepted and followed. The study reported here investigated the factors that may help or hinder the process of implementing guidelines and protocols in the British NHS. Of specific interest were the attitudes and perceptions of those expected to use protocols, with respect to their purpose, usage and usefulness. It was felt that such a study would shed light on the reasons for resistance to protocols and suggest ways in which successful implementation might be achieved.

*Source*: Originally published in *Social Science & Medicine* (1999), 48: 353–361 (abridged).

[...]

Twenty four focus groups were scheduled and run across three hospitals. In total, 126 health care professionals participated in the study. This sample consisted of 33 senior managers, 46 nurses, midwives or technicians, 18 senior nurses, five ward managers, nine consultants, six registrars, eight junior doctors and one senior theatre technician.

[...]

# What is the main purpose of protocols?

Participants in the group discussions were asked for their opinions about the purpose of protocols in the NHS. Responses fell into several categories, the most frequently mentioned of which are summarised in Table 20.1.

Table 20.1   Perceptions of the purpose of protocols

| Purpose | Times mentioned |
| --- | --- |
| To define best practice or standardise behaviour | 20 |
| To protect the Trust and management/to cover the organisation in the face of complaints or litigation | 11 |
| To allow the monitoring and audit of practice required to improve efficiency | 4 |
| For teaching or training | 3 |
| To provide guidance for staff | 3 |
| For insurance reasons | 3 |
| To manage risk and improve safety | 3 |
| To allow for the extension of nurses roles | 2 |
| To protect patients | 2 |

It was largely accepted by all discussion group participants that the primary purpose of procedures was to define best practice and/or standardise behaviour. However, there was also a widespread feeling, mentioned in 11 of the groups, that clinical protocols served as a tool to protect management.

> Cynically, one might say that the hospital is covering their butt gives them a chance to blame the individual rather than the system (senior technician, anaesthetics).

Both medical and nursing staff suggested a fiscal motive for proceduralisation, namely the need to reduce insurance premiums which meant that risk management had become a priority. The increasing willingness of the public to complain and even to litigate was also raised, particularly in relation to obstetrics, as a factor motivating proceduralisation. One consultant obstetrician made this point succinctly:

Our insurance brokers were the stimulus for the managers at a higher level to insist on a number of protocols. Like this is exactly the wrong way to go about it. I mean, we got it all in place because we had to.

Other, less central, but equally important, aspects of the function of protocols were also identified. There was a clear anxiety about the possible use of proceduralisation as a way of shortcutting the need for training, exemplified in the following quotation.

I think part of that is part of de-skilling. If you are going to get Mrs. Bloggs off the street who has just left school and has no nursing knowledge whatsoever you say you follow this protocol and then you don't need the training (consultant, orthopaedics).

On the other hand, the introduction of protocols was sometimes seen as a necessary response to the extension of the role of the nurse, serving to define correct practice in an ever-increasing range of situations.

Significant in its absence from the perceptions of focus group participants was the issue of patient care. Although they were asked directly about the effect of procedures on patient care, only very occasionally was improved patient care volunteered as a motive for the drive to proceduralisation in the NHS. Indeed some staff felt that patient care was being given secondary consideration in the application of some protocols.

I think we think more about the medico-legal implications of protocols than the actual patient risk (consultant surgeon).

In summary, proceduralisation was not perceived by medical and nursing practitioners as being driven by a desire to improve patient care, but rather to avoid financial costs resulting from failures in care.

While risk management, rather than improved patient care, was seen as the driving force behind the proliferation of protocols in the NHS, in subsequent discussion it emerged that many health care professionals also recognised the need to have a protocol, at least in some situations. For example, around 18 comments were made suggesting that protocols are appropriate for new and junior medical staff who have yet to accrue the knowledge necessary to function effectively all the time. Associated with this was the recognition in 13 of the groups that protocols have a role in training staff new to the Trust. It was also suggested that protocols are needed to define correct practice (15), to provide support when challenging the practice of a colleague (6), to support the extension of the nurse's role (6), to help the group function effectively as a team (6) and to change the practice of some of the older members of staff (4).

[...]

# How are protocols actually used? and how useful are they?

For many experienced health care professionals, protocols simply reflect their practice, the information is 'in their heads', so only in novel or unusual situations do they actually find a need to read and follow a protocol. A number of participants (6) suggested that protocols were a particularly useful tool for dealing with uncommon situations that did not arise very often or emergency situations (e.g. cardiac arrest) or where hospitals differed (e.g. antibiotic prescribing regimes). Across specialties and staff groups it was also suggested that while it may be appropriate for more senior and experienced staff to be flexible with protocols, a junior doctor would be expected to explain their reasons for deviating from a protocol.

In general, there was not an expectation that protocols are learned by rote and applied rigidly. Rather, it was suggested that protocols should be made available and referred to when necessary. In this sense they were perceived as an aid to practice rather than a prescription of practice. When protocols have been developed locally to manage particular situations, individuals took it on themselves to make new staff aware of these protocols or policies.

It was noticeable throughout the focus group discussions that nursing and medical staff differed in their approach to protocols. In fact, it was reported that the same procedure may be carried out differently by nursing and medical staff. Nurses, managers, midwives and some clinicians commented on the issue of non-compliance by the medical fraternity. Some 12 comments were made which explicitly referred to the disparity between the practice of nurses and medics. Both doctors and nurses recognised that medical staff are much more likely to 'do their own thing' whereas nurses adhere much more strictly to the protocols in place. In attempting to explain this disparity one manager said

> I think it's historical. Nurses have by and large been used to working with a set of policies, guidelines, protocols, whatever you want to call them, for quite some time now.

This difference in professional cultures was acknowledged by all the professional groups, and was the cause of some unease. A typical comment came from a manager:

> We would probably go through lots of training and accreditation or whatever for nurses to do some things, a junior doctor would walk in and do it without any training at all. They'll just kind of do it and you know that doesn't seem quite right somehow.

Some participants suggested that the result of these differences was that the practice of medical staff may, in some areas, be substandard.

> With us it's very much a case of you learn on the job. I'm sure our technique isn't always up to standard (junior doctor, surgery).

The very different training and culture of the nursing and medical staff means that the introduction of protocols is quite a contentious issue. Indeed it was widely accepted that, in general, the nursing staff show greater willingness to comply with the protocols. For example, the protocols relating to infection control were mentioned repeatedly in the context of non-compliance by medical staff. More senior nurses may feel it necessary to challenge a medical practitioner about a deviation from a protocol. Instances were described in the focus groups in which the necessity for compliance with a protocol appeared to be based on seniority, when in fact there was no rational justification for this e.g. hand washing. The tension between professional groups that this disparity produces was clear in many of the comments made, e.g.

> We came across this incident yesterday in theatres where one of the senior surgeons was able to bend the rules of a protocol that had previously been set in stone, which nurses, porters and

everybody adhered to. But he was able to [...] Is he a specialist in that field? (senior registrar, anaesthetics).

# Problems with protocols

This section will deal with the main theme to emerge from the focus group discussions aside from those introduced by the facilitator. While the majority of focus group participants accepted the need for protocols to establish best practice and guide new staff, there was a general concern that flexibility in practice should be preserved. Health care professionals in the obstetrics specialty were particularly aware of the need to tailor care to the needs of the individual, with five out of the six obstetrics groups raising the issue of individual care. Obstetrics is one area of medicine in Britain in which the public see themselves as consumers rather than as patients. This perception is well recognised by obstetrics practitioners. As one midwife explained,

> We are also aware of choice and you couldn't be dogmatic and say "you have to do this because my protocol says you have to do it". Its not like sort of servicing a piece of machinery is it?

Taking a broader perspective, the overall NHS strategy of developing clinical protocols to manage risk was questioned by some participants, in particular medical staff. The contentious status of much research evidence itself was one reason why protocols were perceived as being problematic, as illustrated in the following extract:

> So protocols as has already been implied, can be seen as tablets of stone and that's what's bad about them. [...] You show me a piece of research which shows us the right way with 100% of people and I'll believe it and I'll go with it I can assure you. So it only tells you it is the best way with the majority of people or the vast majority of people. But there is a percentage still that it's not the best way for. [...] That's the one problem that protocols could bring if you have one only one way of doing a certain thing then you are stopping lateral thinking (consultant anaesthetist).

The latter point made in this quotation was taken up by a number of focus group participants (7), who alluded to the danger that protocols would lead to rigidity and an inability amongst nursing and medical staff to think laterally. As one manager suggested:

> I worry about having putting people into what could be seen as a straight jacket and not allowing the freedom as a professional to be accountable for their practice. You do sometimes begin to generate a culture where people expect everything to be proceduralised and you've actually got to pull back from it and say well we didn't expect you to stop thinking we did want you to actually make judgements and apply your own professional training and judgements in a certain situation we are not going to put a procedure in place for everything.

This comment also covers professional freedom and autonomy and acknowledges that it is recognised that this is an issue which is likely to militate against the implementation of protocols in the health service. Senior staff members repeatedly expressed reservations about proceduralisation, making comments exemplified by the following:

> There are pressures to introduce them which in general are being resisted ... because the perception is that it will restrict clinical practice and that in many areas there is not good proof that a variety of different methods are not equally applicable (consultant, orthopaedics).

A further concern was that the rigidity of protocols might stifle progress:

> One of the problems with standardising things which I think is why another reason why people have gone for guidelines rather than protocols in medical practice, is that you are not necessarily, even though what you do may be quite different from what practically everybody else does, you may not be wrong and of course especially if you are someone who is developing something new you know, there would be no movement forward if you stick to the protocol (registrar, obstetrics).

Other factors were also thought likely to make rigid adherence to protocols extremely difficult. Half of the groups highlighted the problem of limited resources and argued that this in itself could lead to situations in which corners had to be cut and protocols violated. The most frequently mentioned problem was staff shortages, followed by equipment and medical supplies. The two areas of practice that were felt to be particularly problematic in this context were infection control and manual handling, both of which are covered by procedures developed at the level of the Trust, rather than the ward or specialty.

[...]

# What are the barriers to the successful implementation of protocols?

Two main features of the British NHS make the use of protocols as a way of managing risk especially problematic. First, doctors, nurses and midwives are professionals. One of the main issues raised in the focus group discussions was professional autonomy. Medical staff, in particular, were eager to point out the possible negative aspects of proceduralisation. They discussed situations in which applying a protocol would be detrimental to patient care. They were concerned that if staff were unwilling to deviate from the protocols and try new methods, then medical progress would be stifled. It was also proposed that the training of junior doctors benefits from the use, by senior medics, of a range of different techniques and approaches. In general there was a feeling that guidelines and/or protocols threaten the use of initiative and thought in medical and, to a lesser extent, nursing practice. It will be important for those involved in the development and implementation of guidelines to be aware of these worries and deal with them sensitively.

The monitoring of compliance with protocols is also made particularly difficult in the NHS by the fact that a manager may be quite remote from the day-to-day working practice of medical and nursing staff. Traditionally the training and guidance of junior staff is in the hands of the consultant. The focus group discussions revealed that more senior members of the medical profession are often opposed to protocols on the ground that they threaten autonomy and presumably the traditional process of passing on knowledge. Indeed, our findings confirm those of Lloyd (1995, p. 6) who wrote 'it is striking that almost all the opposition to guidelines comes from consultants'.

Distrust of managements motives in introducing procedures may constitute a further barrier to implementation. Lloyd (1995, p. 5) comments that 'clinical guidelines are essential if a department is to provide high quality, cost-effective care that minimises risks to the patient'. In contrast to this, the perception of many staff who participated in the focus groups was that protocols are developed primarily as a means of avoiding and defending litigation. Protocols were perceived to represent paperwork that, while necessary to get ticks in boxes, was tedious and time consuming and of little value in terms of patient care. This pattern of thinking often leads staff to believe that it is not necessary to adhere to protocols. Unfortunately initiatives designed to promote risk management may, by causing a paper blizzard, only serve to exacerbate the problem.

Furthermore, if, because of financial or other pressures (e.g. under-staffing, unavailability of equipment), it is actually extremely difficult for staff to comply, protocols are unlikely to produce changes in clinical practice.

# Conclusion

The successful implementation of protocols designed to govern the behaviour of health professionals will require getting the balance right between standardising practice, to achieve at least some consistency, and allowing for flexibility, so that health care professionals can take responsibility and use clinical judgement where necessary. Most research to date investigating compliance with clinical guidelines has focused on the characteristics of the guidelines themselves. However, the research presented here suggests that in attempting to understand the use of clinical guidelines it may be more useful to consider the culture of the health service and the beliefs, attitudes and norms of its employees. For those people tasked with developing and implementing guidelines the adoption of a social psychological perspective will be helpful in attempting to understand and change clinical behaviour. The participants in the focus group discussions described in this paper needed answers to two key questions: how far do you go (with protocols)? and how should they be used?

# References

Chassin, M. (1990) 'Practice guidelines: best hope for quality improvement in the 1990s', *Journal of Occupational Medicine,* 32: 1199–1206.

Griffiths, R. (1983) *'NHS Management Inquiry', Report,* London: DHSS.

Grimshaw, J., Fremantle, N., Wallace, S., Russell, I., Hurwitz, B., Watt, I., Long, A. and Sheldon, T. (1995) 'Developing and implementing clinical practice guidelines', *Quality in Health Care,* 4: 55–64.

Hunter, D. J. (1994) 'From tribalism to corporatism', in J. Gabe, D. Kelleher and G. Williams (eds), *Challenging Medicine.* London: Routledge, pp. 1–22.

Kelleher, D., Gabe, J. and Williams, G. (1994) 'Understanding medical dominance in the modern world', in J. Gabe, D. Kelleher and G. Williams (eds), *Challenging Medicine*. London: Routledge, pp. xi–xxix.

Kleijnen, J. and Bonsel, G. (1998) 'Guidelines and quality of clinical services in the new NHS', *British Medical Journal,* 316: 299–300.

Lloyd, B. (1995) 'Guidelines to reduce risk and improve the quality and cost-effectiveness of care', *Managing Risk*, April: 5–6.

Robertson, N., Baker, R. and Hearnshaw, H. (1996) 'Changing the clinical behaviour of doctors: a psychological framework', *Quality in Health Care*, 5: 51–54.

# Chapter 21

## How the internet affects people's experience of cancer

*Sue Ziebland, Alison Chapple, Carol Dumelow, Julie Evans, Suman Prinjha and Linda Rozmovits*

The internet is changing the way that people learn about health and illness. Health sites and discussion lists are among the most popular resources on the web (Eaton, 2002). [...]

We know little about what it means to patients to have access to health information on the internet and the subject is well suited to qualitative inquiry (Malterud, 2001). We therefore explored how 175 men and women aged 18–83 with cancer diagnosed in the previous 10 years describe to what extent they used cancer information on the internet. We studied whether participants sought internet information about their cancer and how they perceived and used this information. We identify a broad range of uses and explore how the experience of cancer is being transformed for those with internet access.

## Methods

The interviews we used were collected for research studies for the DIPEx charity, which runs a website (www.dipex.org) based on narratives interviews about people's experiences of health and illness. DIPEx aims and research methods are described in detail elsewhere (Herxheimer et al., 2000) and on its website [...].

[...]

For this study, we used DIPEx interviews with respondents who had had cancer diagnosed after 1992. The interviews included in this study were collected between January 2001 and November 2002. Table 21.1 shows the distribution and age range of respondents. We analysed interviews for five different cancer groups: men with cancer of the prostate or testis, women with breast or cervical cancer, and 17 men and 14 women with bowel cancer.

[...]

Originally published in the *British Medical Journal* (2004), 328: 564–567.

Table 21.1   Reported use of the internet for cancer information and support in men and women interviewed for DIPEx studies and with cancer diagnosed since 1992

| Site of cancer | No of respondents | Mean (range) age at interview (years) | No (%) of respondents with access to internet cancer information | | |
|---|---|---|---|---|---|
| | | | Accessed by self | Accessed by friend or family | Total |
| Breast | 37 | 44 (19–75) | 17 (46) | 2 (5) | 19 (51) |
| Bowel | 31 | 58 (33–80) | 5 (16) | 3 (10) | 8 (26) |
| Cervix | 21 | 40 (23–51) | 6 (29) | 4 (19) | 10 (48) |
| Prostate | 49 | 62 (51–83) | 10 (20) | 7 (14) | 17 (35) |
| Testes | 37 | 39 (21–55) | 17 (46) | 5 (14) | 22 (59) |

# Results

## Why the internet?

The need for health information is not novel, but respondents with access to the internet talked about it having distinctive and appealing characteristics. These included privacy and 24 hour availability:

> So many people have computers nowadays, you haven't actually got to leave your house, it doesn't matter how you're feeling. You don't even have to get dressed; you can just, you know, log on and you can get the information. Which I think is going to do absolutely nothing but help people. (Man with bowel cancer)

Others noted that using the internet removes the embarrassment of face to face or telephone interactions. This feature seemed to appeal particularly to young men who might be worried about their health but reluctant to visit a doctor:

> It's so personal because ... it's your body, but you have to go somewhere. What better place to go than–well certainly in my circumstances, where I have a computer at home that I can switch on, in total privacy. I don't need to feel that I'm asking a dumb question. I don't need to feel that I have to ask all the right questions first time round. (Man with testicular cancer)

People may find it hard to predict when they will want to access different sorts of information about their health. With the internet, they can search for different types and levels of information as and when needed. The following excerpts show how the timing of people's need for information can differ greatly (see also quote by respondent TC07 in Box 21.1):

It's been helpful knowing where to look and being able to sort of follow the evidence and so on, but now I've reached the stage where I'm not looking any more. It kind of comes and goes; to begin with I wanted a whole lot of information, now I feel perhaps I don't want to know too much and I just want to try and keep going and not think too closely about what might happen. (56 year old woman with breast cancer, one year since diagnosis)

I found I became very interested in it afterwards. Like, I'd say, after that first year. Like I started to want to ask different sort of questions and know what it looked like and that sort of thing; I was left thinking "What was that thing?" (33 year old woman, five years since diagnosis)

[…]

# How the internet is changing patients' experience of cancer

We identified two distinct ways in which respondents used the internet to transform roles and change involvement in health care – to covertly question their doctors' advice and to display themselves (to researchers, friends, family, and health professionals) as competent social actors despite serious illness.

Covert questioning    Patients described using the web to check up on their doctor's responses and advice at all stages, from the recognition of symptoms through recommendations for treatment and follow up. Sometimes they looked for information after being given contradictory advice or realising that their doctors found it hard to keep up with a rapidly changing subject. The internet also enables people to investigate the expertise and reputation of a hospital and staff and any evidence of 'postcode rationing.' As the extract from respondent BC41 (Box 21.1) shows, searches on the internet may be used after treatment for reassurance that optimal treatment was given. Other respondents identified treatments they preferred (PC42, CC19) and options that they suspected they would not have been offered (TC05). People differ in how they handle the information they have gained and how it affects their relationship with their doctors. However, the fact that this 'checking up' can be achieved covertly without a doctor's knowledge may avoid threats to 'face' that could endanger the doctor-patient relationship and risk unnecessary conflict (Goffman, 1955; Jadad et al., 2003).

Displaying competence    Another way that the internet is changing people's relationship with their illness is that they can gain, maintain, and display familiarity with a remarkable body of medical and experiential knowledge about their illness. Radley and Billig have pointed out that 'being a good patient means having to fulfil a sociologically ambivalent position. The patient must appear to be more than a patient, a display of healthiness, or normality is also required for the individual to appear worthy of receiving the entitlements' (Radley and Billig, 1996).

The ability to access a wide range of disparate information on the internet, coupled with the opportunity to present themselves as technically proficient and discriminating users of such information, enabled respondents to display a modern form of competence and social fitness in the face of serious illness. Indeed, the following quote suggests that there may almost be an obligation to seek information:

We have one very big advantage ... and that is called the world wide web. Now I use Yahoo ... you go to Yahoo, and you type in testicular cancer, and I guarantee you that for the next two weeks you'll be looking at every site that is different. You have people's experiences, you have drug information, you'll be able to read papers that are published on the web by some of the most eminent doctors around. There is no excuse these days – if you haven't got a computer go down to an internet cafe – there is no excuse whatsoever for not finding out about testicular cancer or all the other things ... The information technology breakthrough of having the internet available is just unreal. You know, we're very lucky because we're at the dawn of something that is quite remarkable ... so there is really no excuse for not becoming totally aware of testicular cancer. (50 year old man with testicular cancer diagnosed in 1992)

If competent patients seek information about their condition and question the treatment they have been offered does this imply that patients who do not do so are being negligent? Although this view was never stated in the interviews, the negative consequences of not doing one's own research were regularly mentioned in the accounts. Examples in Box 21.1 include respondent CRC16, who sought a second opinion when told that a stoma was inevitable and warned that doctors have neither the time nor expertise to be able to provide all the necessary information, and PC42, whose own research identified brachytherapy as the best treatment for his prostate cancer and who explained that specialist advice is too compartmentalised and unbalanced to help decision making. A young woman with cervical cancer (CC19) found an experimental cryopreservation treatment via the internet. Though she was aware that there was no guarantee this would work, she was keen to preserve her fertility and chose to go to another hospital for the treatment. TC29 pointed out that finding one's own information can help one to plan for the consultation and identify appropriate questions, while lack of planning may result in suboptimum consultations and frustrating esprit d'escalier ('an apt retort or clever remark that comes to mind after the chance to make it had gone,' *Concise Oxford Dictionary*).

[...]

---

### Box 21.1 Expressed reasons why people with cancer used the internet for treatment decisions and to supplement medical consultations

**Before the diagnosis**
'During that week I was looking at everything I could find on the subject, on the internet mostly ... I basically just put a search in on testicular cancer, and various sites and pieces of information came up ... it gives you some sort of comfort to know that certain types can be cured fully without too much of a problem, but on the other hand at that time I didn't know what sort of a problem there was. I mean, I didn't even know that it was testicular cancer. I mean it could have been anything'. (TC07, man with testicular cancer diagnosed at 33 years old)

**To research and prepare**
'One can have a better knowledge of how to cope with such major surgery and trauma. I don't expect a surgeon to spend hours on end trying to describes what he was going to perform and what he was

going to make your lifestyle after surgery. I think (the internet) is something which one needs to have access [to] because they are not going to be able to commit themselves to that length of time…Sadly one has to do their own research. In every field of medicine there is an expert somewhere in the country, and they have to locate this person and have a consultation prior to surgery because the GPs don't have access to this information, and even if they do they are not going to spend two or three hours trying to phone round and find out who is the best surgeon … I think a second opinion is something they need to do … it's so important, so important'. (CRC16, 52 year old man who survived bowel cancer without a colostomy after having sought a second opinion)

'The internet was invaluable the second time around when particularly we wanted information on primary cancer, you know, coming after another one, and the particular kind of cancer. I think they were very helpful, they give precise details of the cancers, and I felt that it was extremely helpful to get all the research and the findings and what they can do about it, the prognosis and all the rest of it – yes we did and friends did too. And I think it's very helpful the internet; when anything like that happens, I think that you can immediately go out and see what's going on, other than talking to doctors, and get statistics. I think everyone can be their own researcher now really; you can be in charge of your own affairs and know what's what. Nobody can pull the wool over your eyes'. (BC12, 61 year old woman with ductal carcinoma in situ diagnosed in 2000)

### When choosing treatments

'The problem with the options was that it was very, very compartmentalised. When I went to see the surgeon I think his idea was that radical prostatectomy is the thing, and that's what I heard from everybody else – because all urologists are basically surgeons, and they say 'To a hammer everything looks like a nail' – and I think that's very much the way it is'. (PC42, 51 year old professional man who decided to have brachytherapy at a US clinic despite having been discouraged by the radiotherapist he saw in Britain)

'I didn't know a great deal about testicular prosthesis. I mean, I again looked in the internet, and there were a lot of American websites where people were talking about how difficult it was to get them in America because of silicone and all the scares that there had been, and that in this country at the time it was no particular issue. I don't know whether it's an issue now, but at the time it seemed to me that there was no compelling reason not to, and from what I knew about myself I'd probably feel a bit better about myself if I did have one … I'm quite glad that it was an option. It was an issue I raised, it wasn't an issue that was raised by them, and I think if I hadn't said anything it wouldn't have arisen'. (TC05, man with testicular cancer diagnosed at age 42)

'Basically my mum – because she's great and looking at all these internet sites, she read about having ovarian tissue, basically cryo-ovarian preservation, it's quite new. And so I had read about it, since my mum had found this information, and when I went to the hospital I discussed it with them. And actually they were a bit dismissive about it to be honest, and it certainly wasn't something they would have offered me had I not brought it up. And they said, "Well, you can't have it done here, but you can have it done at another hospital". So I phoned up the other hospital myself, made an appointment, and went in to go and see this woman, and she said to me, "Yes, you can have it done." And she said, "There is, no children have been born as a result of this." But what they do is they take out a portion of either one ovary or both ovaries, and this ovarian tissue is then frozen over a period of six hours by an embryologist and obviously stored in special little tanks'. (CC19, woman with cervical cancer diagnosed at age 27)

### To check that the treatment was optimal

'I've learnt an awful lot – er, maybe too much time on my hands, maybe not, I don't know – but I needed to know. Knowledge is power, and I needed to know that what was happening to me was the right thing … I thought, with being in the UK, when reading about the therapies that the American people were having and the rest of it, I thought, "Wow, what I've had is probably second best." But it isn't. It's up there

*(Continued)*

*(Continued)*

with the best, and I've had the best care that you could possibly imagine – the best surgeon, the best oncologist, the best breast nurse, ever'. (BC41, 47 year old teacher with inflammatory breast cancer diagnosed, who set up her own website to increase awareness)

### To supplement information from the hospital

'Of course, I asked the hospital for any information at all that they had that I could read up on and maybe take home, brochures and stuff like that, leaflets. So I took those home with me … I got books and stuff from my local library and read it up again. And I have medical encyclopedias here, and we read up in those, and then of course on the internet. I went on to American sites and sought information. But it's the practical, uh, day to day dealing with this thing (the stoma) that has to, and making sure that it wasn't going to leak and I wasn't going to smell'. (CRC35, 54 year old with bowel cancer).

### To make sense of medical terms

'I was told I was booked for this 'radical hysterectomy' – which I hated the word, the radical bit, but then read on the internet that it's just the fact that they have to go to the outer limits, as far as they can go with regards to the hysterectomy. 'Radical,' its just such a horrible word isn't it? It just sounds so absolutely dreadful and kind of drastic. And I got a little, she gave me a leaflet about cervical cancer and she said, "You know that you're going to have to have a catheter and you'll probably go home with a catheter," and at that point I didn't really know what that was or, you know, whether that was something in my stomach or how – but it's not through your urethra and bladder that way. But I didn't know that at the time, so I wanted to go looking on the internet, find out about hysterectomy, radical hysterectomy, how the incisions are done, and this catheter'. (CC11, 23 year old student with cervical cancer)

### To find the right questions to ask and avoid esprit d'escalier

'There is some information out there, and I think … that for me one of the things that I needed to know most about was … I needed somewhere I could go to that would say to me, "Well, this is what the circumstance is. This is what's actually happened to you." Um and yes, you can to a certain extent with a doctor, but there are never, you never ask the right questions at the time, um, you're just coming to terms with everything – you need time to consider that, and what better place to do that than at home and looking on the web?' (TC29, 42 year old company director with testicular cancer)

---

## Box 21.2  Use of the internet for social support and living with cancer

### To tackle isolation

'I think that the worst thing about getting a diagnosis like this is a feeling of isolation, because you feel that your world has suddenly shrunk and all you can think about is yourself and you feel very frustrated because nobody has maybe experienced this. And when you're able to talk to other patients it's just very good to know that other people have been through this and to kind of share the experience with other people, and you feel much less isolated … It's not just the medical information aspect, it's just a kind of support, moral support, which is very, very important when you've had a diagnosis of cancer'. (PC42, 51 year old man with prostate cancer)

### To find alternative and complementary treatments

'Quite a lot is written and discussed on the internet about alternative treatments, and if conventional treatments stopped working I would obviously examine some of those, but I don't need to at the moment, I'm delighted with how things are going'. (CRC26, 57 year old man with bowel cancer)

**To access experiential knowledge**
'I mean a silly thing that I found out was that lots of cancer patients actually experience very, very bad mouth ulcers through the chemotherapy, because your body is at a very, very low ebb and unable to fight off all sorts of microbes or whatever which a normal fit person would fight off with no problem. You get ulcers in your mouth. Now one of the sites I found on the internet, it said that one thing they recommend that cancer patients do is even after drinking a cup of tea have a mouth wash and brush your teeth after every meal – mouth wash and brush your teeth, which is what I did. And I didn't have mouth ulcers all the way through my chemotherapy, whereas other men going through the same chemotherapy regime as myself who didn't do that did have mouth ulcers. And that is something that the nurses on the cancer ward didn't even know about'. (TC40, man with testicular cancer diagnosed at 27 years old)

**Social connections**
'I met a lady through an internet site for breast cancer survivors, which is an American site, although there are a lot of British women on there, and we were writing by email for two years, and I went out to see her in July – travelled to America with my husband, my children, er – and that's something that I wouldn't have done before, because we'd have put it off, and the money would have gone to something else. And it felt very important because we had the bond – we'd both had children, we were both in out 30s – and we did it, we went to America and met, and it was such an emotional meeting'. (BC44, 34 year old woman with breast cancer diagnosed in 1997)

**Perceived therapeutic benefits**
'I got on to the internet, which is an amazing media, but it is also full of charlatans so you have to be extremely careful; it's a minefield. There are trillions and trillions of opportunities and people trying to sell you all sorts of cures, and I would say beware of that ... Get involved, be part of your own cure. It's really cathartic, it's, being involved takes your mind off the horror of it, and you immediately begin the process of fighting the disease'. (BC33, 56 year old woman whose son gave her a crash course in using the internet after breast cancer was diagnosed)

**To raise awareness about condition**
[When asked if her would like to be able to talk about testicular cancer more openly] 'Oh yeah, I've, that's why I've sort of started a website to try and spread the news. Er, I think nowadays it's probably, there's a lot more campaigns now to get to build up an awareness of testicular cancer ... the schools, football, schools, campaigns that are basically led by footballers that have got testicular cancer trying to spread the word. There's one or two, but you don't hear of many in the UK of actually people with the disease ... The only people I've found is searching on the internet where you see the news'. (TC16, man with testicular cancer diagnosed at age 44)

# Discussion

This qualitative analysis of narrative interviews with people with a diagnosis of one of five different cancers not only shows the many different ways that people with cancer use the internet but also discusses the meanings that internet health information has for patients. We did not question respondents about why they did not use the internet, and so can say little on this issue. However, lack of familiarity or of access were the main explanations people volunteered when asked if they had sought internet information.

## Use of the internet by patients

Until recently articles in medical journals about the internet have focused on concerns about the quality of health information. Some of our respondents voiced concerns about the difficulty of distinguishing between good and bad information on the web, but it is notable that they only expressed this concern for other, less wary people. In reporting their own internet use, they displayed considerable caution and competence and described techniques (such as comparing different information sources) to ensure that they were not misled.

The main contribution of this study is to show the many different ways in which the internet seems to be used by people with a serious illness, at all stages of their illness and follow up. We have also shown how patients' ability to become expert in their own condition may contribute to changes in relationships between patients and doctors. Patients who are concerned about the effects of cost constraints on health care (concerns that predate the widespread use of the internet) are able to use the web to seek reassurance about their treatment. Patients also want to know more about complementary approaches to treatment, but, as others have shown, may be anxious not to jeopardize their relationship with their doctors by revealing their interest in self treatment (Cant and Sharma, 1999; Stephenson et al., 2003). As Jadad and colleagues recently suggested. 'It will take time and effort to reach the point where the assertive patient is recognized as the 'good' one. Ignorance, fear, inertia, and stubbornness remain to be overcome' (Jadad et al., 2003). The desire to canvass an informal (and therefore face saving) second opinion will be familiar to all who have ever sought supplementary information for friends and family faced with treatment decisions. The internet extends this ability to those whose social circle does not include medical professionals (and probably makes the process more reliable for those whose social circle does include medical professionals).

The internet extends the scope of the best stocked medical library, through access to experiential knowledge as well as medical information. Health professionals in training as well as patients stand to benefit from this, but as yet the internet is rarely used by people who are socially disadvantaged. Unequal access to the internet may increase social class divisions in health care, but this is not inevitable. Indeed, in one UK study socially deprived respondents said they were more inclined to use the internet than more prosperous ones (Mead et al., 2003), and in a US study African-Americans reported higher use of the web for health information than the general population (Cline and Haynes, 2001). On reflection, it is not surprising that such resources have particular appeal to those who suspect (rightly or wrongly) that their ethnicity, age, education, social class, or income may militate against an equal and honest relationship with their doctors (Rozmovits and Ziebland, 2004). The challenge is to ensure that access is broadened through appropriate, supported public channels such as cancer information centres and public libraries.

[…]

# References

Cant, S. and Sharma, U. (1999) *A New Medical Pluralism: Alternative Medicine, Doctors, Patients and the State*. London: University College London Press.

Cline, R. J. and Haynes, K. M. (2001) 'Consumer health information seeking on the internet: the state of the art', *Health Education Research*, 16: 671–692.

Eaton, L. (2002) 'Europeans and Americans turn to internet for health information', *British Medical Journal*, 325: 989.

Goffman, E. (1955) 'On face work: an analysis of ritual elements in social interaction', *Psychiatry*, 18: 213–231.

Herxheimer, A., McPherson, A., Miller, R., Shepperd, S., Yaphe, J. and Ziebland, S. (2000) 'A database of patients' experiences (DIPEx): new ways of sharing experiences and information using a multi-media approach', *Lancet*, 355: 1540–1543.

Jadad, A. R., Rizo, C. A. and Enkin, M. W. (2003) 'I am a good patient, believe it or not', *British Medical Journal*, 326: 1293–1295.

Malterud, K. (2001) 'The art and science of clinical knowledge: evidence beyond measures and numbers', *Lancet*, 358: 397–400.

Mead, N., Varnam, R., Rogers, A. and Poland, M. (2003) 'What predicts primary care patients' interest in the internet as a health resource? A questionnaire study', *Journal of Health Services Research and Policy*, 8: 33–39.

Radley, A. and Billig, M. (1996) 'Accounts of health and illness: dilemmas and representations', *Sociology of Health and Illness*, 18(2): 220–240.

Rozmovits, L. and Ziebland, S. (2004) 'What do patients with prostate or breast cancer want from an internet site? A qualitative study of information needs', *Patient Education and Counselling*, 53(1): 57–64.

Stephenson, F. A., Britten, N., Barry, C. A., Bradley, C. P. and Barber, N. (2003) 'Self-treatment and its discussion in medical consultations: how is medical pluralism managed in practice?' *Social Science and Medicine*, 57: 513–527.

# Chapter 22

## Patients' experiences of accessing their electronic patient records

*Cecilia Pyper, Justin Amery, Marion Watson and Claire Crook*

The electronic health record is a longitudinal record of a patient's health and health care – 'from cradle to grave'. It combines information about patient contacts with primary health care and subsets of information associated with outcomes of periodic care held in electronic patient records.

Patients have been legally entitled to see their health records since November 1991, and at Bury Knowle Health Centre in Oxford patients have previously held their own paper health records (Pyper et al., 2001a). Access to paper records is now fairly common, but rarely is there access to the full electronic record. Previous studies have included research on: patient access to a short record summary (Liaw et al., 1996); access to records on specific or chronic conditions (Liaw et al., 1998; Drury et al., 2000); full access for a limited range of issues (Jones et al., 1992); health professionals' views, without consideration of patient access (Aylward and Parmar, 1999; Wager et al., 2000; Laerum et al., 2001); quality of primary care electronic records (Hassey et al., 2001). Access to electronic records could: support patients in shared decision making and in managing their own care (Coiera, 1996; Homer et al., 1999); improve communication with health care professionals (Fisher and Britten, 1993); offer the opportunity to enter information about health, beliefs, values and wishes for care; and allow patients to review their health history and advise clinicians of any changes to health beliefs and wishes or inaccuracies in their health record (Pyper et al., 2001b).

This paper explores the experiences, concerns and wishes of patients given access to their on-line electronic records.

Originally published in *British Journal of General Practice* (2004), 54: 38–43.

# Method

## Setting

Bury Knowle Health Centre is an Oxford urban practice covering a varied population, including areas of high and low social deprivation (DETR, 2000), with a practice list size of 10,300. [...]

## Recruitment

The first 100 available patients attended to view their own electronic records. They were recruited from a postal survey sent to 10% of the adult practice population. These patients were a randomised sample stratified for age and sex. Computer literacy was not a requirement. The survey elicited patients' views about patient access to health records, including electronic records (Pyper et al., 2001b). A postcard was included with the survey, which could be returned separately to indicate whether patients would like to view their own record. Of the first 100 patients who indicated they would like to view their record and were available, 65 of the respondents were women aged between 18 and 84 years of age (mean = 52 years) and 35 of the respondents were men aged between 19 and 81 (mean = 56 years).

## Facilities

Private viewing booths were installed, together with network, computer, biometric (fingerprint scanning) security, and printing facilities. An easy-to-use screen touch light pen was installed with each computer, in addition to a mouse, to give a choice of means to navigate the screens. Security was maintained by a combination of fingerprint biometrics, password, National Health Service (NHS) number and date of birth. Ninety-five patients viewed their records at the practice and five viewed them in their own homes via a secure link to the NHSNet accessed by one of the researchers.
   [...]

# Results

## Navigation

Most patients found they could navigate around each section of their electronic record and between sections with ease (Table 22.1). Some patients, especially left-handed people, had problems with using the mouse and opted for the touch screen light pen. Those with little or no computer experience needed a very brief verbal explanation of how and where to 'point and click' or 'point and touch'. Patients spent between 18 and 75 minutes viewing

Table 22.1   Level of patient agreement with questions about accessing their electronic patient record (n = 100)

| Question | % |
|---|---|
| Found it easy to find your way around the record | 73 |
| Found registration section useful | 85 |
| Found record summary useful | 94 |
| Found consultation details useful | 90 |
| Found medication details useful | 59 |
| Found referrals section useful | 42 |
| Found at least one section useful | 99 |
| Found registration section easy to understand | 94 |
| Found record summary easy to understand | 84 |
| Found consultation details easy to understand | 80 |
| Found medication details easy to understand | 61 |
| Found referrals section easy to understand | 41 |
| Found record easy to understand overall | 73 |
| Found record difficult to understand overall | 5 |
| Worried about security – before seeing record | 48 |
| Confident of security in use – after seeing record | 61 |

their electronic records while simultaneously being prompted for their opinions. The mean time patients took to view was 33 minutes and the interquartile range was 28 minutes to 40 minutes, with 71% of participants taking 35 minutes or less. The time patients took varied owing to multiple factors, including the quantity of information held within the health record and the patients' level of interest and dexterity. Times were not adjusted to allow for the impact of the interviews, although our observation was that people did not stop and talk, but browsed as they talked:

I think that the light pen is excellent for older patients. (User 31)

I don't believe it is user friendly. (User 28)

The layout and design is excellent and it is very user friendly. (User 47)

## Usefulness

Ninety-nine per cent of patients found at least one section useful, particularly their record summaries and consultation details (Table 22.1). The main benefits as perceived by the patients are listed in Box 22.1:

---

**Box 22.1  Patient views on advantages of accessing electronic health records**

- Improves doctor–patient relationship by reassuring, improving consultations, and encouraging patients to be better informed about their own health and health care
- Improves accuracy by identifying errors and omissions and improving the completeness of the electronic patient record, and being clear and legible and avoiding the need to read doctors' handwriting. It will also help doctors if records are complete and accurate
- Promotes easier access to information. Patients can review healthcare episodes, dates, and which doctors were seen, including locum doctors. It assists access for emergency services — this is useful when travelling or when moving out of the area
- Improves shared management by facilitating self-monitoring of long-term conditions, by enabling access to vaccination dates, prompting when boosters are needed, clarifying medication details, and clarifying why long-term medication has been prescribed

---

Clearer than expected, very easy to understand, very easy to access. (User 30)

On the whole, I think it would prove excellent in building relationships between health professionals and patients. (Focus group attender)

Great — looks good and I believe it will save time, money, and even lives in the long run. (User 47)

Will people start diagnosing themselves? Will that be detrimental to people's health? (User 100)

I can't believe how many times I have actually been to see my doctor! (User 47)

## Understanding

Most patients found it easy to understand their records. Where problems arose it was with the record summaries or consultation details (Table 22.1). Many patients requested explanations of medical terms (42%), abbreviations and acronyms (13%), and information on tests or results (17%) and metric weight measurements (5%). Clinical questions were referred on to a GP via the routine appointment system. In the early stages the researchers dealt with non-clinical queries. During the course of the study a glossary was developed to explain frequently used terms and tests. In addition, a directory of relevant websites was compiled:

I am sometimes confused and can't remember what doctors said. (User 71)

It is very clear, easy to understand. (User 87)

Medical jargon could lead to misunderstanding and cause worry. (Focus group attender)

## Accuracy

Seventy per cent of patients found at least one error or omission. The majority were trivial, especially those in the registration section, such as missing postcodes or outdated telephone codes. Twenty-three per cent of patients found an error or omission that could be described as important (Box 22.2). Other 'errors' noted by patients were misunderstandings; for example, thinking that 'DNA' referred to genetic tests rather than being an abbreviation for 'did not attend', and differing interpretation of information between patients and health professionals, such as what constitutes 'heavy' smoking:

> You can check up on your details and make sure that they are correct. (User 8)

> I broke my collar bone years ago, should that be on 'significant past problems'? (Focus group attender)

> I was not born in 1910. (User 72, aged 42 years)

> I wish the health visitor had written in my record. (User 3)

> I would like to see my record from time to time to check, especially as another person with the same name is registered here. (User 52)

---

**Box 22.2  Significant errors and omissions identified by patients, and causes of misunderstandings**

- Significant errors: out-of-dates personal data; wrong medication or discontinued medications; consultations listed under the wrong patient; dates and frequencies of recurrences of conditions wrong; referral dates wrong; incorrect site of amputation recorded
- Missing information: medication, vaccinations, allergies, test results, and patient records from before the practice became electronic
- Missing consultations: nurse, health visitor, out-of-hours doctor
- Missing events: adverse reaction to medication, breast screening, operations, tuberculosis, childbirth, premature childbirth, miscarriage, sterilisation, irritable bowel syndrome, severe migraine, glaucoma, fracture, repeated episodes, and minor surgery
- Missing referrals: cardiology, urology, endoscopy, orthopaedic, physiotherapy
- Misunderstanding of terminology: acronyms being misconstrued; medical terms that may have different meanings in common use — for example, one patient understood phlebitis to mean that a flea had bitten her leg!
- Poor patient recall: patients unable to remember what operations were for and their outcomes
- Differences of opinion: about diagnosis, especially for depression; what constitutes heavy smoking; which past events are considered significant and which are listed in the patient summary
- Misunderstanding how information is managed in the NHS: the practice administrative recording system, administrative prompts, transfer of information — for example, from genito-urinary medicine clinics, out-of-hours services and emergency services

---

# Printing

Nearly all were in favour of having print facilities. Thirty-seven per cent used the print facility for printing the following: the entire record (6%); consultation details (21%); summary (15%); medication (4%); and referrals (2%). Two patients considered printing to be a risk to confidentiality.

Three said they would take printouts with them when travelling out of the area. One commented that internet access to electronic records would make printing unnecessary:

> I would prefer to have a printout of my records as due to eye problems I would not be able to read them on a computer screen. (Focus group attender)

> Good idea to keep hard copy — easy to read at a later date. (User 54)

> I am concerned about the security of printing out a copy, it could fall into wrong hands. (User 84)

## Security and confidentiality

Prior to viewing their electronic records, 47% had concerns about security. Most were reassured by the use of biometrics, passwords and NHS numbers, with only 4% being concerned after using the system.

Patients' views were solicited concerning future accessibility of their electronic record via the internet. Fourteen per cent were extremely enthusiastic and had no security concerns, 54% expressed some concerns about security, but felt the concept was acceptable if the security matched that of the NHSNet, and 10% of patients were very unhappy about any use cf the internet. Twenty-two per cent did not respond:

> I'm worried about hackers — you hear all sorts of horror stories don't you. (User 47)

> Everyone has concerns about computer security. Nothing is really secure whether paper or a computer file. (User 43)

> Too much security might make it unnecessarily difficult. (User 81)

> What would people want with my health records anyway? (User 71)

> I am also concerned about security of paper records in reception and receptionists seeing my records. (User 49)

> I would be concerned at the possible lack of security with computer-held records, employers, insurance companies, etc., being able to access supposedly confidential information. (Focus group attender)

> I don't care who sees them, in fact it would be helpful to me, as a cardiac patient, if they were easily accessible. (Focus group attender)

> [...]

## Exploitation of the electronic patient record

Patients expressed concerns about the potential commercial use and exploitation of their data. Concern focused predominantly on data being accessed outside primary care by non-medical staff, other patients, employers, insurance companies, pharmaceutical companies, the government, police, social services, and computer hackers. Use for research or epidemiology was acknowledged as legitimate and acceptable, but patients wanted to be informed. They wanted to trust the process of anonymisation and to be assured that if the NHS sold their data the revenue would be used to benefit patients:

> If patients do participate in research for companies then perhaps money should be put into the NHS. (Focus group attender)

> Insurance companies are going to know anyway, they have to tell them about your health now. (Focus group attender)

> What if access was given to their employer and there were things they would rather that their employer didn't know about them? (Focus group attender)

## Receiving new information or bad news

Many patients have concerns about receiving new information; for example, test results or correspondence between health professionals. They were especially concerned if the information contained abnormal results or bad news. In the focus groups, patients said they would like to state how new information should be managed. The majority would prefer bad news to be held back until they could be informed by a health professional:

> I believe this is a good idea, and to have access via the internet, however I would prefer getting any bad news from a doctor rather than from a computer. (Focus group attender)

## Additional patient electronic patient record requirements

All patients were asked what else they would like to have seen in their electronic records (Box 22.3). In particular, they wished to write more personal statements about their wishes for care and the level of intervention in the event of serious health conditions, as well as their donor wishes. Patients wished to give a trusted individual access to their electronic patient record and authority to act for them if they were unable to make decisions owing to ill health:

> I would like details on whether test readings are normal. (User 39)

> I would like my records to show that in the event of serious loss of quality of life due to old age, injury or disease, I do not wish to be kept alive by medical intervention but would want to let nature take its course. (Focus group attender)

> I have a condition which I self manage with medication from the chemist, I would like to enter that information on the system. (User 11)

> I would like links to other useful health websites and more information about symptoms, etc. (User 34)

---

**Box 22.3. Patient requests**

- Additional registration details: next of kin, home circumstances, if widowed, details of children and dependents, cross references to family members' records, workplace details, patient consent, e-mail address
- Improved understanding: explanation of medical terms, use of easy-to-understand language, glossary of acronyms, imperial conversion for weight and height, normal ranges (for example, body mass index) for test results
- On-line services: repeat prescription orders, patient accessed appointment booking, results requests
- Additional health record information: histories going further back in time, blood group, reasons for medications, previous medications
- Options to add information about self-medication, nominated trusted individuals, wishes regarding living wills or wishes in the event of a serious illness regarding care or consent

---

[...]

# Discussion

## Key findings

Almost all patients found their session useful and could navigate around their health record easily. The majority found it easy to understand, although nearly half required clarification via a glossary. Most took about half an hour to view their record for the first time, although this depended on the length of the record and skill using computers. A third of patients used the print facility, but very few printed large amounts.

The advantages perceived by patients include: being better informed about their own health care and medication; being able to identify and correct errors and omissions, thus improving the accuracy and completeness of the electronic patient record (nearly a quarter found significant errors); being reminded of appointments and screening; that life wills, next of kin, and donor wishes could be added; that access to electronic patient records will assist NHS professionals caring for patients outside their own health centre. Before receiving abnormal results or bad news electronically, most patients would prefer to be told by a health professional first.

Patients have concerns about the security and confidentiality of electronic patient records, especially via the internet. However, provided they are confident of the security, two thirds of patients would like to able to access their record via the internet. Patients wish to be able to give consent as to who can access their electronic patient record.

[...]

## Implications for primary care

It had been anticipated that the computer literate would be the group most eager to view their records. However, it was the frequent users of health care who were the first patients, particularly older people, many of whom had no experience of computers.

Many patients are worried by the idea of seeing their own electronic patient record, but their concerns can be alleviated by effective communication of the advantages and by demonstration of the technology involved. … The participants may be a biased group who, in being willing to discuss their views, may also be more open minded to changing those views than others.

Patient access to electronic records is set to become routine within a few years. Patients needed time and explanations from the non-clinical support workers recruited specifically for this study. Widespread patient access will require the NHS to review its present workforce. Existing non-clinical personnel (Pyper, 2002) will require training and reallocation to work with patients if they are to become actively involved in the management of their electronic records and their health care.

Patients' access to their electronic patient records needs to be developed in partnership with patients and health professionals. Our experience is that working with patients keeps us focused on what matters to them. An electronic record based on internet technology that meets the legal, security and Caldicott standards could facilitate the delivery of a more efficient information infrastructure where the electronic record is linked with evidence-based health information sites on the internet.

# References

Aylward, G. W. and Parmar, D. N. (1999) 'Information technology in ophthalmology – experience with an electronic patient record', *British Journal of Ophthalmology*, 83(11): 1264–1267.

Coiera, E. (1996) 'The internet's challenge to health care provision', *British Medical Journal*, 312: 3–4.

DETR (2000) *Indices of Local Deprivation*. London: Department of the Environment, Transport and the Regions. Available online at: www.oxfordcity-pct.nhs.uk/vitalstats.pdf (accessed 28 Nov 2003).

Drury, M., Yudkin, P., Harcourt, J. et al. (2000) 'Patients with cancer holding their own records: a randomised controlled trial', *British Journal of General Practice*, 50(451): 105–110.

Fisher, B. and Britten, N. (1993) 'Patient access to records: expectations of hospital doctors and experiences of cancer patients', *British Journal of General Practice*, 43: 52–56.

Hassey, A., Gerrett, D. and Wilson, A. (2001) 'A survey of validity and utility of electronic patient records in a general practice', *British Medical Journal*, 322: 1401–1405.

Homer, C. S., Davis, G. K. and Everitt, L. S. (1999) 'The introduction of a woman-held record into a hospital antenatal clinic: the bring your own records study', *Australian and New Zealand Journal of Obstetrics and Gynaecology*, 39(1): 54–57.

Jones, R. B., McGhee, S. M. and McGhee, D. (1992) 'Patient on-line access to medical records in general practice', *Health Bulletin*, 50: 143–150.

Laerum, H., Ellingsen, G. and Faxvaag, A. (2001) 'Doctors' use of electronic medical records systems in hospitals: cross-sectional survey', *British Medical Journal*, 323: 1344–1348.

Liaw, T., Lawrence, M. and Rendell, J. (1996) 'The effect of a computer generated patient-held medical record summary and/or a written health record on patients' attitudes, knowledge and behaviour regarding health promotion', *Family Practitioner*, 12: 289–293.

Liaw, S. T., Radford, A. J. and Maddocks, I. (1998) 'The impact of a computer generated patient held health record', *Australian Family Physician*, 27 Supplement 1: S39–S43.

Pyper, C. (2002) 'Knowledge brokers as change agents', in R. Lissauer and L. Kendell (eds), *New Practitioners in the Future Health Service*. London: Institute of Public Policy Research, pp. 60–70.

Pyper, C., Amery, J., Watson, M. et al. (2001a) *Patient Access to Online Medical Records: Background Report*. Birmingham: NHS Information Authority (2001–1a–609). Available online at: www.nhsia.nhs.uk/erdip/pages/demonstrator/bury/bury_(2).pdf (accessed 10 Dec 2003).

Pyper, C., Amery, J., Watson, M. et al. (2001b) *Survey of Patient and Primary Health Care Team Perceptions and Attitudes on Electronic Health Records*. Birmingham: NHS Information Authority. Available online at: www.nhsia.nhs.uk/erdip/pages/demonstrator/bury/bury_(13).pdf (accessed 28 Nov 2003).

Wager, K. A., Wickam, L. F., White, A. W. et al. (2000) 'Impact of an electronic medical record system on community based primary care practices', *Journal of the American Board of Family Practice*, 13: 333–348.

# Chapter 23

## Positive action

*Vijay K. P. Patel*

*Consideration needs to be given to the needs of 'children affected adversely by the disability of another person in the family.'*

The emergence of HIV/AIDS has over the last fifteen years led to the development of some innovative practice and collaboration between health and social care agencies, with the focus primarily on HIV positive adults. As a result, there is a substantial range of literature and research on issues for adults living with HIV. It is an illness that impacts just as hard on their partners, children and extended family. Families as a whole have to come to terms with the potential losses and 'face up to the complex issues of how the virus was acquired, often with associated feelings of parental guilt, and involving subjects we least like to talk to children about: drug use; sexuality and death. All of this within a climate of stigma (Morton and Johnson, 1996).

The experience of working with adults with HIV/AIDS has been well documented. The voices and experiences of children affected are rarely heard and they are less likely to be supported. Batty, writing in 1993, said that 'children are especially vulnerable to the stigma' and support needed to be made available to them. This included the provision 'of a safe space in which they can ask questions and express feelings without risk of breach of confidentiality' (Batty, 1993).

In this context, lobbying led to the inclusion of children affected by HIV/AIDS as part of those affected by disability, and therefore considered to be in need within the Children (Scotland) Act 1995 (s. 93). Subsequent research demonstrated there were 741 known children affected by HIV in Scotland, of whom 52% were primary school age, and 76% lived with a parent or carer who was HIV positive (Children in Scotland, 1996). Other research by Imrie and Coombes (1995) calculated there were 3,000 children in the UK affected by HIV/AIDS and they concluded that 'children affected by HIV have distinct needs, which differ from those experienced by children affected by other life threatening illnesses,' primarily because of the social stigma and the unpredictable nature of the illness.

Originally published in *In on the Act – Barnados projects implementing the Children (Scotland) Act 1995*. London: Barnados, pp. 33–48.

The groupwork described below and carried out by a Barnardo's project is one attempt at working within a complex area. Secrecy, stigma, isolation, children's rights and parents' rights have made it hard to access these children, let alone create an environment in which children can express their fears and worries.

## Work of the project

The project works with affected families and aims to provide a flexible package of support services for families infected and affected by HIV/AIDS. The project was set up in 1993 as part of Barnardo's Agenda for Action programme, which had as one of its themes work with children affected by HIV/AIDS. It is based in two major Scottish cities[1] with two practitioners in each location. Working in partnership with parents, it is responsive to the practical and emotional needs of children.

The package can include all or some of the following:

1   Supporting and enabling parents to communicate with their children on HIV related issues e.g. lifestyle changes, preparation for bereavement, HIV disclosure, long-term care planning. Advising and supporting parents who may be experiencing difficulties coping with their children's responses to changed/stressful circumstances.
2   Assisting families to make appropriate short, medium and longer term care plans for their children.
3   Provision of pre- and post-bereavement support for children, individually and in group settings.
4   Provision of post-bereavement support for new carers, especially relatives, to enable them to support the bereaved child.
5   Provision of flexible respite care and practical support services for children, using carers and volunteers.
6   Developing in other agencies awareness of the needs of affected children, and acting as advocates for children in the agency network.

## Rationale and aims

As Dwivedi (1993: 5) notes, 'Latency age children, as a function of their particular stage in life, are very group orientated.... For them groupwork is an effective therapeutic approach, as it recreates the important social aspect of the child's life which occurs among the siblings, with the parents, at school, in the neighbourhood, and so forth'.

The isolation experienced by affected children is physical, social and psychological. One-to-one work with an adult allows a child to have some of their physical needs met in terms of being comforted and being able to find out information. There is, however, a strong need for a child to have his or her feelings normalised and or validated by their peers. 'The small group is a natural and highly attractive setting (Dwivedi, 1993:10) which can simulate the real world. In planning this group, the aims were worked out around a shared group of values which incorporated the rights of children to be informed, involved and listened to, in accordance with the UN Convention on Children, and the principles of the Children (Scotland) Act 1995. The aims were:

- **To provide activities/experiences which enhance a child's self esteem and make them feel good about themselves**. The impact of HIV/AIDS within the family can, and does, lead to a reduction in a child's confidence. The isolation experienced by a family impinges heavily on the children and can lead to a belief that they are not 'normal'. Unless a child is able to have some feelings of self worth, they are unlikely to be able to engage with any adult, no matter how well intentioned the person is.
- **To enable children to mutually support themselves and be aware they are not alone**. The secrecy within the family, along with the isolation outwith, does lead to the very clear belief that they are the only child in the world who is facing this.
- **To support children in identifying, understanding and expressing feelings**. The lack of self esteem and isolation may mean that the child does not have the know-how to communicate their feelings. The project needed to ensure that children were given a variety of tools to encourage self expression.
- **To provide appropriate information on HIV/AIDS**. Previous experiences had highlighted that whilst children may be able to use sophisticated language to talk about HIV/AIDS, this may not necessarily mean that they understand the concepts.
- **For the children to have fun wherever possible**. It is important that whilst working with difficult issues, we ensure that children clearly see that it is not all doom and gloom. If they enjoyed themselves in an easy and relaxed manner, they were more likely to reveal their fears and worries in the sessions.

# Value base

The community at large still commonly views HIV positive people as being 'bad, irresponsible and deserving their come-uppance'. This societal value and belief is one that these children share combined with a general failure by society to value children as individuals. Consequently there is an unwillingness to listen to or acknowledge their views.

This group was run on the basis that each person should be valued for who they are. Their different experiences should be acknowledged, and they should be accorded respect, listened to and supported equally. Within this area, issues of race, gender, language and disability needed to be challenged, especially as two of the three workers were male, whilst two were white Scottish, and one was British Asian.

If the children were to feel comfortable, then they needed to pick up a clear message, that in this group they were to be respected for being brave enough to come and face a topic that was frightening. They also needed to know that they would not be discriminated against because of the situations in which they lived. Whilst adults would be in charge to ensure the group's physical safety, the group would set the agenda and the pace at which it worked. This, as anybody who has run a group knows, is a challenging task.

# Referrals

The process for referrals in this area is complex because of the nature of secrecy, confidentiality and the potential conflict between an adult's right to confidentiality and a child's need to understand.

For obvious reasons, any child referred needed to be aware that there was someone in their family who was HIV positive. However before getting access to the children, the parent's trust and support needed to be gained. In talking with the parents/carers, the pain of coming to terms with the virus and the uncertainty that it brings to their lives was fully acknowledged. Time needed to be spent with the adults, not only to get their consent, but to ensure that such a group is something that they would value for their children. The quality of relationships that workers had with parents/carers was important in ensuring that the children understood that the important person/people in their lives trusted the workers and actively gave permission for the children to come knowing that HIV/AIDS would be mentioned and talked about. This element of partnership between parents and workers was vital in terms of the group starting on a good footing.

This whole process required a lot of time and even more flexibility. Fears around children being able to cope, children asking 'awkward questions' or telling everybody, all had to be resolved. Throughout, a clear message was given to parents and children, that it was alright to be scared or uncertain, and that it was *OK to say no*. The choice had to be with the parent and child.

Referrals could come directly from families, or via other helping agencies. A specific leaflet was produced for parents, with a different one for children. Both clearly stated that the group was for children who knew someone who was HIV positive.

Step one was talking to the parent/s and ensuring that there was written consent from the positive person for information to be disclosed. Parents were asked to describe what they thought the child understood about HIV/AIDS. Step two involved two of the co-workers meeting the parents and ensuring they understood the purpose and the potential not only for their confidentiality to be compromised, but also for problems as their child made sense of some of the issues. Step three was speaking to the child alone and ensuring that it was their choice to come to a group for children affected by HIV/AIDS.

Out of eight initial enquiries, five boys agreed to come: one was eight, two were ten and the other two were eleven. One of the boys who was HIV positive changed his mind because he felt he was not ready to be in a group where HIV was to be mentioned openly.

The remit of this [chapter] precludes discussion as to why only one girl was identified. We knew that the numbers of affected boys and girls was roughly equal. However one clear reason for the lack of referrals seems to be the perception that girls seem to cope much better and therefore require less input.

# Group structure

Children's lives are generally very dynamic and ever-changing. This is especially true in relation to affected children, where from week to week they may have to cope with an ill parent, living with an aunt/uncle, or experiencing difficulties in school, all of which may or may not be HIV-related.

A fixed structure, whilst meeting the aims of the group, would not necessarily meet the needs of the children. Previous experience with another group had highlighted the need for a lot of flexibility in programming. As a result, the initial programme plan was kept loose, within which broad themes were identified to be incorporated. In reviewing each week, we considered what may be needed to be addressed in the next session and how that could be done whilst continuing with the themes around change, loss, HIV and self-esteem.

Within each session, time was set aside at the beginning for food and general chat about events over the week and the plan for the session. Time would be left at the end to play some game, normally chosen by the group following protracted discussion and disagreement!

There were three co-workers. This provided flexibility, and the potential to provide a lot of attention to each child. It also meant that the group could continue if one worker had to deal with an emergency. The programme is described below:

Week 1   Games, self portrait, city map, question box, visit to hill-top view of city
Week 2   Graffiti wall, city map
Week 3   Video exercises
     (a) miming feelings,
     (b) role play of scenes directed by the boys
Week 4   All about me, Simon Says, video role plays related to family settings including illness, rules and family conflict.
Week 5   Trust game, quiz on worries and concerns about HIV, preparing questions for the doctor and nurses session.
Week 6   Survey of boys in city, video interview with paediatrician and nurse
Week 7   Visit to HIV organisation, certificate ceremony, trip to hill-top view for photos and a bag of chips. Goodbyes, final thoughts and feelings.

# Methodology, process and symbolism of the sessions

Forgetful memories meant for the first two weeks only two children attended. By week four, all had Tuesday afternoons associated with being together and would be waiting at their front doors. The child who was HIV positive decided to come to the last session, after having listened to his brother rave about the group. He was warmly welcomed by the others and said he regretted not having gone to the other sessions.

In considering the benefits of this group, much of the learning for the boys came not from direct input but from the symbolism behind the work. This ties in with a point made by Dwivedi (1993) about experiential groups, that the 'effective therapeutic element occurs through the situation each child creates within the group', (Keepers, 1987) and that these situations can then go on to create positive learning experiences, either naturally, or with the guidance of the therapist.

## Conflict

Throughout the life of the group, there was continual conflict either between the boys or between the boys and co-workers. At the time, it felt that there was no progression. Given their ages, a certain amount of fighting was to be expected, especially as they needed to establish their own identities within this group. Group members were also very skilful at defending themselves emotionally. As a result fighting was used as a way of avoiding or deflecting some thing they perceived to be 'hurtful'.

The subject of HIV is 'terrifying' and consequently, the boys used challenging behaviour to avoid the subject. This could take the form of demands to play 'games' and the regular comment that 'this is boring'. This required a lot of management in terms of continually having to reaffirm the reason for this group, whilst being sensitive to the feelings that were being raised. Part of this was dealt with by taking the conflict back to the group and with choices of continuing or stopping because they were unable to manage. Whilst it looked as though some sessions would finish prematurely, all the sessions went to time and the tasks were achieved.

This required a lot of control and appeared contrary to the aim of the boys taking the lead. However it was important to give them a message that the adults in this group were neither scared of HIV, nor of talking about it. The adults had to support them in dealing with their fears, by being open, explicit and at times continuing with a task rather than going with the wishes of the group. This was very important in terms of the boys seeing that there were adults who were prepared to deal with this 'monster'.

## The city map

This was a poster about 3m by 3m in which workers drew the boundaries of the boys' home city. They drew places they liked, where they lived, places they would go to etc. This drew together the commonalities for the boys such as schools, family, places they like. It also showed visually that HIV was not related to one area or one family, but affected a number of families throughout the city. It allowed us to state at a very early stage, in a clear and safe manner, the reason why all the boys were there: they all knew someone living in their city who had the virus.

## Poster

This was a blank sheet with the words HIV & AIDS written on it. The seemingly straight-forward task was to write or draw anything that you knew or had heard about the virus. In doing this there was a lot of embarrassment and giggling along with graphic penile drawings. This was important at a later stage in terms of creating the environment where the boys could use their own language to talk about condoms, women, gay men, needles etc. Much of the language was used to test the co-workers to see if they would blush or get embarrassed. While acknowledging that the boys were testing, the adults also had to challenge some of the comments made about gay men and about women in a manner which encouraged them to think about their views. The poster demonstrated that although they knew certain words, they did not necessarily understand their meanings.

## Question box

Throughout the life of the group, a box was always left in a fairly visible place, into which anybody could place statements or questions. Whilst only used once by a child, it acknowledged that there are a lot of things which they might want to find out about but were too afraid/embarrassed, or did not know how, to ask directly. One boy used this strategy with his carer after the group finished as his way of letting her know what was on his mind and what he needed to talk about.

## Video

A camcorder was used in sessions three, four and six. At one level, using an expensive piece of equipment demonstrated trust in them especially as the group could be very active. The trust was fully repaid in terms of the care they showed and the skill that was developed in using it. The process of acting on camera and then watching, is very risky, especially if users have little belief in themselves. By first of all playing and then moving onto role plays, the boys developed confidence and were able to watch themselves and laugh genuinely at their antics. In the latter sessions, each in their own way was able to demonstrate their understanding about family dynamics, and feelings that parents and children especially have towards illness. The session with the paediatrician demonstrated not only their concern about HIV, but also their progression, to be able to ask a stranger very direct questions and to be filmed doing so.

## Survey

By week six, workers were able to identify common threads. Out of them they made up a survey, including such statements as 'Some boys feel they are to blame for their parent/s becoming ill' and 'Some boys feel confused because no one has explained about HIV/AIDS to them'. This allowed all the boys to be able to identify their concerns, without having to make a personal statement. The discussion around these statements, proved to be heated, and surprisingly, everyone did make their own personal identification. One boy decided to write another one up which the rest of the group agreed with, which was 'Some boys and girls feel bad because their mum or dad has HIV'.

## Doctor's visit

The group had been building up towards a visit by a paediatrician and a specialist HIV community nurse who were going to be filmed answering questions prepared by the group. This was seen as being very important by the boys and the feeling of letdown and frustration was clearly evidenced in the chaos that resulted from the visitors being late. The following twenty minutes were the quietest in the life of this group as everybody clearly concentrated on the responses of the visitors to their questions. In arriving at this point, the boys were symbolically receiving a number of messages. The fact that two people, who traditionally hold a high position within the community, were coming to their group (the opposite of normally having to go to the surgery). The two visitors were prepared to be interviewed and listen to their questions and took time to answer them as honestly and as clearly as possible. The agenda had been set and was being controlled by the boys, their worries, fears and concerns were being valued and responded to. Everybody received a copy of the video at the end of the group. Feedback from parents highlighted the learning they had acquired. An unforeseen benefit was that the child could watch the video again and again to refresh or check out specific information.

## Ending

Given the potential losses these children were going to face, it was important that the final session be finished properly. It took place in Body Positive (a centre for HIV positive people) where they were welcomed and introduced to the facilities. There was a ceremony in which each child received two certificates, one for their parents and one for them to keep. The certificates were awarded for each child 'For coming along to the Tuesday Group, For being brave enough to take part, For trusting other boys and adults', along with commendations for skills such as painting, juggling and asking questions. They also received a card which reminded them that if they had a question or a worry either ask someone you trust or ring – ****** on 123456. The group then went to the chippie before heading onto a major hill in the city. This had become a favourite place not only for the view, but because it symbolised that they were not the only children coping with HIV in this city. As part of the ending, they were asked to say one thing they liked and one thing they enjoyed. It proved very hard to end, as none of them wanted to say goodbye.

## Outcomes

The boys at the end of the group, all stated that this was a group which they had enjoyed and one which they would wish to continue. The value they placed was in the fact that they could play, but around that was the fact that they learnt something about HIV/AIDS as well.
  In referring to the aims:

*To provide activities/experiences which enhance a child's self esteem and make them feel good about themselves:* At the end each person received a certificate (including workers) highlighting successes such as learning to juggle, acting and a copy of the video. All the carers reported the enjoyment in their children especially as they sat through the video.

*To enable children to mutually support themselves and be aware they are not alone:* The boys felt that they belonged to and owned this group in terms of agreeing/disagreeing on what games to play, who should take what role when they were role playing etc. In one session, a ball landed on the roof and the boys were determined to recover it, not because it gave them a chance to do some climbing, but because it belonged to one of the co-workers. The city map highlighted their commonality, as the football highlighted their common interest.

*To support children in identifying, understanding and expressing feelings:* Some of the video role plays, along with the survey, provided the opportunities for each of them to learn and to express their feelings. The active discussion around the survey highlighted the fact that they had been aware of the issues and were able to express the feelings they had as affected children.

*To provide appropriate information on HIV/AIDS:* Through the sessions, the words HIV/AIDS, sex etc. became more public, more acceptable and the group were able to move beyond the 'giggling stage', to talk about illness, HIV prevention and sexual behaviour. An unforeseen bonus was the video which allowed children to go back and check information if they felt uncertain.

*The children to have fun wherever possible:* A year later the boys are still talking about the group. During its life there was a lot of hilarity, especially with the video role plays, as well as conflicts. The clearest indicator that the boys enjoyed it was the fact that by week four, they were waiting at the door to be picked up and they hated finishing.

There were some processes which enabled this group to work:

1   The structure allowed the boys to create their own opportunities to bring their concerns to the attention of either the workers or the other boys, in their own time.
2   Through all of this there was a clear message by co-workers that they would deal with any difficulties and try to take appropriate action. This meant that there was a lot of policing, but this was important for some members as they had not experienced adults being prepared to stop them. This needs to be emphasised, because for one boy it provided him with the clear message that in this setting, there were adults who were not scared of him and could deal with his feelings no matter how strong they were.
3   Four out of the five who attended had at least some experience of 'work' which was related to their feelings, which was not in a classroom context. Consequently the boys came knowing that as part of the session they would have to 'work', no matter how much they denied it. The one who did not have the experience of one-to-one, however came with a clear and verbalised agenda of waiting to find out more about HIV and AIDS.
4   Having a boys' group was seen as advantageous with hindsight, although that was not the intention. Developmentally boys and girls tend to stick to same sex groups at this age and potentially the different emotional responses may have caused the group to become to divided. The experiences that some of the boys came with and the behaviours exhibited could perhaps not have been as well accepted in a mixed gender group.

Visits to the boys and their parents/carers a month after the group finished highlighted some differences that parents perceived, which they attributed as being positive and coming directly from attending the group. In considering the benefits it would be useful to provide two case studies. (Names have been changed to maintain anonymity)

**Martin** aged 9, had a number of poor experiences of exclusion in school, and he was someone who was perceived to need a lot of adult supervision as he was hard to manage in groups. His behaviour within the group did ameliorate, but the significance for Martin was how the behaviour was interpreted. He found it hard to concentrate for long periods of time, or if the subject was uncomfortable or distressing. As a result he would want to do something else, normally distracting everybody else. Martin had developed a very skilful defence that protected him and his family which primarily meant that he acted up to deflect everybody's attention from the real concerns. Within this group setting, Martin was able to pick up two messages: that there were adults who were not scared; and who would look after him. As a child who was labelled as being 'out of control', this was vital in order to ensure he could cope. This would also free him up in knowing that there were adults who would give clear messages to him that they were not confused or had a hidden agenda. As a result through the course of the group, whilst he would stop doing an activity himself, he did not stop others and would play or take a walk outside.

Following the end of the group, feedback from Martin and his parents highlighted several significant changes. He has 'slowed' down and appeared calmer and more relaxed. Martin himself missed going on Tuesday nights. He had enjoyed it and although he wanted to keep going, he accepted that it was more important for other children to be given the chance. His parents felt that his behaviour had changed markedly and that he looked less troubled and was talking to them much more. As a result they were more relaxed and consequently able to focus on all the positives that Martin had. Over the course of the group Martin was able to grow, instead of remaining stuck as a 'problem child'.

**Anthony**, aged 10, was experiencing instability during the group sessions. His parent was ill and he was being moved between relatives until he finally settled with a grandmother. He had already experienced the loss of one parent to HIV/AIDS. He had identified that a group for children would be a good idea and came charging in every week. He was accepted within it and valued as part of it. Anthony was very desperate for information but was unable to accept attention focused on him. For him the activities were important as they allowed him to participate and have his concerns raised indirectly. The camcorder was invaluable for him as it allowed him to listen whilst having the excuse that he 'wasn't really listening, he was just filming'. In one role play where he was the social worker talking to an ill parent, he was clearly able to demonstrate his understanding of the situation that he was experiencing in reality, and his awareness of how adults around him were trying to make decisions. Anthony found himself making very clear and powerful statements such as 'boys and girls feel bad because their parents are HIV positive'. After the group finished, he started leaving notes for his granny with questions or worries that he could not express directly.

Since the group finished, each child has either had ongoing or follow up contact with one of the co-workers. There have been clear benefits in terms of how the relationship between child and worker has strengthened, as has the relationship between child and parent/carer and parent and worker. The Tuesday Group seemed to symbolically represent a safe space to talk. Consequently the children now talk far more freely, and meaningfully about the virus. HIV seems to have lost its former power. Instead of being talked about in hushed tones, it is something more commonplace. As a result the boys have individually chosen specific people (in most cases parents) in whom they will confide alongside the worker.

## Conclusions

As noted earlier, the Tuesday Group was seen as being of value both to the boys who attended, and their parents. A year on, the boys who attended still refer to it as being a positive and important experience.

The group was both risky and exciting. By encouraging them to take some risks, they were asked to face some of the pain that many other people would choose to avoid. The risk of going into these 'uncharted waters' was well worth it for the group in terms of the learning and fun they experienced. In the process, the children were also able to develop some respect for themselves and each other. They also had the opportunity to make informed choices. For many, they were also able to take information home and that could form a safe basis from which to talk to their parent/carer about their worries.

In reflecting on this process, parents and carers were not involved as much as originally planned, partly because the programme was being directed by the group, and partly due to lack of time. In planning for a future group, it would be invaluable for parents to be given the opportunity to meet and to discuss their concerns and strategies for coping. A useful model would be the one set up by a hospice where parents/carers met in one room whilst children were in another. A natural progression would have been for some joint meeting where the boys could present their material. However in working with these children it was important to have a defined ending and allow them to see that it was possible to finish something you did not want to end, and still cope with it.

The strength of this group lay in its value base of acknowledging how painful this subject is and according everybody involved the respect they deserved. The parent's involvement and courage was crucial in allowing their children to attend, especially as they were not to know what the child might come home and ask. In moving on, the boys were able to express that this was a group that would be good for other children to attend, as did their parents.

To quote from Anthony

*The Tuesday Group is for somebody who knows people with HIV/AIDS and it was only for boys and girls. \*\*\*\*\* managed to get a doctor to tell us about the virus, how to catch it and there are three different ways, one is injecting needles, two sex with some one who has the virus and three babies who get it through their mother. We play games and video film [camcorder] and we got a bag of chips and then went up to the [hill in the city].*

# Note

1   The cites involved have not been named in order to protect the anonymity of the individuals quoted in the report.

# References

Batty, D. (ed.) (1993) *HIV Infection and Children in Need*. British Association for Adoption and Fostering, p. 135.

Children in Scotland (1996) *Children Affected by HIV and AIDS in Scotland*. Children in Scotland.

Dwivedi, K. N. (ed.) (1993) *Groupwork with Children and Adolescents: A Handbook*. London: Jessica Kingsley.

Imrie, J. and Coombes, Y. (1995) *No Time to Waste: The Scale and Dimension of the Problem of Children Affected by HIV/AIDS in the UK*. Essex: Barnardos.

Keepers, T. D. (1987) 'Group treatment of children: practical considerations and techniques', in P. A. Keller and S. R. Heymen (eds), *Innovations in Clinical Practice 6*. Sarasota, FL: Professional Resources Exchange, pp. 165–175.

Morton, S. and Johnson, D. (eds) (1996) *Children and HIV*: *Supporting Children and Their Families*. London: HMSO.

# Section 4
## Ideas

## Introduction

The final section of the book focuses on some of the ideas that underpin the provision of health and social care in the 21st century. Chapter 28, for example, deals with ethics and evidence based care, ideas which have created much debate in health and social care in recent years.

It may seem strange that the opening anthology chapter combines the writings of psychologists John Bowlby on attachment and Abraham Maslow on human motivation with the feminist writings of Janet Finch and Hilary Graham about care and the pioneering work of Vic Finkelstein in relation to disability rights. If one looks at teaching materials in relation to health and social care, however, one finds that Bowlby and Maslow invariably feature: their work has had an enduring impact, as has the work of feminists and disability rights activists.

Chapter 26 by Bytheway and Johnson provides a broader context for the extract by Janet Finch. It focuses on the concept of 'carers', one now central to health and social policy and practice but which some 30 years ago barely existed. Drawing on ideas around social construction, it traces the development of the carers' movement. Interestingly, since this chapter was first written, the term 'carer' has been extended to paid workers as well as 'informal carers' and this, understandably, has led to strong objections from carers' organisations as it threatens their political base.

Jan Walmsley's chapter (27) traces the history of policies for people with learning difficulties between 1971 and 2001. She detects a shift from services being underpinned by the notion of care to being underpinned by the notion of citizenship. The final section of the chapter includes an interesting comparison of the two White Papers *Better Services for the Mentally Handicapped* (1971) and *Valuing People* (2001). Walmsley concludes that whilst there has been some progress, it is varied, with some categories of people with learning difficulties benefiting more than others.

The other chapters in this section are also about the development of social policies: policies which are based in ideas that derive from philosophy, politics and economics about how society and its institutions should be organised. Chapter 25 discusses reactions to the Beveridge Report of 1942 which laid the foundations of the British welfare state. The accounts from nonagenarians contained in the anthology in Section 1 of this book are a reminder of what life was like before Beveridge set out his plan to tackle the five giants of want, ignorance, disease, squalor and idleness. Later in the section, we have included a chapter by Vic George and Paul Wilding about the New Right, or what at that time they referred to as the 'anti-collectivists'. This chapter is taken from the first edition of their book *Ideology and Social Welfare*, published in 1985 when the radical change in direction of social policy was beginning to bite. It is interesting to look back to this analysis of Thatcher's Britain 20 years on. The following chapter (30) by David Coates reflects on the legacy inherited by the new government in 1997 when the Labour Party was returned to power after 18 years. He presents the reader with a society that has become more polarised between the 'haves' and the 'have nots', a society with an infrastructure suffering from years of underinvestment and with health and welfare services inadequate to meet the needs of an ageing population. The final chapter brings us into the 21st century. Drawing on the notion of the 'Inverse Care Law' proposed by the socialist general practitioner, Julian Tudor Hart, which argues that health care is provided in inverse proportion to need, Mary Shaw and Danny Dorling propose a 'Positive Care Law' which states that where informal care is most needed it is provided. Based on research, these two complementary laws are something of an indictment of the health and welfare services in Britain today and demonstrate the continuing inequalities in service provision in the 21st century.

# Chapter 24

## Anthology: ideas

*Compiled by Julia Johnson and Andy Northedge*

The extracts in this anthology reflect just some of the ideas that have had an enduring influence on developments in health and social care. Two writers, John Bowlby and Abraham Maslow, are psychologists whose ideas still feature in the education of health and social care workers. Bowlby's work on attachment has been particularly influential in the field of child care while Maslow's work on human motivation is still used as a framework for understanding the concept of need. Janet Finch and other feminist academics were instrumental in bringing the plight of women carers to public attention and Vic Finkelstein was a founder member of the Union of the Physically Impaired Against Segregation (UPIAS) and the disability rights movement.

Although this is only a tiny selection of important writers, what they have in common is that their work has been not only extremely influential but also highly controversial and the subject of much academic and political debate.

## 24.1   The influence of Abraham Maslow

Abraham Maslow's book, *Motivation and Personality*, first published in 1954, became the foundation of his life's work in humanistic psychology. The extract below is taken from the Foreword to the third edition (published in 1987). It is written by Robert Frager, who explains Maslow's influence.

[...]

When Maslow began his career, there were only two major forces in psychology: the experimental, behaviorist approach and the clinical, psychoanalytic approach. These models were not sufficient for Maslow. 'On the whole ... I think it fair to say that human history is a record of the ways in which human nature has been sold short. The highest possibilities of human nature have practically always been underestimated' (1971: 7).

In his intellectual career Maslow sought to balance this underestimation with ground-breaking investigations of the highest possibilities for human growth and development.

He was instrumental in the emergence of two major new forces in psychology: the humanistic and the transpersonal. Both explore the full, rich complexity of human nature without restricting human behavior to a mechanistic or pathological model.

Maslow's greatest strength was in his ability to ask significant questions. He posed questions for psychology that are central to the lives of all of us: What is it to be a good human being? Of what are human beings capable? What makes for happy, creative, fulfilled human beings? How can we determine that a person has fully actualized his or her potentialities unless we know what those potentialities are? How can we truly transcend the immaturity and insecurity of childhood, and under what circumstances can we do so? How can we develop a complete model of human nature, honoring our extraordinary potentional, without losing sight of our nonrational, nonaccomplishing side? What motivates psychologically healthy individuals?

[...]

The creative questions that Maslow asked continue to inspire important insights into human nature and encourage farther exploration.

Maslow's life was dedicated to the study of people that he considered to be psychologically healthy: 'indeed, self-actualizing people, those who have come to a high level of maturation, health and self-fulfillment, have so much to teach us that sometimes they seem almost like a different breed of human beings' (Maslow, 1968: 71).

He discovered that human functioning is different for people who operate in a state of positive health rather than a state of deficiency. Maslow called this new approach 'Being-psychology.' He found that self-actualizing people were motivated by 'Being-values.' These are values that are naturally developed by healthy human beings and are not imposed by religion or culture. He maintained that 'we have come to the point in biological history where we are now responsible for our own evolution. We have become self-evolvers. Evolution means selecting and therefore choosing and deciding, and this means valuing' (1971: 11). The values that self-actualizers appreciate include truth, creativity, beauty, goodness, wholeness, aliveness, uniqueness, justice, simplicity, and self-sufficiency.

Maslow's study of human nature led him to many conclusions, including these central ideas:

1   Human beings have an innate tendency to move toward higher levels of health, creativity, and self-fulfillment.
2   Neurosis may be regarded as a blockage of the tendency toward self-actualization.
3   The evolution of a synergistic society is a natural and essential process. This is a society in which *all* individuals may reach a high level of self-development, without restricting each others' freedom.
4   Business efficiency and personal growth are not incompatible. In fact, the process of self-actualization leads each individual to the highest levels of efficiency.

In 1968 Maslow commented that the revolution inside psychology that he spearheaded had become solidly established. 'Furthermore, it is beginning to be *used,* especially in education, industry, religion, organization and management, therapy and self improvement ...' (p. iii) Indeed, his work is an integral part of the dominant intellectual trends of this century. [...]

## References

Maslow, A. (1968) *Toward a Psychology of Being*, 2nd edn. New York: Van Nostrand.

Maslow, A. (1971) *The Farther Reaches of Human Nature*. New York: Viking Press.

*Source*: Abraham H. Maslow (1987) *Motivation and Personality*. New York: Harper & Row, pp. xxxiii–xxxvi. First published 1954.

# 24.2    John Bowlby on the beginnings of attachment behaviour

In his two volumes on *Attachment and Loss*, first published in 1969, Bowlby set out his ideas about the immense significance of the relationships infants form with their primary carers. In Chapter 14, from which this first extract is taken, he describes the way attachment behaviour develops in infants. At the time he wrote this it was the convention to refer to the infant as 'he'.

... [I]t is convenient to divide this development into a number of phases, though it must be recognised that there are no sharp boundaries between them.

### Phase I: Orientation and signals with limited discrimination of figure

During this phase an infant behaves in certain characteristic ways towards people but his ability to discriminate one person from another is limited to olfactory and auditory stimuli. The phase lasts from birth to not less than eight weeks of age, and more usually to about twelve weeks; it may continue much longer in unfavourable conditions.

The ways in which a baby behaves towards any person in his vicinity include orientation towards that person, tracking movements of the eyes, grasping and reaching, smiling and babbling. Often a baby ceases to cry on hearing a voice or seeing a face. [...] After about twelve weeks the intensity of these friendly responses rises. Thenceforward he gives 'the full social response in all its spontaneity, vivacity and delight' (Rheingold, 1961).

### Phase 2: Orientation and signals directed towards one (or more) discriminated figure(s)

During this phase an infant continues to behave towards people in the same friendly way as in Phase I, but he does so in more marked fashion towards his mother-figure than towards others. [...] The phase lasts until about six months of age, or much later according to the circumstances.

### Phase 3: Maintenance of proximity to a discriminated figure by means of locomotion as well as signals

During this phase not only is an infant increasingly discriminating in the way he treats people but his repertoire of responses extends to include following a departing mother, greeting her on her return, and using her as a base from which to explore. Concurrently, the friendly and rather undiscriminating responses to everyone else wane. Certain other people are selected to become subsidiary attachment-figures; others are not so selected. Strangers become treated with increasing caution, and sooner or later are likely to evoke alarm and withdrawal.

[...]

Phase 3 commonly begins between six and seven months of age but may be delayed until after the first birthday, especially in infants who have had little contact with a main figure. It probably continues throughout the second year and into the third.

### Phase 4: Formation of a goal-corrected partnership

During Phase 3 ... the mother-figure herself comes sooner or later to be conceived as an independent object, persistent in time and space and moving more or less predictably in space-time continuum. ... [H]owever, we cannot suppose that a child has any understanding of what is influencing his mother's movements to or away from him, or of what measures he can take that will change her behaviour. [...]

Sooner or later, however, this changes. By observing her behaviour and what influences it, a child comes to infer something of his mother's set-goals and something of the plans she is adopting to achieve them. From that point onwards his picture of the world becomes far more sophisticated and his behaviour is potentially more flexible. To use another language, it can be said that a child is acquiring insight into his mother's feelings and motives. Once that is so, the groundwork is laid for the pair to develop a much more complex relationship with each other, one that I term a partnership.

[...]

*Source*: J. Bowlby (1997) *Attachment and Loss: Volume 1, Attachment.* London: Hogarth Press, pp. 266–268. [abridged]. First published 1969.

---

# 24.3    John Bowlby on focusing on a figure

In Chapter 15 of *Attachment and Loss*, from which this second extract is taken, Bowlby discusses the different figures to which a child may become attached.

---

[...]

... almost from the first many children have more than one figure towards whom they direct attachment behaviour; these figures are not treated alike; the role of a child's principal attachment-figure can be filled by others than the natural mother.

### Principal and subsidiary attachment-figures

During their second year of life a great majority of infants are directing their attachment behaviour towards more than one discriminated figure, and often towards several. Some infants select more than one attachment-figure almost as soon as they begin to show discrimination; but probably most come to do so rather later.

Of fifty-eight Scottish infants studied by Schaffer and Emerson (1964a), 17 (29 per cent) are reported to have been directing attachment behaviour towards more than one figure almost from the time they started showing it to anyone. After another four months not only had half the children more than one attachment-figure but a number of them had as many as five or more different attachment-figures. By the time these children had reached eighteen months of age, those who still restricted their attachment behaviour to only one figure had fallen to 13 per cent of the sample; which means that for a child of eighteen months still to have only one attachment-figure is quite exceptional. Ainsworth's findings for the Ganda show a comparable state of affairs: all but a tiny minority were showing multiple attachments by nine or ten months of age.

Nevertheless, although by twelve months a plurality of attachment-figures is probably the rule, these attachment figures are not treated as the equivalents of one another. In each of the two cultures considered the infants show clear discrimination. In the case of the Scottish sample a scale was devised for measuring the intensity of protest that a child exhibited on being left by each figure. Results showed that for most children there was regularly more protest when he was left by one figure than by another, and that a child's attachment-figures could be arranged in hierarchical order. Using a broader range of criteria Ainsworth found than Ganda children tended to focus most of their attachment behaviour on one special person. Up till about nine months of age, she observed, a child with more than one attachment-figure nevertheless tended to confine actual following to a single figure. Moreover, when a child was hungry, tired, or ill he usually turned specifically to that figure. Other figures, on the other hand, were sought when a child was in good spirits: such a figure might be an older child who was in the habit of playing with him.

[...]

## The principal attachment-figure

It is evident that whom a child selects as his principal attachment-figure, and to how many other figures he becomes attached, turn in large part on who cares for him and on the composition of the household in which he is living. As a matter of empirical fact there can be no doubt that in virtually every culture the people in question are most likely to be his natural mother, father, older siblings, and perhaps grandparents, and that it is from amongst these figures that a child is most likely to select both his principal attachment-figure and his subsidiary figures.

In both the Scottish study and the Ganda study only those children who were living with their natural mother were selected for observation. In those circumstances it is not surprising that in an overwhelming proportion of cases a child's principle attachment-figure was his natural mother. There were, however, a few exceptions. Two Ganda children of about nine months, one a boy and one a girl, were said to be attached to both mother and father but to prefer father, in the boy's case even when he was tired or ill. A third Ganda child, a girl, showed no attachment to her mother even at twelve months, but instead was attached to her father and a half-sister.

Amongst the Scottish infants mother was almost always principal attachment-figure throughout the first year of life, but in some cases came to share the role, usually with father, during the second year. There were, however, three out of fifty-eight Scottish infants whose first attachment-figure was said to have been someone other than mother: two chose father and a third, whose mother was in full-time work, chose grandmother who looked after him most of the day. [...]

Observations such as these and many others make it abundantly clear that, although it is usual for a child's natural mother to be his principal attachment-figure, the role can be taken effectively by others. Such evidence as we have is that, provided a mother-substitute behaves in a mothering way towards a child, he will treat her as another child would treat his natural mother. Just what comprises a 'mothering way' of treating a child is discussed in the next section. Briefly, it appears to be engaging in lively social interaction with him, and responding readily to his signals and approaches.

Though there can be no doubt that a substitute mother can behave in a completely mothering way to a child, and that many do so, it may well be less easy for a substitute mother than for a natural mother to do so. For example, knowledge of what elicits mothering behaviour in other species suggests that hormonal levels following parturition and stimuli emanating from the newborn baby himself may both be of great importance. If this is so for human mothers also, a substitute mother must be at a disadvantage compared with a natural mother. On the one hand, a substitute cannot be exposed to the same hormonal levels as the natural mother; on the other, a substitute may have little or nothing to do with the baby to be mothered until he is weeks or months old. In consequence of both these limitations, a substitute's mothering responses may well be less strong and less consistently elicited than those of a natural mother.

### Subsidiary figures

It has already been remarked that we may need to distinguish more carefully than has hitherto been done between attachment-figures and playmates. A child seeks his attachment-figure when he is tired, hungry, ill, or alarmed and also when he is uncertain of that figure's whereabouts; when the attachment-figure is found he wants to remain in proximity to him or her may want also to be held or cuddled. By contrast, a child seeks a playmate when he is in good spirits and confident of the whereabouts of his attachment-figure; when the playmate is found, moreover, the child wants to engage in playful interaction with him or her.

If this analysis is right, the roles of attachment-figure and playmate are distinct. Since, however, the two roles are not incompatible, it is possible for any one figure at different times to fill both roles: thus a child's mother may at times act both as playmate and as principal attachment-figure, and another person, for example an older child, who acts mainly as playmate may on occasion act also as a subsidiary attachment-figure.

[...]

*Source*: J. Bowlby (1997) *Attachment and Loss: Volume 1, Attachment*. London: Hogarth Press, Pimlico edition, pp. 304–307. [abridged]. First published 1969.

## 24.4    Janet Finch on non-sexist alternatives to community care

In her article 'Community care: developing non-sexist alternatives' published in *Critical Social Policy* in 1984, Janet Finch reiterated the thesis that community care means care by the family, which means care by women. She explores alternative ways of providing care that would not involve the exploitation of women. In this extract she discusses Hilary Graham's reservations about this approach.

---

[...]

Hilary Graham's article[1] is an exploration of the concept of caring. Her central theme is that caring is both labour and love. Social policy analyses of caring have tended to emphasise the labour involved, but rather overlooked the fact that caring means caring *about* as well as caring *for* in our culture. In both senses, she argues that the relationship is defined in gender terms: women *are* the people who care (in both senses), the activity of caring significantly defines women's identity, and it takes place in the 'private' sphere where women are found. The experience of caring is 'the medium through which women are accepted and feel they belong in the social world'. Caring most certainly *is* labour for women, but (unlike the labour-contracts negotiated through the cash-nexus) it is work whose form and content is shaped by our intimate social and sexual relationships. Recent feminist work on caring, she argues, whilst it has correctly shown the exploitation of women's labour and the benefits to the state which it entails, has tended to 'underplay the symbolic bonds which hold the caring relationship together.' [...]

Graham's perceptive and sensitive analysis pushes us away from any slick solutions to the problem of women-as-carers. We may profoundly disapprove of women's social identity being so significantly defined by their relationships with other people, but while that remains the case, the prospects for non-sexist forms of caring remain bleak. Further, a recognition that caring *about* is frequently (although not necessarily) intertwined with caring *for* a dependent person should make us wary of any proposals for non-sexist forms of care which overlook the dimension of affection, which of course is not confined to people who are related through kinship or marriage. That is not to argue that, because I care 'about' someone I must necessarily care 'for' them; but it is to argue that I may *choose* to do so. Of course, that 'choice' can be real only if other alternatives actually exist; and, because at the present time most people do *not* have a range of alternatives, it is profoundly insulting to claim that many thousands of women now caring for their relatives have 'chosen' to do so. But in a future in which women were *not* required to provide care merely through want of alternatives, it might well be that both women and men would sometimes want to care 'for' those people whom we also care 'about' – not because care by relatives or friends is inherently superior to other kinds of care, but because it has a dimension of continuity on the affectional level which strangers can never provide. Any alternative policy for looking after highly dependent people would have to take account of the dimension of love as well as labour. But again, it is difficult to see how one could then avoid sliding into a situation where, *de facto*, women were the ones who 'chose' to provide care, unless the whole argument is to assume fundamental change in the cultural designation of women as carers.

Graham's work also casts some doubt upon the solution to the impasse of community care to which I had been previously attracted: the residential alternative. Of course, residential care as it exists now also exploits women in low-paid, often part-time work, and is an alternative that many dependent people and their relatives actively resist, if at all possible. Nonetheless, it is possible to envisage different forms of residential provision which would not exploit women in low-paid jobs, and which would be organised to give the cared-for maximum privacy and autonomy, to leave them less isolated from the healthy, and so on: that is, forms of residential facility which avoid the worst features of 'institutions.' Given that kind of provision, we might hope that the legacy of the workhouse could be overcome, and that residential provision could become acceptable – even popular – with the dependent population in need of care, just as sheltered housing has so proved with fit elderly people. [...] Graham's identification of the importance of the relational aspects of care, however, at least should make us pause before opting for this solution because, as she puts it, discussions of this issue, by underplaying the affectional aspects of caring, have tended to lose sight of 'people's deep resistance to the socialisation of care.' If her analysis is correct, the barriers to that resistance cannot be removed straight-forwardly by providing better facilities and proper paid staff, but we have to take some account of that dimension of resistance which derives from people's desire to care and be cared 'for' by those whom they also care 'about.'

### Note

1  H. Graham (1983) 'Caring: a labour of love', in J. Finch and D. Groves (eds), *A Labour of Love: Women, Work and Caring*. London: Routledge & Kegan Paul.

*Source*: Janet Finch (1984) 'Community care: developing non-sexist alternatives', *Critical Social Policy*, 9: 6–18. [Extract].

## 24.5   Vic Finkelstein on uniting physically impaired people against segregation

In a keynote address at the Disability History Week in June 2002, which is reproduced on the Leeds University Disability Studies website, Vic Finkelstein describes his South African upbringing and experiences as a political prisoner under the apartheid regime. At the age of 15 he broke his neck while pole vaulting and, as he puts it, 'left the world as I was and then re-entered as a "disabled person"'. In the extract from his address, reproduced below, he describes how, as a political exile, he became involved in disability politics in Britain.

### Role models

For me arriving in Britain was a liberation, a new beginning. Despite all the daily restrictions imposed on disabled people in this country I felt far less trapped than I had ever felt in SA [South Africa]. Here I met my future wife who introduced me to the services and facilities that were available. She also persuaded me to attend meetings and during one of these gatherings we met Paul and Judy Hunt. Talking to them was a revolution in thinking and suddenly the segregation imposed on black South Africans by apartheid and the universal segregation imposed on disabled people seemed identical.

Aside from the year I spent at Stoke Mandeville Hospital I never had the opportunity of associating with other disabled people. My heroes and role models were all non-disabled people. In a great rush soon after arriving in Britain, in addition to Paul and Judy, I now also met up with Ken and Maggie Davis, Ken and Anne Lumb, Dick Leaman, Brenda Robbins, Anne Rae, Kevin Hyett and Sian Vasey, to mention just a very few; some of whom joined together in setting up the Union of the Physically Impaired Against Segregation (UPIAS). We all shared common experiences of systematic segregation and prejudice, and we all believed in campaigning for an integrated society. Like most people I had started with a negative perception and understanding of disabled people and now, amongst my new-found friends I began a process of reworking my role models.

Using the language and experience of apartheid I wrote a cartoon series for the Link television programme that Rosalie Wilkins presented on Sunday mornings. Overcoming apartheid involved turning the racist world upside down and in my story disabled people living in an apartheid-like village become the dominant group, design the social and physical environment exclusively for themselves and then oppress people who deviate from themselves. The story ends with alliance building for a society in which everyone can participate as an equal citizen.

As an emancipatory organisation UPIAS opposed all forms of oppression and we insisted that our group be open to people with different physical impairments (despite comments about UPIAS now). Focusing on society as a whole we avoided becoming a 'single-issue' group and we opposed segregation in housing, education and employment. We also advocated alliance building with other disability and non-disability organisations. By the late 1970s and early 1980s UPIAS members were working with a wide range of people in different local and national organisations. [...]

When I applied for a psychology course at university I was confronted by a professor who put forward a string of arguments why I, as a disabled person, was unsuited to studying psychology. When I applied for a teaching course at university I was confronted by a special education inspector who put forward a string of arguments why I, as a disabled person, should not get involved in special education – she maintained that it was not a good idea for disabled teachers to teach disabled children because we get too involved! On that basis, I countered, women should not teach girls: her argument collapsed and she did not openly oppose my entry into that profession.

But human diversity has a habit of confounding exceptions and I was warmly welcomed and supported by Vida Carver at The Open University when she recruited me to what I believe was the world's first course in disability studies. This course was clearly different to the existing medical and rehabilitation courses and in an important way provided 'establishment legitimacy' to our emancipatory wishes. The course provided a nation-wide platform from which stereotypes about disability could be questioned and new perspectives on services and lifestyles could be raised. It also gave disabled people an opportunity to study and tutor a course which had started to make real sense of their lives.

I now found myself actively engaged with UPIAS, the British Council of Disabled People, Disabled People's International and The Open University, as well as other local and national disability associations. In the light of this activity I came to recognise that the 'soul' expressed by all these groups could be found in the growing sense of identity.

This was no less than an emergent culture of disabled people and I joined … in forming a steering group to set up the London Disability Arts Forum (LDAF) to support and promote our own culture …

## Emancipation

If there is one thing I have learnt in travelling through life's adventures it is that the cultural values now worshipped by non-disabled people and imposed on the rest of us are flawed. The deeply human values cherished by disabled people are where I believe humanity needs to go, otherwise it will destroy itself. It seems to me that mainstream culture has horribly lost touch with reality. People running round and round a track in circles, or kicking an air-filled leather bag up and down a grass field, is not just regarded as healthy enjoyable fun but held up as the height of achievement!

With such an unreal culture that worships physical perfection it cannot be an accident that euthanasia has once again been raised to a level of legitimacy in able-bodied society to deal with suffering and difference. In contrast the aspirations and culture expressed by disabled people over the past thirty years is an affirmation of human validity in all its forms.

We have repeated over and over again, and at every level in society, that disabled people are not just 'dependent' beings, a drain on resources who need to be made 'normal', institutionalised or provided with perpetual 'care' (however 'excellent' such provision might be). Society needs emancipated disabled people because non-disabled people will depend on us to take a leading role in humanising the health and community support services and in returning mainstream culture to its fundamental roots – the sanctity of human life.

[…]

When I went pole-vaulting at school that fateful day I left behind one destiny and replaced this with another more fulfilling, more rewarding and more human than I could ever have hoped as I made my way under a sun that we all share.

*Source*: Vic Finkelstein (2002) 'Whose History???' Keynote address at the Disability History Week, 10 June 2002 [Extract] Available online at: www.leeds.ac.uk/disability-studies/archiveuk/archframe.htm

# Chapter 25

## An introduction to the Beveridge Report

*John Jacobs*

## Why Beveridge?

The impetus for what was to become the Beveridge Report came from the TUC, who had for some time been pressing the Government for a comprehensive review of social insurance. In February 1941 they sent a deputation to the Minister of Health to draw attention to the existing anomalies in health insurance and the response was to set up a committee of civil servants to consider the problems. In June the Minister for Reconstruction, Arthur Greenwood, invited Sir William Beveridge to chair the committee and the Beveridge Report was under way.

Beveridge was an obvious choice. He was eminently suited to the task by virtue of his long association with the world of national insurance and the problems of unemployment, and because he combined the skills of the social investigator with those of the practical administrator.

After Charterhouse and Oxford, Beveridge gave up the prospect of a career at the bar and for two years took on the unlikely post of sub-warden of Toynbee Hall, a university Settlement in Whitechapel, in 1903. Here he encountered the realities of the effects of unemployment in London's East End and became actively involved in both investigating the problems and administering the schemes to deal with them. As a result of his experiences there he was to write in 1909 *Unemployment, A Problem of Industry*, an influential book which helped to create the system of labour exchanges as a means of combating unemployment. He then spent three years as a leader-writer on social issues at the *Morning Post*, where he continued to involve himself in matters to do with social security. From here he moved directly into a civil service post in the Board of Trade in 1908 to implement his ideas about labour exchanges and to assist in framing legislation for unemployment insurance which reached the statue book in 1911. During the First World War he continued to work in various departments and chaired a committee on unemployment insurance.

From: J. Jacobs (1992) *Beveridge 1942–1992*. London: Whiting & Birch, pp. 5–19 [abridged].

Beveridge had made a favourable impression on the Webbs when they were working on the review of the Poor Laws which culminated in the *Minority Report* of 1909. When they needed a full-time Director for their brainchild, the London School of Economics, they offered the job to him. In 1919 he took up his post there where he stayed until 1937. During that time he continued to write on social security issues and for ten years from 1934 he chaired the Unemployment Insurance Statutory Committee, which strengthened his contacts in the TUC, which were to be invaluable when he came to write his Report, and kept him involved in insurance matters. He left the LSE for the mastership of University College, Oxford where he was when called upon to chair the committee on social insurance and allied services. By that time he had had almost forty years of more or less continuous experience with the problems of poverty and unemployment.

## The Report: 'a momentous document'

When it was published on December 1st 1942 *Social Insurance and Allied Services*, or as it was universally called, the Beveridge Report, was an instant and phenomenal success. Legend has it that a queue a mile long formed outside the Government Stationery Office in Kingsway; it sold over 635,000 copies, and the press and public were nothing short of ecstatic in its praise. *The Times* called it 'a momentous document which should and must exercise a profound and immediate influence on the direction of social change in Britain' (Beveridge, 1954, p. 117); it pushed the war news off the front pages, and hundreds of clubs, groups, and associations of all kinds met to discuss the Report and to send resolutions to their MPs demanding its immediate implementation. Cartoonists and sub-editors had a field day referring to this 'rare and refreshing Beveridge' and invoking images of a brave new world to come. Beveridge himself became an overnight celebrity.

On the face of it, a report about social insurance is an unlikely candidate for such adulation; it is 300 pages of closely argued discussion about the complexities of the administration of benefits and the knotty problems of the principles of social security policy, full of historical references and statistical tables. Tommy Handley, referring to the Report on ITMA, said 'I've been up the last three days and nights reading the first chapter of a book called 'Gone with the Want' by that stout fellow Beveridge' (Calder, 1971, p. 609) and indeed one could see that it might have taken him three days and nights to get to grips with it. What was it about this unpromising material that so spectacularly caught the imagination of the people?

To answer this question we have to see both what the Report promised in respect of social security and what it symbolised to a beleaguered nation in the middle of a terrible war for survival.

## Freedom from want

First, the Report was a plan for a better system of social security. Beveridge promised nothing less than freedom from want for everyone from the cradle to the grave. Compulsory insurance for all would bring benefits for all, and because these benefits were to be set at a level which would provide for basic needs there would be no need for anyone ever again to be in want. As the scheme relied upon insurance benefits there would be no need for reliance on means tests except for a few and diminishing number of people who fell outside the scheme. The days of the inter-war years, where many had gone hungry and had been forced to suffer the indignities of the household means test, were to go for ever. For a weekly contribution of 4/3d all one's needs would be taken care of, whether in unemployment, sickness or old age.

The combination of the comprehensiveness of the scheme, its simplicity and the contrast it offered to what for millions of people was a very recent memory of humiliating poverty during the long depression of the thirties ensured its success. On December 2nd *The Daily Mirror*'s front page headline could catch the essence of the plan in a few words: 'Beveridge tells how to banish want; Cradle to Grave plan; all pay – all benefit'. It was a promise that was easy to understand and went to the heart of what for many people had been their deepest fears.

Of course, the plan was much more complicated than the headlines suggested. In essence it tidied up many anomalies under the existing schemes, proposed a simple system of compulsory insurance against all the main events which lead to loss of income, and added in some new features. It built upon the existing pattern of benefits which it rationalised and extended to include almost everyone.

The existing schemes of benefits had grown up piecemeal since the turn of the century. Appendix B of the Report sets out the history of the existing schemes of insurance and other cash benefits from which it can be seen that by 1942 there were major anomalies and gaps in the schemes. For example, while unemployment benefit could include additional payments for the wife and children of the unemployed insured man, sickness benefit could not. (It was this kind of anomaly which had led the TUC to ask for a review of social security in the first place.) The rates of benefit differed between unemployment benefit and sickness benefit even though the needs of the man and his dependants were much the same, and between these and old age pensions. There were six different central government departments involved in the administration of the various benefits and many different local agencies involved in making the payments. Beveridge aimed to sweep most of these agencies away and replace them with a single Ministry of Social Security, and to clear away as many of the different rates of benefit as possible and replace them with uniform rates based solely on his assessment of what was needed for a minimum income.

There were three crucial elements to his Plan. The first was that everyone was included; second, they were covered 'from the cradle to the grave' and third was the promise that the benefits would be at a level which enabled a family to live without recourse to other means. He divided the population into six different groups classified according to age, marital status and place in the workforce and set out the contribution conditions and the benefits for each group. These six groups included almost everyone, the notable exceptions being single parents (a relatively small group at that time) unmarried women not in work and caring for dependents, and divorced or separated wives. Those normally employed, in whatever occupations, were all to be compulsorily insured against unemployment and sickness and were to contribute to their retirement pension. Married women were given the option of being insured on their husbands' contributions or, if they were in work, of paying contributions and earning entitlement to benefits, which would then be at a higher rate, on their own account. The 'cradle to grave' promise was to be met by the introduction of maternity benefits, children's allowances and funeral grants, all of which were new departures in social security payments.

Whereas it could be said that these measures were for the most part simply a rationalisa-tion and extension of existing benefits Beveridge's insistence that the benefits should be at a high enough level to ensure that an individual or a family could live on them without recourse to other means was a crucial break with existing policy. He wanted to establish a national minimum income level, and devoted fourteen pages in his Report to an explanation of how he came to arrive at the figure he proposed. He claimed that 'social insurance should aim at guaranteeing the minimum income needed for subsistence' (Beveridge, 1942, para. 27) and '… the scheme of social insurance outlined in this Report provides insurance ben-efit adequate to all normal needs, in duration and in amount' (Beveridge, 1942, para. 29).

The reference to the duration of benefit is also important; Beveridge wanted benefits to continue in payment for as long as was necessary, without limit of time, though he did expect that anyone who was in receipt of unemployment or sickness benefit for any length of time would be prepared to undergo training or other tests of their willingness to work as he said that prolonged dependence on benefits was demoralising and not to be encouraged.

[…]

# The insurance principle

Beveridge was adamant that his scheme must be based on the principle of insurance, as opposed to payments out of general taxation. 'Benefit in return for contributions, rather than free allowances from the State, is what the people of Britain desire' (Beveridge, 1942, para. 21). He believed it was wrong in principle to relieve the insured from the burden of contributions so that they 'should not feel that income for idleness, however caused, can come from a bottomless purse' (Beveridge, 1942, para. 22). This meant that benefits could only be set as high as the poorest members of the community could pay for with their con-tributions, which meant that while benefits should not be set any lower than was needed for subsistence they should not be set any higher, otherwise the poorest would not be able to afford the contributions. But he wanted benefits to be set at the minimum level for another reason; he believed that the State should not remove from individuals the will to improve their lot by hard work and thrift, so he deliberately set the benefits at the mini-mum to allow individuals to provide for themselves above this if they so wished. Thus he decided that his Plan would be based upon a system of one flat-rate benefit for everyone which would be financed by flat-rate contributions. In deciding this he decided against the schemes, which were common abroad, of relating the benefits and therefore the contribu-tions to the previous earnings of the insured.

His insistence on sticking to the insurance principle also meant that he was in some difficulties when it came to retirement pensions. If pensions were paid at the new higher rate immediately then many pensioners would benefit without having made the contribu-tions. He therefore proposed that the full pension should be phased in over a period of twenty years and that in the meantime only part of the subsistence level benefit would be paid. For millions of pensioners, however, having seen the promised jam, twenty years seemed far too long to wait for it, even if in the case of sound insurance, and this was the one proposal in the Plan which met with general condemnation.

[…]

# National assistance

While most people would be insured under his comprehensive scheme, either on their own account or as dependants of the insured worker, Beveridge recognised that some people would inevitably fall through the holes in the system and would not be eligible for insurance benefits. For those people Beveridge proposed that the existing scheme of national assistance, paid for out of general taxation, as opposed to insurance benefits, should continue. As with all other benefits, he proposed that this assistance should also be paid at subsistence level, the difference being that assistance would be subject to a means test.

He envisaged that there would be a number of people in the first years after the introduction of his scheme who would still need assistance because he anticipated that his higher level of benefits for pensioners would be phased in over time and until they reached their full amount pensioners might need their income supplemented by national assistance, but he expected that as his higher level of benefits came in so the need for assistance would diminish. Other groups of people who might need assistance because they would be outside the scope of his insurance scheme were some disabled people who would never be able to pay sufficient contributions to qualify for benefits, some of the unemployed who had been disqualified from benefit for failing to take jobs offered to them or who had left their last job without good cause or who had refused to attend a training centre after six months without work, and deserted or separated wives.

Given that this group consisted largely of pensioners, the disabled and deserted wives it is curious to find Beveridge in punitive mood in his proposals for national assistance. While accepting that it must be at subsistence level he goes on to say:

> It must be felt to be something less desirable than insurance benefit; otherwise the insured persons get nothing for their contributions. Assistance therefore will be given always subject to proof of needs and examination of means; it will be subject also to any conditions as to behaviour which may seem likely to hasten restoration of earning capacity. (Beveridge, 1942, para. 369)

It is reasonable that assistance has to be given on proof of need and after examination of means, but why he should want to make the receipt of assistance 'less desirable' and subject to more conditions than insurance benefit is hard to explain given that it is not the fault of the pensioners that he set their pension below subsistence level for the first twenty years, nor the fault of the disabled that they are unable to work to pay the insurance contributions, nor that he decided not to include deserted and separated wives in his scheme for insurance, as he could have done. One can only assume that he was too steeped in the traditions of the prevailing poor law orthodoxy, where assistance was often deliberately given under degrading conditions, to see that there was no need to treat these groups of claimants any differently from the insured population.

These then were the main proposals of Beveridge's Plan. He summarised them at the beginning of the Report in one paragraph as follows:

> The main feature of the Plan for Social Security is a scheme of social insurance against interruption and destruction of earning power and for special expenditure arising at birth, marriage or death. The scheme embodies six fundamental principles; flat rate of contribution;

unification of administrative responsibility; adequacy of benefit; comprehensiveness; and classification. Based on them and in combination with national assistance and voluntary insurance as subsidiary methods, the aim of the Plan for Social Security is to make want under any circumstances unnecessary. (Beveridge, 1942, para. 17)

It was this promise of comprehensive coverage and adequate benefits that created the vision that after the war there would be no return to the bad old days of the Depression and that no-one need ever be poor again. This was the 'rare and refreshing Beveridge' that intoxicated press and public.

# The brave new world

The promise to abolish poverty once and for all was a message which by itself might have ensured the Beveridge Report the public acclaim it received, but the Report was much more than just a scheme of social security. In Beveridge's mind it was merely a part of a grand scheme of reconstruction that he foresaw after the war was over, and it came to symbolise for millions of people their hopes for a better Britain. It was this symbolic content, superimposed on the reform of social security, that gave the Report its electrifying power.

The Report came at a time when Britain was just beginning to believe that the war could be won. November 1942 was the month when the allies had their first major strategic victories of the war when Monty's Eighth Army routed Rommel at El Alamein and a combined force of British and Americans regained control of North Africa. The Russians had surrounded the German army at Stalingrad and were about to win a decisive victory which turned the tide of the war on the eastern front. Into this mood of optimism came Beveridge's message about the kind of society we should look to have once the war was over. And his message had the smack of revolution about it.

> Now, when the war is abolishing landmarks of every kind, is the opportunity for using experience in a clear field. A revolutionary moment in the world's history is a time for revolutions, not for patching. (Beveridge, 1942, para. 7)

True he later qualified this by calling it a 'British revolution', by which he meant a 'natural development from the past' (Beveridge, 1942, para. 31), but it was stirring stuff nevertheless, and a far cry from the merely technical tidying up job the Minister had expected when setting him to work eighteen months before.

In the most quoted paragraph in the Report he made it clear that his Plan was only one part of a comprehensive set of plans that would need to be ready when the war ended if society was to be refashioned on new lines:

> Organisation of social insurance should be treated as one part only of a comprehensive policy of social progress. Social insurance fully developed may provide income security; it is an attack upon Want. But Want is only one of five giants on the road of reconstruction and in some ways the easiest to attack. The others are Disease, Ignorance, Squalor and Idleness (by which he meant unemployment). (Beveridge, 1942, para. 8)

To this apocalyptic vision of a society where all these giants would be slain he added some very real and tangible policy proposals which he said would have to be implemented if his Plan was to work. His three assumptions, as he called them, were that there would have to be a system of family allowances for all children apart from the first in each family; that there would have to be a comprehensive health service for everyone, and that the Government should take steps to intervene in the economy to ensure the avoidance of mass unemployment. Taken together, all these measures held out the promise of a world free from not just want but from the terrifying fear of old age and ill health that haunted millions of people before the war, and where unemployment would be abolished. It was this grand vision of a brave new world that articulated the deeply felt needs of the vast majority of the population and to which they responded with such enthusiasm. It made the war almost seem worth it, if after it, the old order could be swept away and a world free from poverty, fear and unemployment, could take its place.

# References

Beveridge, W. (1942) *Social Insurance and Allied Services* (The Beveridge Report), Cmnd 6404. London: HMSO.
Beveridge, W. (1954) *Beveridge and His Plan*. London: Hodder and Stoughton.
Calder, A. (1971) *The People's War*. Granada.

# Chapter 26

## The social construction of carers

*Bill Bytheway and Julia Johnson*

In this chapter we trace the dramatic history of this concept and attempt to explain how it has acquired its statutory status. There are two distinct threads to this history: that of pressure groups seeking to improve the situation of those looking after disabled and older people, and that of researchers and policy-makers who have been concerned to develop the policies and practices of service and support agencies. Both interest groups have focused primarily on the policies of central government and have frequently collaborated. Nevertheless, as will become apparent, their distinct interests have also generated tension in the course of the category of carer being constructed and promoted.

## Constructing the 'carer'

In 1995 the Carers (Recognition and Services) Act entered the statute book: carers now have legal status. It is perhaps difficult to appreciate that, less than forty years before this Act, the term 'carer' was barely in the English language, and particularly difficult for those many people who perceive themselves to be carers and who are indeed devoting themselves to the care of sick or disabled people. For people with such experience, the idea that 'being a carer' is a recent social invention will seem absurd. Yet people who were in the same situation in the 1950s would not have used the word 'carer' and, more to the point, would not have thought of themselves as distinctive in the sense of belonging to a special category of people. It is for this reason that we can think of the concept of 'carer' as a social construction, a category created through the interplay between individual experience and various interest groups – policy-makers, researchers and pressure groups.

The literature on care has grown rapidly since the emergence of this concept, and in this there is no ambiguity: 'the carer' is one particular person providing care for one other particular person. The care relationship so conceived is essentially asymmetric and one-to-one: A cares for B. In the development of care services in the community, policy

Originally published in A. Symonds and A. Kelly (eds) (1998) *The Social Construction of Community Care*, Basingstoke: Macmillan, pp. 241–253 [abridged].

has focused on the needs of B, the person receiving care. This means that the role of carer often appears in practice guidelines to be taken for granted, not unlike that of 'the GP', an individual – not indeed necessarily always the same individual – who is always 'there'. Other people are incidental in the conceptualisation of this relationship and the multiplicity and reciprocal nature of many caring relationships are overlooked.

# The emergence of the individual female carer

To a large extent, comtemporary policy and research is being developed by people who graduated in the social sciences in the 1960s and the 1970s. Many current beliefs about the value of community and family can be traced back to Townsend's seminal text, *The Family Life of Old People* (1957). In the 1950s the term 'carer' did not figure in either research or policy but, in a chapter titled, 'The Family System of Care', Townsend created an image of how care was provided by relatives within the context of ongoing family life. He argued for the central importance of the *family* rather than *individuals* (that is, carers) in the conceptualisation of how care was routinely provided within the community. However, he made it quite clear that the responsibility to provide care in London families of the 1950s fell primarily on women, although he also emphasised that older women played an active part in the early adult lives of their children: they provided care as much as they received it. We return to this point later in this chapter.

Townsend also discussed the various roles of unmarried adult children and was particularly interested in the extent of co-residence among older siblings. Many women were of course unmarried or widowed because of the huge numbers of men who had been killed in the First World War. With time, many had taken up a caring or supporting role within their (extended) families but, in the 1950s, some in turn were beginning to need support themselves. It was in the context of such demographic trends and changing pressures that the National Council for the Single Woman and Her Dependants was formed to campaign on behalf of single women. [...] In our view, it is important to the history of 'the carer' that this organization initially directed attention on one particular category of – largely middle-class – individuals: 'single women'. In so doing it challenged Townsend's more diffuse focus on care needs within the working class family.

# The impact of feminism

The concern of the Labour governments of the 1960s and 1970s with social security and the financial welfare of chronically sick and disabled people led, in 1975, to the introduction of Invalid Care Allowance (ICA). This was intended to 'protect the current incomes and future retirement pensions of members of the labour market whose full-time employment was prematurely terminated by the care of elderly relatives' (Glendinning, 1988: 131). Arguably this was the first significant gesture made by central government towards people providing care. However, being focused upon the financial cost of leaving employment, it was not payable initially to married and cohabiting women who it presumed would be at home anyhow (Baldwin 1994: 187). After a long and active campaign ICA was eventually in 1986 to include them. It was only then that it could be construed to be a payment for care rather than a benefit to (partially) replace lost earnings.

In 1981, in the course of the campaign to extend the ICA to married women, the Association of Carers was formed. It defined a carer as 'anyone who was leading a restricted life because of the need to look after a person who is mentally or physically handicapped, or ill, or impaired by old age', and among its aims was 'to encourage carers to recognise that their own needs are just as important as those of the person they are looking after'. One year later, the National Council for the Single Woman and Her Dependants reconstituted itself as the National Council for Carers and Their Elderly Dependants. Although clearly competing with the Association for Carers to represent married women carers, it maintained its focus on the needs of the 'elderly infirm relatives'. The competition was short-lived, however, and in 1986 the two were merged to form the Carers National Association.

The campaign to extend ICA to all women politicised the issue of care and, as a result, the assumption that women 'naturally volunteer' to provide family care began to be seriously questioned. In particular, attention was drawn to how this expectation denied middle-aged women opportunities to gain paid employment, or to regain it when children had left home (Finch and Groves, 1980). Responding to this concern, the Equal Opportunities Commission produced the first authoritative assessment of the unpaid and unacknowledged contribution of women to informal care. Following its own research, it concluded that:

> it remains the case that families are expected to provide care for the vast majority of the handicapped, the sick and the elderly, and, as is demonstrated in this study, it is the closest female relative to whom the task of caring usually falls. (EOC, 1980: 1)

This report also provided another early definition of carers: 'those adults who are responsible for the care of the sick, handicapped or elderly' (p. 1). The author of the report suggested that the term 'carers' was not entirely satisfactory, but was 'probably the best available'. The conclusion that the task of caring fell on the 'closest female relative' implies that the EOC conceptualisd care as an asymmetric one-to-one relationship, and that it saw individuals as the social unit that was primarily involved in the provision of care. The author, in noting that the majority of carers were women, added the words 'of course' and went on to explain that, because of this, the feminine pronoun would be used throughout the report. This, we would argue, was a crucial step in the feminisation of the concept of carer in the UK, one reinforced by the publication of Finch and Groves (1983) influential collection of studies of women and caring. Effectively, by definition, a male carer had become anomalous. But more significantly, so too had the idea that caring might be produced collectively by 'relatives' as part and parcel of ordinary family life.

The White Paper *Growing Older* (DHSS, 1981), reflecting the priorities of the newly elected Conservative government, issued the now famous decree that: 'care *in* the community must increasingly mean care *by* the community'. Far from confirming the importance of the role of the carer, this policy document did not refer to carers. Rather, it associated the concept of informal care with 'the community', not just the family but 'kinship, friendship and neighbourhood' (p. 3), although it acknowledged that caring 'may involve considerable personal sacrifice, particularly where the "family" is one person, often a single woman, caring for an elderly relative' (p. 37).

The government's conceptualisation and promotion of 'care by the community' was widely interpreted to mean 'care by women'. A series of research studies developed out of this and many reports and seminars were given titles such as 'Caring for the Carer'. In this way the term 'the carer' became established in the professional vocabulary.

In much of this research, carers were identified through the users of services. For example, the study of Charlesworth et al. (1984) was based on a sample of older people who had been referred to specialist services in two urban areas in the North West during 1979 and 1980: 'Wherever possible a principal carer was identified (following initial contact with the specialist service and an assessment by a psychiatrist) and this person was interviewed by a social scientist' (Charlesworth et al., 1984: 8).

Through this procedure, a sample of carers was obtained, each caring for one of the older people in the initial sample. Likewise, the sample for the well-known and influential study of Nissel and Bonnerjea (1982) was located primarily through the health services and voluntary agencies in Oxford. There were many other similar local studies that identified carers through the users of formal services. This sampling strategy was appropriate at that time in that two widely expressed concerns were the adequacy of the support provided by the formal sector, and the suspicion that men were offered support more readily, and more generously, than were women. The effect, however, was to define carers as one more 'newly discovered' element in the system of support that surrounded service users: people living in the community who were already receiving health or social services. This dependence on the 'service provider route' meant not only that the ability of the researchers to generalise to all carers was limited (Twigg and Atkin, 1994: 157), but also that policy began to be related to the apparent needs of such carers – needs that the service agencies that were already involved could and should be taking into account.

Overall, the extensive body of small-scale research undertaken in the 1980s reinforced the assumption that informal care is largely about the relationship between one carer, a middle-aged woman, and one dependent person – usually an older parent. It could be argued that the feminist critique, intended to expose the 'burden borne' by middle-aged women, only served to reinforce the expectation that, despite the apparent injustice, women would continue to provide the care that was required. As Arber and Ginn comment: 'caring has been portrayed primarily as work done by daughters for parents.... There has been little examination of the concept of caring, or questioning of the stereotype of "carers as middle-aged women"' (1991: 130).

Many commentators concluded from the early research studies not only that women provided by far the greater proportion of informal care, but also that the contribution of men was negligible. In fact, the percentage of male carers in these samples ranged from 23 per cent to 41 per cent (Arber and Gilbert, 1989: 73) – certainly under 50 per cent, but not negligible percentages at all.

The first authoritative national survey of the population to address the question of care was the 1985 General Household Survey (Green, 1988). On the basis of this, it was estimated that there were 6 million carers in Great Britain, of whom 40 per cent were male. Both statistics came as a shock to the policy world. [...]

Doubts about the legitimacy of the huge number of carers ... were raised by Parker (1992), who undertook a secondary analysis of the data. She suggested that accepting the figure of 6 million was 'not helpful' and that a more appropriate figure would be between 1.3 and 1.7 million. By examining findings on caring activities and taking some account of the time spent in caring, she distinguished between *informal care* defined as being heavily involved in personal and physical assistance and *informal help* defined as practical support, often provided 'as part of a network where others take main responsibility' (1992: 14) ...

Not surprisingly, Pitkeathley, the director of the Carers National Association, disputed Parker's revised conceptualisation. [...] Whereas Parker's concern was to assist policy-makers and service agencies to target those primary carers who should be given practical support, Pitkeathley's concern was to sustain the strength of the carers movement and to develop a powerful case for the contribution of all carers to the overall provision of care to be properly recognised.

Regarding the explanation of the unexpectedly high proportion of male carers identified in the General Household Survey, Arber and Ginn (1990) focused attention on 'spouse care'. Their analysis showed that four in ten carers were spouses, mainly 'elderly', and half of these were men. They suggested that the high percentage of males in the General Household Survey was due largely to the contribution of older husbands caring for ill wives. In doing so they also pointed to the ageism implicit in much of the earlier informal care literature:

> The prevailing view of elderly people as a 'social problem' emphasises the 'burden' of elderly people and concentrates on the problems for the rest of society of the increasing number of elderly people in the population. This negative and blinkered vision has almost entirely neglected the provision of care by the elderly themselves. (Arber and Ginn, 1990: 446)

This same point was made by Townsend thirty years earlier: 'In previous surveys the fact that old people perform services for others has had less attention than the fact that others perform services for them' (1957: 62).

# Disaggregating carers

With the extension of ICA to all carers, the formation of the National Carers Association and the impressive national statistics from the 1985 survey, the category of 'carer' was secured. A 'generic' approach to research on carers began to be adopted (Twigg, 1992). The archetypical question was no longer 'who *provides* care?' but 'who *are* the carers?' Paradoxically, however, this new question meant that the category of 'carers' required disaggregation. Arber and Ginn had started this by challenging the stereotype of the carer as a middle-aged daughter and drawing attention to 'the forgotten male carer'. The implications of this for social workers were developed by Fisher (1994: 677):

> We will have to develop a new appreciation of the caring capacities of men, particularly older husbands. There are circumstances where men accept the obligation to care, undertake intimate personal care, and derive identity and reward from their caring work.

Similarly, Atkin (1992) argued that 'differences need to be recognised if appropriate services are to be developed' and to that end he distinguished between: spouse, parental, filial, sibling, child and non-kin carers. The King's Fund Centre established a carers unit in the late 1980s which specialised in supporting projects focused on work with carers in ethnic minorities.

Meantime the Carers National Association had been campaigning effectively in Parliament. Malcolm Wicks MP, previously director of the influential Family Policy Studies Centre, introduced a Carers' Bill. Against many expectations he was successful and, in 1995, the Carers (Recognition and Services) Act entered the statute book. Under this Act a carer is defined as 'an individual [who] provides or intends to provide a substantial amount of care on a regular basis for the relevant person', the latter being a person (child or adult) whose needs for community care services are being assessed under other legislation. Although, in introducing his Bill, Wicks indicated that he was concerned that it should 'include all carers', he identified three particular groups (House of Commons, 1995: 424). First he referred to 'adults looking after a frail elderly relative', and he accepted that they 'represent the bulk of caring by family carers'. But he then went on to draw attention to two other groups which he sought to include in the legislation: 'parent carers' and 'child carers'. He referred to the latter as 'a newly recognised group' and much of the debate which followed was referenced to these two groups. Although he was concerned to include 'all carers', Wicks also indicated that the policy intention, following the argument of Parker, was to 'target that group of carers who carry the major burden'. So, having begun with a reference to the total estimated number of 6.8 million carers in Britain, he moved on to discuss in more detail the 1.5 million 'who provide care for 20 hours a week or more' and who he described as 'a caring army' (House of Commons, 1995: 426). What this review has done is focus on the way in which the category of 'carer' has emerged over the last twenty years. It began as an operational concept enabling the Equal Opportunities Commission to assess the impact on women of community care policies. It has now become a social identity written into the nation's statutes.

# Discussion

Robbert (1990) has focused on the part played by researchers, medical practitioners, ordinary people and the media, in defining the characteristics of Alzheimer's disease. She presented a modified version of the sequential model of the social construction of illness, first put forward by Conrad and Schneider (1980). It is not difficult to modify this still further to account for the social construction of 'carers' (Johnson, 1994). On the basis of our review of the literature we would tentatively suggest the following:

1   *Recognition*. Certain situations are recognised as not normal and as a cause for concern. Graham (1983: 14) identifies Leonard, Barker and Allen as feminists who raised questions about care and family life in the mid 1970s.
2   *Definition*. The situation is 'discovered', and the discovery is reported in a professional journal or monograph. It is defined and named. The first EOC report (1980) is a good example.
3   *Claims making*. Champions and 'moral entrepreneurs' start to make claims for the new discovery and to develop or reorientate interest groups. Finch and Groves (1983) and the early promotional material of the two carers organisations exemplify this stage.

4  *Legitimacy*. Positive reports from, and official recognition by, regulatory and professional bodies (such as the EOC and the British Association of Social Work) follow. The General Household Survey, undertaken by the government's Office of Populations, Censuses and Surveys, was a major contribution. Increased funding for research specifically into informal care followed (for example, Bytheway, 1987).

5  *Institutionalisation*. The name and definition become formally recognised as an accepted classification. Agencies are established and developed which provide organised support for local groups, and which issue guidelines to practitioners (such as the King's Fund Centre Carers Unit and the Carers National Association). The future of these projects and the continued employment of those working on them depend on the continued acceptance of the classification.

A model of this kind helps us understand the historical development of the carers movement, but it does not explain why it was so successful. Like Robbert, Gubrium (1986) has also studied the development of the Alzheimer's disease movement in the USA. His analysis demonstrates how it was necessary for the campaigning groups to organise the description of Alzheimer's as a distinct disease entity 'separate from the varied experiences of normal ageing' (Gubrium, 1986: 3). It is not difficult to see the parallel here with the need for the carers groups to make care distinct from normal family life. Gubrium argues that this is achieved by strategically organising the definition and description of the condition. To a significant extent this is accomplished through attention being given to the experiences of individual carers. For example, in introducing his Bill, Wicks recounted that:

> The Minister and I had an opportunity yesterday to meet a small delegation of carers from various parts of the country. They had an opportunity to talk with us about their needs. (House of Commons, 1995: 424)

Gubrium brings out how the Alzheimer's movement used both the experience of celebrities (Ronald Reagan, for example), and the personal testimonies of members of local support groups:

> The cultural apparatus for revealing the disease penetrates and incorporates diverse personal experiences. Those closest to the victim, who are the 'real experts' in the care and management of the disease – the caregivers – are taught or teach each other that they all share the same travail, all in combat with the same enemy. Each comes to know, by one set of interpretive rules or another, that the experiential minutiae of the 36 hour day, as observed and felt, is part of the silent epidemic. Thus Alzheimer's is not only 'over there' in the slogans, crusade, and celebrities, but right at home. (Gubrium, 1986: 209)

[…]

Compared with community care policies, there has been little critical discussion of the strategies and actions of the carers movement. A wide range of groups covering a broad political spectrum have supported it and agreed that carers have had a raw deal. The one significant exception to this is the independent living movement. Representing primarily the interests of disabled people, this is driven by three basic principles:

- Those who know best the needs of disabled people, and how to meet those needs, are disabled people.
- The needs of disabled people can best be met by comprehensive programmes which provide a variety of services.
- Disabled people should be fully integrated into their community (Morris, 1991: 172).

It is not difficult to see how these principles conflict with the concept of the carer. This came out into the open in 1990 when Wood began his contribution to a seminar on 'the needs and resources of disabled people' with the simple statement: 'Let us state what disabled people do want by first stating what we don't want. WE DON'T WANT CARE!!!!' (Wood, 1991: 201).

[...]

Morris (1991) was particularly critical of the contribution of feminist researchers to the development of care policies. In particular, Finch (1984) and Dalley (1988) had advocated collectivist, non-community-based policies of care as a way of relieving women of the 'burden' of providing care in the community. Morris rejected their implicit distinction between 'us' (women) and 'them' (disabled or dependent people), and in a particularly powerful passage she tackled the anti-familist stance expressed by Dalley:

> There is no recognition here that disabled people have often been denied the family relationships that she takes for granted. Insult is then added to injury by the assumption that for a disabled person to aspire to warm, caring human relationships within the setting where most non-disabled people look to find such relationships is a form of false consciousness. We are denied not only the rights non-disabled people take for granted, but when we demand these rights we are told that we are wrong to do so. (Morris, 1991: 160)

Keith and Morris (1995) returned to the attack over the issue of young carers. ... What is particularly interesting in regard to their arguments is how they explain their concerns over this issue in social constructionist terms:

> The research studies of, the campaigning on, and the media interest in 'young carers' have tended to repeat two things which were common in the earlier debate and research on carers generally. They have defined and named a role ('young carers') which, until the children and young people came into contact with researchers or professionals, was not how they described themselves. And secondly, both researchers, campaigners and journalists alike have defined the main policy issue to be that of providing services to 'young carers' which would ease the 'burden of caring'. (Keith and Morris, 1995: 38–39)

From the Equal Opportunities Commission through to the 1995 Act, it is clear that the campaign for carers' rights has been driven by personal accounts of caring which have reinforced the distinctiveness of the carer role, which have neglected the experience of the person receiving care, and which have drawn upon a limited set of key words such a 'restricted' and 'burden'. In this way the descriptive organistion of accounts of the carer's experience have fostered the asymmetric and one-to-one nature of the care relationship.

[...]

# Conclusion

In proposing, in conclusion, that care should be reconceived as part of ordinary family and community life, there is of course an obvious danger that we are thought to be indulging in a certain kind of communitarian nostalgia. To counter this, we would argue that anyone with first-hand experience of care will know that although, for the individual, care implies active involvement in a number of one-to-one relationships (and that this number may well be just one), these relationships are normally set in the context of 'ordinary' networks of personal relationships, networks which normally include a complexity and multiplicity of care needs. Typically care is provided outside paid working hours and, for this reason, is often provided by people not in employment: people who are retired, disabled, of school age or unemployed. The person with first-hand experience of care will know that care relationships are often mutual, that most people who are involved are actively involved in both receiving and providing care, albeit perhaps in very different ways. Lastly it will be widely recognised that while care is thought of within the framework of family relationships (one incidentally in which in legal terms the primary person is 'the next of kin': the person who stands to inherit), the care system often draws heavily upon old friendships and current patterns of day-to-day neighbouring. This is particularly true for those people whose family relationships have never been important or have become tenuous with time.

The carers movement and policy researchers, while bringing to our attention the real plight of many isolated and unsupported caring individuals, have obscured to some extent the realities of informal caregiving and, therefore, appropriate ways of supporting those who provide care in the community.

# References

Arber, S. and Gilbert (1989) 'Transitions in caring: gender, life course and the care of the elderly', in B. Bytheway, T. Keil, P. Allatt and A. Bryman (eds), *Becoming and Being Old*. London: SAGE, pp. 72–79.

Arber, S. and Ginn, J. (1990) 'The meaning of informal care: gender and the contribution of elderly people', *Ageing and Society*, 10(4): 429–454.

Arber, S. and Ginn, J. (1991) *Gender and Later Life*. London: SAGE.

Atkin, K. (1992) 'Similarities and difference between informal carers', in J. Twigg (ed.), *Carers: Research and Practice*. London: HMSO.

Baldwin, S. (1994) 'The need for care in later life: social protection of older people and family caregivers', in S. Baldwin and J. Falkingham (eds), *Social Security and Social Change*. Hemel Hempstead: Harvester Wheatsheaf.

Bytheway, B. (1987) *Informal Care Systems*. Report to the Joseph Rowntree Memorial Trust.

Charlesworth, A., Wilkin, D. and Durie, A. (1984) *Carers and Services: A Comparison of Men and Women Caring for Elderly People*. Equal Opportunities Commission.

Conrad, P. and Schneider, J. (1980) *Deviance and Medicalization: From Baldness to Sickness*. St Louis: Mosby.

Dalley, G. (1988) *Ideologies of Caring: Rethinking Community and Collectivism*. London: Macmillan.

DHSS (1981) *Growing Older*. London: HMSO.

EOC (1980) *The Experience of Caring for Elderly and Handicapped Dependants*. Manchester: Equal Opportunities Commission.

Finch, J. (1984) 'Community care: developing non-sexist alternatives', *Critical Social Policy*, 9: 6–18.

Finch, J. and Groves, D. (1980) 'Community care and the family: a case for equal opportunities', *Journal of Social Policy*, 9(4): 487–511.

Finch, J. and Groves, D. (eds) (1983) *A Labour of Love: Women, Work and Caring*. London: Routledge & Kegan Paul.

Fisher, M. (1994) 'Man-made care: community care and older male carers', *British Journal of Social Work*, 24: 659–680.

Glendinning, C. (1988) 'Dependency and interdependency: the incomes of informal carers and the impact of social security', in S. Baldwin, G. Parker and R. Walker (eds), *Social Security and Community Care*. Aldershot: Avebury.

Graham, H. (1983) 'A labour of love', in J. Finch and D. Groves (eds), *A Labour of Love: Women, Work and Caring*. London: Routledge & Kegan Paul.

Green, H. (1988) *General Household Survey 1985: Informal Carers* (Series, GH5, no. 15, suppl. A). London: HMSO.

Gubrium, J. F. (1986) *Oldtimers and Alzheimer's: The Descriptive Organization of Senility*. Greenwich, CT: JAI Press.

House of Commons (1995) *Carers (Recognition and Services) Bill*, Parliamentary Papers 422–478. London: HMSO.

Johnson, J. (1994) 'Social responses to need', *An Ageing Society* (Unit 10). Milton Keynes: The Open University.

Keith, L. and Morris, J. (1995) 'Easy targets: a disability rights perspective on "the children as carers debate"', *Critical Social Policy*, 44–45.

Morris, J. (1991) *Pride against Prejudice*. London: Women's Press.

Nissel, M. and Bonnerjea, I. (1982) *Family Care of the Handicapped Elderly: Who Cares?* London: Policy Studies Institute.

Parker, G. (1992) 'Counting care: numbers and types of informal carers', in J. Twigg (ed.), *Carers: Research and Practice*. London: HMSO.

Robbert, R. (1990) 'The medicalization of senile dementia', 2nd International Conference on the Future of Adult Life, Leeuwenhorst, The Netherlands.

Townsend, P. (1957) *The Family Life of Old People*. London: Routledge & Kegan Paul.

Twigg, J. (1992) 'Introduction', in J. Twigg (ed.), *Carers: Research and Practice*. London: HMSO.

Twigg, J. and Atkin, K. (1994) *Carers Perceived: Policy and Practice in Informal Care*. Buckingham: Open University Press.

Wood, R. (1991) 'Care of disabled people', in G. Dalley (ed.), *Disability and Social Policy*. London: Policy Studies Institute.

# Chapter 27

## From care to citizenship?

*Jan Walmsley*

This chapter examines organisations and structures during a momentous period in learning disability history. Organisations and structures alone can be rather dry, so the chapter's theme will be the extent to which citizenship was furthered by the various frameworks in place. We are discussing a basically positive period in learning disability history. …[I]t was a period when life improved overall for people with learning difficulties, when people had greater opportunities for an ordinary life, and social inclusion, and when citizenship emerged as a policy theme. It saw the virtual ending of large state-run long-stay hospitals as a residential option and the inclusion of children of all abilities in mainstream schools as an attainable goal. However, the chapter will also explore some considerable continuity beneath the rhetoric of policy. The authors of the 1971 White Paper said to their proposed shift from hospital to community care that 'no new policy is involved for local authority services. What is needed is faster progress to overcome the present deficiencies' (DHSS, 1971: 43). Similarly, in 2004, a review of independent living and community care concluded that whilst much of the policy framework was in place to offer independent living to disabled people, including people with learning difficulties, there were major organisational, financial and attitudinal barriers to achieving the vision for individuals (Morris, 2004). Moreover, although it was a period of intense optimism, of a belief that the disadvantages of impairment could be overcome if the right policies, services and attitudes were in place (Walmsley and Johnson, 2003), the same problems as have dogged learning disability policy and services remained, with commentators dubbing some of the aspirations articulated in *Valuing People* 'romantic'. That is, that they represent a model of individualised consumer choice which was ill-suited to the needs of many people whose impairments would always render them vulnerable without strong societal support.

[…]

## The big change: deinstitutionalisation

If it is remembered for anything in learning disability, the last 30 years of the twentieth century will be remembered as the period when most of the large hospitals closed.

From: John Welshman and Jan Walmsley (eds) (2006) *Community Care in Perspective: Care, Control and Citizenship*. Basingstoke: Palgrave Macmillan, pp. 77–96 [abridged].

Although institutional care had been widely criticised since the NCCL campaign of the early 1950s, in practice the long-stay hospitals had continued to expand in numbers, albeit gradually, until the late 1960s (DHSS, 1971: 19) giving the NHS a near monopoly in residential provision. Indeed, several major hospitals actually opened in this period. It took a long time for the institutional momentum to slow down. Although the 1971 White Paper did not visualise the closure of long-stay hospitals, in the period 1971–2001 those community care solutions advocated throughout the preceding half century became a reality on the ground.

[...] The location of learning disability in social care is not entirely secure – recent proposals are but the most recent of a series of identified threats to social services as the 'lead agency' for community care (Means et al., 2003).

The large NHS hospitals were replaced by a host of community-based hostels, later group homes, supported living, independent living funded through Direct Payments, supported employment, along drives to improve access to leisure, to friendships and to sexual relationships. In sum, these were associated with the type of life most people took for granted, an 'ordinary life' (King's Fund, 1980). Fashions about the type of accommodation thought appropriate also changed, with smaller units increasingly preferred over large. Whereas in the 1970s large hostels were the norm, by 1988 the Wagner Review of Residential Care was of the view that 'although new hostels are still being planned and built, it could be that the present generation of purpose-built hostels is the last. There is a growing feeling that a buildings based service is inflexible' (Atkinson, 1988: 127). These predictions proved accurate. Hostels fell into disfavour, and the later 1980s, 1990s and early twenty-first century saw trends to smaller units – group homes for up to seven people, individual flats and even owner-occupied houses for some under shared ownership schemes. [...]

The main beneficiaries of the thrust to residential care were the residents of former hospitals. The Wagner Report (1988) noted that little progress had been made towards providing for people who had remained with their families, thus:

There is now an accumulation of adults, some middle aged, with ageing and elderly parents, whose futures are still unplanned and uncertain, and who are at risk of being admitted to a residential setting during a major family and personal crisis. (Sinclair, 1988: 131)

Not much changed in this regard. It was estimated in 2005 that 29,000 people lived at home with parents over 70 (*Viewpoint*, 2005: 18). Similarly there was in 1988 little opportunity for young people to leave home as they reached adulthood (Sinclair, 1988: 131). A lack of statistical data makes it hard to establish a clear picture, though anecdotal evidence suggests that parents in 2005 expected that provision for residential care would be made as their young people approached adulthood (Dumbleton, 2005).

Not only were people living with families not catered for, there has been an increasing acknowledgement that the specific needs of families from black and minority ethnic and cultural groups have been neglected. Following a number of key studies which researched the experiences of such groups (Shah, 1992), concerns began to be voiced regarding the double discrimination often encountered. Families' experiences of being socially excluded by language barriers and racism, negative stereotypes and attitudes (Baxter et al., 1990; Mir et al., 2001) have emerged as important issues for policy makers, most noticeably in *Valuing People*. However, although there is at the policy level a greater awareness of the needs of people with learning difficulties from Black and

Minority Ethnic (or other minority) groups, there is little in place to ensure that steps are taken to address the issues (*Viewpoint*, 2005).

# Economic factors

[...]

In the 1970s, spending on mental handicap lagged well behind spending on health services for the general population. In 1975–76, for example, per capita funding on beds in mental handicap hospitals was £8.96 per day, compared to between £20.37 and £31.41 in acute hospitals (Ryan and Thomas, 1987: 167). Institutions were increasingly catering for more severely handicapped patients which also increased costs; at the same time the number of mildly handicapped patients who had earlier assisted in the running of the hospitals had dropped (DHSS, 1971: 19).

The 1971 White Paper set aside cash for improvements in community services, £40m for each year 1971–75, but ominously intoned 'the main responsibility lies with local authorities themselves', given that, as it said 'no new policy is involved for local authority services' (DHSS, 1971: 43–44, paras 198, 206). No money was ring-fenced for the expansion of learning disability services which meant that, as ever, they were subject to considerable local variation.

During the 1970s, hospital closures moved very slowly. Whereas in 1971 there were 58,850 people in hospitals, this figure had fallen only to 51,500 in 1980 (Wright et al., 1994). [...] One of the major barriers to closure was financial. Not only was it almost as expensive to run a half-full hospital as it was to run a fully occupied one, it did not benefit local authorities who were therefore unable to adequately fund new services. Cash savings from hospital closures accrued to Health Authorities whilst the cost fell on local authorities (Johnson, 2005). It was the 1980s which saw acceleration so that by 1990 there were 32,700 hospital beds, 37 per cent fewer than in 1980 (Wright et al., 1994). The acceleration is explained in part by financial factors. [...] Money continued to be an issue throughout the period and undoubtedly will be so for the foreseeable future. Government-funded research has shown that high quality community care is not cheaper than hospital care. Researchers found that while some types of living accommodation were cheaper than a hospital place, on average new types of accommodation were more expensive. At 1992 prices, hospital had cost an average £514 per person per week, whilst after five years, average costs for the same population in community-based housing was £598 per person per week (Cambridge et al., 1993: 72). Local authority responsibility for learning disability services has meant that there has continued to be a wide variation in the type and quality of services available, and the pace of change has been inconsistent (Fryson and Ward, 2004).

Furthermore, financial pressures on the private care sector have led to many smaller providers going out of business, to be replaced by larger firms. In 1992 there were only six private sector providers with 1000 beds on more; in 1998 there were 17 (Laing and Buisson, 1998, 1999). This has implications for service user choice.[1] Further individualisation of care services, under schemes like Direct Payments, are argued by governments to be cost neutral, though it is argued that 'deconstructing a 20 bed care home offering 24/7 intensive support and dispersing that into 20 individual services will require more money, staff time and adapted housing stock' (Churchill, 2005: 18).

# Markets, quasi-markets and care management

One major development in terms of organisation was the shift from monolithic provision of services by the NHS or Social Services to the creation of purchasers (later commissioners) and providers of services initiated by the 1990 NHS and Community Care Act. This was one of the most far-reaching and significant organisational changes of the period, affecting all health and Social Services activity. In 1971, virtually all services were directly provided by statutory agencies, funded either by taxation collected by central government in the case of health, or local taxes (successively rates, Poll Tax and Council Tax) in the case of Social Services. [...]

The 1990 Act is one of the landmark pieces of legislation behind the organisation of community care. Although it draws on the moral superiority of community care ideas (Walmsley, 1997) it was in large part motivated by the need to curb social security payments for residential care. The open-ended, nationally funded and controlled Department of Social Security budget for care was replaced by a cash-limited, locally administered budget only for those users who were individually assessed as requiring support. Purchasers purchase care on behalf of clients who have been assessed as requiring them. The services are provided by organisations which tender under a competitive process (initially Compulsory Competitive Tendering, subsequently Best Value) for the privilege. Thus a quasi-market is created. The rhetoric of choice has been extensively deployed to justify this marketisation ...

... [Choosing] done on behalf of individuals by care managers, drawn from a number of existing professional roles (such as social work and nursing) who undertake the assessment, hold the budget and negotiate the care package. Where block contracts are negotiated for a large number of places in care homes or in day services, the semblance of choice is even less convincing, given that in any specific area there are likely to be large-scale providers who dominate provision. Since the introduction of the quasi-market in the 1990s, there have been further developments which emphasize consumer sovereignty. Although hearing service users discussing the price of housing is a marked advance in terms of social inclusion and citizenship, there are indications that people living alone in their own homes can be left to cope with minimal support services, and if they do not have reliable support from family or friends can struggle with maintenance.

[...]

# 'Users'

[...] The user movement of people with learning difficulties began in the UK around the mid-1980s with the establishment of People First London Boroughs. A survey undertaken in 1989 found a considerable number of groups, some 'independent', that is, supported by advisors who were outside services, but many were part of the service system in ATCs and residential care (Crawley, 1989). The user movement in learning disability has been associated with the broader Disability Rights Movement which began in the 1970s, with the struggle for self-determination and an end to 'dependency born of powerlessness, poverty, degradation, and institutionalisation' (Charlton, 1998: 3). Disabled people led a campaign for disability rights legislation arguing, via the social model, that it is society, and not a person's impairment, that is disabling (Finkelstein, 1980; Oliver, 1983). The vocabulary of services, and of people's expectations, became more rights based. The right to Direct Payments won in legislation in 1996 can be attributed to effective campaigns by disabled people and their organisations, something from which a few people with learning disabilities benefited.

Self-advocacy organisations have to a limited extent followed the lead of disabled people's organisations in demanding and expecting rights for people with learning disabilities, and for them to be at the centre of the decision-making process, as illustrated by slogans such as 'We are the Experts' and 'Nothing About us Without Us' (Chapman, 2005). [...]

The role of users has been enhanced by Government interest in supporting a consumer voice in the development of policy and the running of services. This accompanied the marketisation of services in the 1990s, with service users redefined as consumers or customers (Davies et al., 2005). In line with a general move to increase the 'user' or 'patient' voice in the development of services, the Government has been broadly supportive of this development. The active inclusion of people with learning difficulties in the development and implementation of *Valuing People* is the most obvious manifestation of the recognition of the user movement, and Government's positive stance towards it.

There has been criticism of the incorporation of the self-advocacy movement into the organisations and structures of community care. The requirement of *Valuing People* for representation on Partnership Boards (DOH, 2001) has intensified the workload for organisations representing people with learning difficulties, without any obvious practical benefit to the majority (Fryson and Ward, 2004). Issues or representation remain fraught with difficulty, particularly as only the most able and vocal of service users are able to participate meaningfully, and their ability to effectively speak for others, often more severely disabled, has yes to be proven (Concannon, 2004). Furthermore, 'carers' and 'users' do not often speak with one voice. Indeed, there appears to be an inherent tension between the interests of family members in protecting their sons and daughters (care), often through the maintenance of paternalist service models (such as full-time placement at Day Centres), and the demands of the more radical end of the user movement for independent living (citizenship). Several studies indicate that parents are weary of consultation and fear that change actually means less resource (Tilley, 2001; Concannon, 2004). ... User organisations rarely express such concerns as clearly, though there are indications that the value people accord to their current services is greater than the rhetoric implies (Rolph and Walmsley, 2006), with the role they play in sustaining friendship networks being particularly important (Walmsley, 1995; Rolph et al., 2005).

[...]

# From *Better Services* to *Valuing People*

This period, 1971 to 2001, is framed for England by the publication of the two White Papers. ... As we have noted, it was a period when 'community care' finally triumphed as a policy option, both in rhetoric and in reality, and during which public perceptions of learning disability were at their most optimistic for well over a century. The aspirations of people with learning disabilities to be taken seriously, to be active citizens participating in society and to have a voice both reached the surface and were to some extent fulfilled during this period. Whereas in 1971, the fight was to close hospitals and replace them with hostels and Training Centres (for adults) with a strong 'care' message, and the views of people with learning disabilities were assumed, by 2001, those views were actively canvassed in the preparation of, and follow-up to, *Valuing People*. It is, in short, a quite remarkable story of change.

The background to the White Papers differs. Whereas *Better Services* was in part prompted by revelations of appalling neglect and abuse in long-stay hospitals, which had brought services for people with learning disabilities into the media eye, and put pressure on the Government, by the end of the twentieth century, learning disability was more of a policy backwater. There are indications, however, that this was a success for a group of academics and professionals who had been looking for mechanisms to hasten reform, and who finally found a responsive minister. Civil servants had been making the case for a new strategy in a relatively low key manner. […] The other important point to note is that it was originally only a strategy, and not a White Paper. As such, it was fairly low profile, low risk. It was only when it became clear that the work had substantial support from the learning disability field, and would be seen as a positive news story, that there began to be political support for its being a White Paper.[2]

…[T]he development and writing of the *Valuing People* strategy was the first attempt by Government to include the voices of carers and individuals with learning difficulties. A Task Group was set up of people with learning difficulties who travelled the country visiting self-advocacy groups and collecting evidence of the quality and often, disparity, of local services. Following on from the launch of the strategy, a National Forum of people with learning difficulties was set up with four representatives elected to the Task Force, the body set up to oversee the implementation of the strategy. This put the voice of people with learning difficulties into the centre of the government process. The force behind *Valuing People* was therefore the active engagement with carers and people receiving services in the development of national policy and the encouragement at the same time of an inter-departmental approach to moving services for people with learning disabilities onto a more mainstream basis. The strategy represented a change in attitude to 'person-centredness', and a more participative approach to policymaking.

[…]

As far as the themes of this book are concerned, *Valuing People* came out championing 'Rights, Independence, Choice, and Inclusion' (DOH, 2001: 3). … While both White Papers commit to greater spending, their objectives bear close scrutiny. The first and second objectives of *Better Services* (to explain why services needed to be extended and improved and to invite greater sympathy and tolerance on the part of the general public for the 'mentally handicapped') were closely linked to a 'care' theme. The aims of *Valuing People* are not set out as clearly. Rather we are presented with 'A New Vision' and some aspirations which might loosely be called aims. Under the overall heading of 'Better Life Chances for People with Learning Disabilities', we find

- more choice and control for people with learning disabilities,
- supporting carers,
- improving health,
- housing, fulfilling lives and employment and
- quality services. (DOH, 2001: 4–8)

This quite marked difference in approach carries through into the body of the White Papers. *Better Services* is a lengthy document which attempts to set out the situation regarding services in some considerable detail. Whilst one might take issue with the medical framing of some of the data, and the prescription of types of service – no acknowledgment of ethnic diversity, no aspirations for supported living or employment – it is undeniable that setting out an evidence base of whom we are talking about, and what their needs may be, is reassuring. In effect, *Better Services* set out some concrete objectives for local authorities, namely 43,500 more places in ATCs than were in use in 1971; 24,100 residential places for adults; and 2800 for children (DHSS, 1971). We know that these targets were not met in the timescale set (see above). They did, however, set up a major expansion in provision of Day Centre and community-based residential placements.

*Valuing People* had a more challenging job if it was attempting to map provision, for, whilst in 1971 there were few providers which were not either NHS or local authority, by 2001 services were provided by a bewildering array of organisations – private, voluntary and statutory, not to mention hybrids such as Direct Payments, or family carers. Its authors made little attempt to chart this complex picture. Whilst it is stronger on values than its predecessor, *Valuing People* is surprisingly devoid of statistics (DOH, 2001: 15, figure 1). ... However whereas in 1971 there were clear and measurable targets for what was then regarded as improvement, in 2001 any target was vaguely worded, and by any standards hard to measure. Probably the most concrete performance indicator in the White Paper is the aspiration to empty NHS long-stay hospitals by April 2004. This was achieved, though not by the target date. Moreover although commendable, this has not necessarily led to community inclusion or participation for all those who might once have found themselves in hospitals. It also does not address those long-established institutions run by non-NHS bodies which continue to flourish to this day. This means that for some, citizenship is an abstract and distant goal – care and control remain the philosophy.

# Conclusion

This chapter has been an overview of the organisations and structures, primarily in England and Wales, which supported community care for people with learning difficulties between 1971 and 2001. It has, of course, told an over-simplified story. As other social policy analysts have pointed out, the pace of change has been such that it is hard to write a coherent account of policy changes (Means et al., 2003). [...] Rather we are more hesitant about the idea of 'progress', acknowledging that while some 'improvements' have been made, in other respects the picture is more mixed. For many, particularly those with more severe impairments or with 'challenging behaviour', there was less change.

# Notes

1   Personal communication with the editors.
2   Ibid

# References

Atkinson, D. (1988) 'Residential care for children and adults with mental handicap', in Sinclair (ed.), *The Research Reviewed*. pp. 125–156.

Baxter, C., Poonia, K., Ward, L. and Nadirshaw, Z. (1990) *Double Discrimination: Issues and Services for People with Learning Disabilities from Black and Ethnic Minority Communities*. London: King's Fund.

Cambridge, P., Hayes, L. and Knapp, M. (1993) *Care in the Community: Five Years On*. Aldershot: Ashgate.

Chapman, R. (2005) 'The Role of the Self-Advocacy Support-Worker in UK People First Groups. Developing Inclusive Research'. Open University Unpublished PhD thesis.

Charlton, J. (1998) *Nothing About Us Without Us: Disability, Oppression and Empowerment*. Berkeley, CA: University of California Press.

Churchill, J. (2005) 'Don't be deluded by Green Paper', *Community Care*, 21 July.

Concannon, L. (2004) *Planning for Life: Involving Adults with Learning Disabilities in Service Planning*. London: Routledge.

Crawley, B. (1988) *The Growing Voice: A Survey of Self-advocacy Groups in Adult Training Centres and Hospitals in Great Britain*. London: Campaign for the Mentally Handicapped.

Davies, C., Hudson, B. and Hardy, B. (2005) 'Working towards partnership', Workbook 4, *K202 Care Welfare and Community*, 2nd edn. Milton Keynes: Open University, pp. 59–104.

DHSS, Welsh Office (1971) *Better Services for the Mentally Handicapped* (Cmnd. 4683). London: HMSO.

DOH (2001) *Valuing People: A New Strategy for Learning Disability for the 21st Century* (Cm. 5086). Norwich: The Stationery Office.

Dumbleton (2005) 'On Being a Parent in the Twenty First Century', paper given at the Social History of Learning Disability Conference. Open University, Milton Keynes.

Finkelstein, V. (1980) *Attitudes and Disabled People: Issues for Discussion*. New York: World Rehabilitation Fund.

Fryson, R. and Ward, L. (eds) (2004) *Making Valuing People Work: Strategies for Change in Services for People with Learning Disabilities*. Bristol: Policy Press.

Johnson, J. (2005) 'Funding matters', Workbook 4, *K202 Care Welfare and Community*, 2nd edn. Milton Keynes: Open University, pp. 7–57.

King's Fund (1980) *An Ordinary Life*. London: King's Fund.

Laing and Buisson (1998, 1999) *Care of Elderly People: Market Survey*, 10th and 11th edns. London: Laing and Buisson.

Means, R. Richards, S. and Smith, R. (2003) *Community Care: Policy and Practice*, 3rd edn. London: Palgrave.

Mir, G., Nocon, A., Ahmad, W. with Jones, L. (2001) *Learning Difficulties and Ethnicity: Report to the Department of Health*. London: DOH.

Morris, J. (2004) 'Independent living and community care: a disempowering framework', *Disability and Society*, 19(5): 427–442.

Oliver, M. (1983) *Social Work and Disabled People*. Basingstoke: Macmillan.

Rolph, S. and Walmsley, J. (2006) 'Oral History and New Orthodoxies: Narrative Accounts in the History of Learning Disability', *Oral History*, vol. 34, no. 1: 81–91.

Rolph, S., Atkinson, D., Nind, M. and Welshman, J. (2005) *Witnesses to Change: Families, Learning Difficulties and History*. Kidderminster: BILD Publications.

Ryan, J. with Thomas, F. (1987) The Politics of Mental Handicap (revised edn). London: Free Association Books.

Shah, R. (1992) *The Silent Minority: Children with Disabilities in Asian Families*. London: National Children's Bureau.

Sinclair, I. (ed.) (1988) *Residential Care: The Research Reviewed (Literature Surveys Commissioned by the Independent Review of Residential Care Chaired by Gillian Wagner)*. London: HMSO.

Tilley, E. (2001) 'Advocacy Organisations for People with Learning Difficulties'. University of Cambridge: Unpublished dissertation.

*Viewpoint* (2005) 'Older carers urged to plan for the future', *Viewpoint*, May: 18–19.

Walmsley, J. (1995) 'Life history interviews with people with learning disabilities', *Oral History*, 23(1): 71–77.

Walmsley, J. (1997) 'Telling the history of learning disability from local sources', in Atkinson, Jackson and Walmsley (eds), *Forgotten Lives*, pp. 83–94.

Walmsley, J. and Johnson, K. (2003) *Inclusive Research with People with Learning Disabilities: Past, Present and Futures*. London: Jessica Kingsley.

Wright, K., Haycox, A. and Leedham, I. (1994) *Evaluating Community Care*. Buckingham: Open University Press.

# Chapter 28

## Ethics and evidence-based medicine

*Ian Kerridge, Michael Lowe and David Henry*

Evidence based medicine is founded upon an ideal – that decisions about the care of individual patients should involve the 'conscientious, explicit and judicious use of current best evidence.' (Sackett et al., 1996). Several publications are dedicated to evidence based medicine, and, at an international level, the Cochrane Collaboration has been formed to gather, analyse, and disseminate evidence derived from published research (Chalmers et al., 1992). Several practical approaches to evidence based medicine in clinical decision making have also been described (Rosenberg and Donald, 1995; Henry, 1992).

Evidence based medicine, it is claimed, leads to improvements in clinicians' knowledge, reading habits, and computer literacy; provides a framework for teaching; enables junior team members to contribute to decisions; and allows better communication with patients and more effective use of resources. From an ethical perspective, the strongest arguments in support of evidence based medicine are that it allows the best evaluated methods of health care (and useless or harmful methods) to be identified and enables patients and doctors to make better informed decisions (Bastian, 1994; Hope, 1995).

However, the presence of reliable evidence does not ensure that better decisions will be made. Claims that evidence based medicine offers an improved method of decision making are difficult to evaluate because current practice is so poorly defined. Medical decision making draws upon a broad spectrum of knowledge – including scientific evidence, personal experience, personal biases and values, economic and political considerations, and philosophical principles (such as concern for justice). It is not always clear how practitioners integrate these factors into a final decision, but it seems unlikely that medicine can ever be entirely free of value judgments.

We review ethical concerns associated with evidence based medicine – in particular that it invites a simplistic approach to the role of evidence in medicine, which can be misinterpreted and may not allow for the complexity of clinical decision making.

Originally published in the *British Medical Journal* (1998), 316: 1151–1153.

# The philosophical basis

[...]

## Immeasurable outcomes

The first philosophical criticism of evidence based medicine is that many important outcomes of treatment cannot be measured. This arised from the fact that evidence based medicine claims to provide a simple, logical process for reasoning and decision making – look at the evidence and decide accordingly. But to make balance decisions, all the relevant consequences of an action must be considered. Unfortunately, current measures of some outcomes of medical treatment (such as pain) are inadequate; some (such as justice) may not be measurable; and other complex outcomes (such as quality of life) may not even be adequately definable (Guyatt et al., 1994; Evidence-Based Care Resource Group, 1994).
[...]

## Deciding between competing claims

The second philosophical criticism, that it may be impossible to decide between competing claims of different stakeholders, is emphasised by the manner in which patients continue to have little influence over the priorities of research. Evidence based medicine claims to reject the power of expert opinion but it is still mostly doctors who determine research objectives, who interpret research data, and who implement research findings. A number of commentators have called for greater involvement by consumer groups in setting research agendas, but how conflicts between the agendas of the different stakeholders are to be resolved remains unclear (Chalmers, 1995; Oliver, 1995). Evidence based medicine is unable to address political concerns because the values of different stakeholders, and hence the way in which they interpret evidence, cannot always be made congruent with each other.

## At odds with common morality

The third philosophical criticism, that evidence based medicine may lead to activities that seem at odds with common morality, arises from the fact that evidence based medicine assesses interventions solely in terms of evidence of efficacy. An example of the difficulties that may arise from this approach occurs in the field of meta-analysis. Researchers performing meta-analyses are generally urged to search as widely as possible for data and to use unpublished studies if they are methodologically sound. However, valuable research findings may arise from unethically conducted research and data from unpublished studies may not meet the ethical safeguards that are demanded by publishers. In such cases it may be under whether results should be used or discarded.

Most of the discussion of this topic has focused on Nazi experimentation, (Samei and Kearfott, 1995), but there are many more recent examples of unethical research (Berger, 1990).

The *New England Jouranl of Medicine* has stated that it will not publish results of unethical research, regardless of scientific merit; but what these standards mean in practice is not entirely clear (Samei and Kearfott, 1995; Angel, 1990; Smith, 1997). For example, the Gruppo Italiano per lo Studio della Sopravvivenza nell'infarto miocardio (GISSI-2) trial, published in the *Lancet* in 1990, did not require the informed consent of trial subjects (Gruppo Italiano, 1990). Although few present day ethics committees would accept this standard, this study has been widely quoted and included in many meta-analyses. Ethically it seems clear that both researchers and publishers should consider the ethical basis of studies that are included in meta-analysis, but the extent of this obligation remains uncertain.

# Collecting evidence

## Randomised controlled trials

Proponents of evidence based medicine emphasise the value of some forms of evidence over others, placing particular emphasis upon the results of randomised controlled trials (Mulrow, 1994). For example, the United States Preventive Services Taskforce (1995) rates the value of evidence from randomised controlled trials as 'grade I', evidence from non-randomised trials as 'grade II', and evidence from the opinions of respected authorities as 'grade III'.

## Ethical concerns

Randomised controlled trials have the potential to prevent the propagation of worthless treatments and confirm the value of effective treatments. They raise a number of issues that cause ethical concern, including: the selection of subjects, consent, randomisation, the manner in which trials are stopped, and the continuing care of subjects once the trials are complete.

# Using evidence

[...]

## Systematic bias

Governments and health funds find the notion of allocating health resources on the basis of evidence attractive (Downey, 1997). Eddy has suggested that healthcare funds should he required to cover interventions only if there is sufficient evidence that they can be expected to produce their intended effects (Eddy, 1996). The Australian health minister, Dr Michael Wooldridge, who is a strong supporter of evidence based medicine, has adopted a similar position, stating '[we will] pay only for those operations, drugs and treatments that according to available evidence are proved to work' (Downey, 1997).

Given the complexities of the issues surrounding resource allocation, the drive to seek certainty and simplicity at the policy level is understandable. However, the large quantities of trial data required to meet the standards of evidence based medicine are available for relatively few interventions. Evidence based medicine may therefore introduce a systematic bias, resulting in allocation of resources to those treatments for which there is rigorous evidence of effectiveness, or towards those for which there are funds available to show effectiveness (such as new pharmaceutical agents). This may be at the expense of other areas where rigorous evidence does not currently exist or is not attainable (such as palliative care services). Allocating resources on the basis of evidence may therefore involve implicit value judgments, and it may only be a short step from the notion that a therapy is 'without substantial evidence' to it being thought to be 'without substantial value' (Evidence-Based Care Resource Group, 1994).

## Individual versus population health

Evidence based medicine, as described above, concentrates upon the efficacy of individual treatments. Physicians must not only address the needs of individual patients, but should also be concerned with issues of efficiency and population health (Maynard, 1997). Proponents of evidence based medicine argue that these issues can be resolved by the use of 'evidence based purchasing'. However, decisions reached rationally at the population level will at times conflict with those made in the interests of the individual. Evidence based medicine does not provide a means to settle such conflicts. Even attempts to replace evidence based medicine with other quantitative methods such as 'decision-analysis based medical decision-making' seem unlikely to remove from medicine the need for reasoning that is based on value (Dowie, 1996).

## Simplistic solutions

According to Williams (1972), 'there is great pressure for research into techniques to make larger ranges of social value commensurable. Some of the effort should rather be devoted to learning – or learning again – how to think intelligently about conflicts of values which are incommensurable'. This is particularly the case where it comes to making decisions about allocation of health resources. Those charged with making these decisions are seeking simplistic solutions to inherently complex problems – the danger is that through evidence based medicine we will supply them.

# References

Angel, M. (1990) 'The Nazi hypothermia experiments and unethical research today', *New England Journal of Medicine*, 322: 1462–1464.

Bastian, H. (1994) *The Power of Sharing Knowledge: Consumer Participation in the Cochrane Collaboration*. Oxford: UK Cochrane Centre.

Berger, R. L. (1990) 'Nazi science – the Dachau hypothermia experiments', *New England Journal of Medicine*, 322: 1435–1440.

Chalmers, I. (1995) 'What do I want from health researchers when I am a patient?', *British Medical Journal*, 310: 1315–1318.

Chalmers, I., Dickersin, K. and Chalmers, T. C. (1992) 'Getting to grips with Archie Cochrane's agenda', *British Medical Journal*, 305: 786–788.

Dowie, J. (1996) '"Evidence-based", "cost-effective", and "preference-driven" medicine: decision analysis based medical decision making is the pre-requisite', *Journal of Health Services Research & Policy*, 1: 104–113.

Downey, M. (1997) 'Trust me I'm a doctor', *Sydney Morning Herald*, 10 May, p. 1.

Eddy, D. K. (1996) 'Benefit language; criteria that will improve quality while reducing costs', *Journal of the American Medical Association*, 275: 650–657.

Evidence-Based Care Resource Group (1994) 'Evidence based care. 1. Setting priorities: how important is this problem?', *Canadian Medical Association Journal*, 150: 1249–1254.

Gruppo Italiano per lo Studio della Sopravvivenza nell'infarto miocardio (1990) '1 GISSI-2: a factorial randomised trial of alteplase versus streptokinase and heparin versus no heparin among 12,490 patients with acute myocardial infarction', *Lancet*, 336: 65–71.

Guyatt, G. H., Sackett, D. L. and Cook, D. J. for the Evidence-Based Medicine Working Group (1994) 'Users' guides to the medical literatures', *Journal of the American Medical Association*, 271: 59–63.

Henry, D. (1992) 'Economic analysis as an aid to subsidisation decisions. The development of Australian guidelines for pharmaceuticals', *PharmacoEconomics*, 1: 54–67.

Hope, T. (1995) 'Evidence-based medicine and ethics', *Journal of Medical Ethics*, 21: 259–260.

Maynard, A. (1997) 'Evidence-based medicine: an incomplete method for informing treatment choices', *Lancet*, 349: 126–128.

Mulrow, C. D. (1994) 'Rationale for systematic reviews', *British Medical Journal*, 309: 597–599.

Oliver, S. R. (1995) 'How can health service users contribute to the NHS R and D program?', *British Medical Journal*, 310: 1318–1320.

Rosenberg, W. and Donald, A. (1995) 'Evidence based medicine: an approach to clinical problem-solving', *British Medical Journal*, 312: 1122–1126.

Sackett, D. L., Rosenberg, W. M. C., Gray, J. A. M., Harnes, R. B. and Richardson, W. S. (1996) 'Evidence based medicine: what it is and what it isn't', *British Medical Journal*, 312: 71–72.

Samei, E. and Kearfott, K. J. (1995) 'A limited bibliography of the federal government-funded human radiation experiments', *Health Physics,* 69: 885–891.

Smith, R. (1997) 'Informed consent: the intricacies', *British Medical Journal*, 314: 1059–1060.

US Preventive Services Taskforce (1995) *Guide to Clinical Preventive Services*, 2nd edn. Baltimore: Williams and Wilkins, p. 862.

Williams, B. (1972) *Morality*. Cambridge: Cambridge University Press.

# Chapter 29

## The anti-collectivists

*Vic George and Paul Wilding*

In Britain, criticism of the expanded role of government has been a central element in New Right arguments. … Mrs Thatcher has stressed the damage done to the economy through over-government, the wounds to a sense of individual, family and community responsibility which result and the way in which, as government has expanded, it has become less effective and less efficient (Thatcher, 1977). Reduction of the role of government was one of the central themes of Mrs Thatcher's first government – through exportation of responsibilities from central government to local government and from central government to private industry, through the privatisation of services, through stress on the role and responsibility of family and neighbourhood.

## Attitudes to the welfare state

As might be anticipated from the values of the anti-collectivists, their faith in the spontaneous order of the market system, and their suspicion of government activity, their attitude to the welfare state is fundamentally hostile.

This is not to suggest that anti-collectivists deny government any role in welfare. 'It would be quite false', Barry has argued, 'to say that liberals in general and Hayek in particular are opposed to the idea of a Welfare State' (Barry, 1979). Anti-collectivists, however, are apprehensive about such a role. They see welfare state policies as threatening or damaging to central social values and institutions – the family, work incentives, economic development, individual freedom, for example – and in general they are opposed to provision which is more than minimal.

Hayek has perhaps made most effort to define which welfare activities can be regarded as legitimate for government. Such activities, he has suggested, are entirely compatible with liberal principles so long as three conditions obtain – that government does not claim a monopoly, that resources are raised by taxation on uniform principles and taxation is not used as an instrument for income redistribution, and that the wants to be satisfied are

From: V. George and P. Wilding (1985) *Ideology and Social Welfare*. London: Routledge & Kegan Paul, pp. 35–43.

collective wants of the community as a whole and not merely collective wants of particular groups (Hayek, 1978).

Hayek accepts that is a responsibility of government to guarantee a social minimum. He speaks of the need for some such arrangement as 'unquestioned' (Hayek, 1960: 285). When it becomes 'the recognised duty of the public to provide for the extreme needs of old age, unemployment, sickness etc.', Hayek sees it 'as an obvious corollary to compel them to insure (or otherwise provide) against those common hazards of life' (Hayek, 1960: 286). Guaranteeing a basic minimum income, in Hayek's view, 'appears not only to be a wholly legitimate protection against a risk common to all, but a necessary part of the great society in which the individual no longer has specific claims on the members of the particular small group into which he was born' (Hayek, 1979). Minimal state provision may be unproblematic, but as Hayek sees it, 'a government dependent on public opinion, and particularly a democracy, will not be able to confine much attempts to supplement the market to the mitigation of the lot of the poorest ... it is certain to be driven on by the principles implicit in the precedents it sets' (Hayek, 1976). A concern for a minimum leads on to a concern about inequality and the pursuit of the mirage of social justice. Anti-collectivists see such expansion as inevitable because of two factors – firstly, because of the nature of democratic government which leads to competition between parties for votes and so contributes to an expansion in the promises and activities of governments and, secondly, because of the pressures for expansion generated internally by welfare bureaucracies. To amateur and inexpert politicians the arguments they advance for expansion are compelling. State action leads, by its own inherent logic, therefore, to a situation which is quite unacceptable to anti-collectivists. Welfare state policies, if not tightly limited in a way which the anti-collectivists recognise as politically almost impossible, represent a dangerous shuffle down the road to egalitarianism and socialism.

When government moves beyond minimum provision anti-collectivist anxieties increase. It is possible to categorise their anxieties and objections under seven headings. The first and in some sense the major concern is the threat to freedom implicit in welfare state policies. Seldon puts it in extreme terms. 'The welfare state', he fulminates, 'has gradually changed from the expression of compassion to an instrument of political repression unequalled in British history and in other Western industrial societies' (Harris and Seldon, 1979: 204).

What precisely is the basis of this threat to freedom? One element emphasised by Seldon is the way in which, *de facto*, the welfare state imposes maximum standards on people. Having paid the taxes which finance collective welfare, most people cannot then afford to make private provision. They therefore have no real alternative but to accept the standard of service provided by the state. In Seldon's view 'the British welfare state has logically and ineluctably become the main instrument for the creation of equality by coercion' (Seldon, 1967: 18).

Another blow to freedom inflicted by the welfare state is the way it allows or enables majorities to coerce minorities and individuals. Even if they might not wish to do so, minorities and individuals have to pay through taxation for particular services of a particular standard. Such services may be intended for their use but individuals might still prefer to do without them and spend their money in other ways. In a welfare state they cannot do this. The majority decides what shall be spent on particular goods and services. Minorities who object or who have other priorities cannot escape.

Freedom is also threatened by government monopolies in service provision and the lack of choice which results. Inevitably, too, public provision of services gives immense power to the bureaucrats and professionals who make judgments about need because, in Friedman's words, such services 'put some people in a position to decide what is good for other people. The effect is to instill in the one group a feeling of almost god-like power; in the other a feeling of childlike dependence' (Friedman and Friedman, 1980: 249).

Anti-collectivists are deeply pessimistic about the chances of genuine democratic control of government activities. 'It is sheer illusion to think', Hayek argues, 'that when certain needs of the citizen have become the exclusive concern of a single bureaucratic machine, democratic control of that machine can then effectively guard the liberty of the citizen' (Hayek, 1960), in contrast to the dispersed power characteristic of the market.

A second anxiety which disturbs anti-collectivists is the effect of welfare state policies on government. A government committed to more than a minimum of welfare provision inevitably becomes a focus of pressure from a range of interests seeking action to redress grievances and injustices. In democracies, governments depend on support. Inevitably, therefore, governments seek to satisfy particular interests. They cease to be simply makers of general rules and umpires of the spontaneous order. [...]

A third broad area of criticism is that welfare state policies are destabilising to the economic and social system. ... The argument that the welfare state contributes to the destabilising of the social system is based on ideas about the implications of the politicisation of issues of resource use and distribution. Welfare state policies feed the notion that these processes are susceptible to modification and alteration. Political pressure inevitably follows such a realisation. 'Social conflict is intensified by the welfare state', says Seldon, 'because it uses the political process to decide the use of resources, though "representative institutions" that are in practice controlled by *un* representatives who happen to be politically endowed' (Seldon, 1967: 40).

A fourth, more specific charge against state welfare provision is that it is not responsive to individual and group needs because of the nature of such provision. A public service provides what officials, professionals and politicians *think* people need. Judgments are made not by consumers but by other people on their behalf. Anti-collectivists contrast this situation with a market system where consumers choose what they want from a range of goods and services provided by producers who stand or fall by their ability to provide the products that consumers want. If one believes, as do the anti-collectivists, that the consumer knows best, then 'the supply of goods and services, including medical care, should as nearly as possible be based upon individual preferences' (Lees, 1961: 14). That means a market system rather than publicly organised services.

A fifth charge levelled by the anti-collectivists is that state provision of welfare is fundamentally inefficient. Because bureaucratically provided services are less responsive to particular needs than market systems they will be less efficient at meeting those needs. The lack of competition in welfare provision will lead to ossification and a lack of experiment and innovation. Lees describes the absence of competition in the National Health Service as one of the service's most serious weaknesses. Because of the importance of experiment and innovation in the progress of health services, he regards medical care as 'one of the last commodities that should be monopolised by the state' (Lees, 1961: 30). Writing of pension provision Friedman argues that 'individual freedom to choose, and competition of private enterprises for custom would provide improvements in the kind of contracts available and foster variety and diversity to meet individual need' (Friedman, 1962: 186).

Friedman argues that the very nature of welfare spending makes for inefficiency. All welfare spending falls into two categories of expenditure – spending someone else's money on yourself which makes for extravagance and a lack of concern to keep costs down, and spending someone else's money on a third person which again leads to a lack of concern for economy and, in addition, provides a lack of incentive to obtain for the third party the service he will value most highly. 'These characteristics of welfare spending', in Friedman's view, 'are the main source of their defects' (Friedman and Friedman, 1980: 146–147). Public services lack the two basic disciplines of the market – close concern with costs and sensitivity to consumer preferences. Inefficiency and ineffectiveness are therefore inevitable.

Another aspect of the inefficiency attacked by the anti-collectivists is the way in which the benefits of welfare programmes accrue only to a limited extent to those to whom they are directed. This is because of the strength of forces making for their misdirection. Interest groups press for services and legislation for their particular benefit – and the more successful groups are seldom groups of the poorest and the most needy. Universal, free services are often of most benefit to middle- and upper-income groups. The weaker and poorer members of society are as disadvantaged in the political market as in the economic market. In addition a major slice of all welfare programmes goes to those who staff and administer the programmes (Friedman, 1962: 147–148).

There are two other related points in the charge of inefficiency. The first is that free services lead either to an excessive consumption of resources or to unsatisfactory and unacceptable attempts by bureaucrats to assess the validity of claims and pronounce on the relative importance of needs. This excess demand exacerbates another fundamental difficulty for state welfare services – raising the revenue required. The problem is a simple one – people's reluctance to pay taxes for services they do not or may not need when they could be using their money to meet real, current needs. Anti-collectivists see as fundamental the problem that the state will never be able to raise sufficient revenue to provide services equivalent in quality to those which would be supplied by the market system (Seldon, 1967: 68).

The sixth charge which is levelled by anti-collectivists is that the welfare state has led to the neglect of other sources and systems of welfare and inhibited and hindered their development. They would see three sources and systems of welfare as more important than state services – the family, the voluntary sector and the market. They argue that all three have been damaged by the welfare state.

In the past, Friedman argues, 'Children helped their parents out of love and duty. They now contribute to the support of someone else's parents out of compulsion and fear. The earlier transfers strengthened the bonds of the family; the compulsory transfers weaken them' (Friedman and Friedman, 1980: 135). The same thesis is implicit in Mrs Thatcher's argument that 'if we are to sustain, let alone extend, the level and standard of care in the community, we must first try to put responsibility back where it belongs: with the family and with the people themselves' (Thatcher, 1977: 83).

Seldon has argued strongly that when assessing the supposed achievements of the welfare state we must not forget the array of welfare services it prevented from developing (Seldon, 1981: 7). Specifically, he argues that

The NHS has done the health of the people a 'dis-service' because it has prevented the development of more spontaneous, organic, local voluntary and *sensitive* medical services that would have grown up as incomes rose and medical science and technology advanced. If it were not for the *politically*-controlled NHS we should have seen new forms of medical organisation and financing that better reflected *consumer* preferences, requirements and circumstances (Bosanquet, 1983: 162).

The primacy of family, voluntary and market services – the supposedly 'natural' sources of welfare – has been a continuing theme in New Right apologetics in Britain. As Patrick Jenkin put it when Secretary of State for Social Services, 'The Social services departments should seek to meet directly only those needs which others cannot or will not meet … Their task is to act as a safety net, the final protector for people for whom there is no other, not at a first port of call (*Guardian*, 21 January 1981). 'I believe', Mrs Thatcher told the National Conference of the Women's Royal Voluntary Service, 'that the voluntary movement is at the heart of all our social welfare provision, that the statutory services are the supportive ones, underpinning where necessary, filling the gaps and helping the helpless (*Guardian*, 19 January 1981).

The last charge we need to consider is the accusation that the welfare state is damaging to people. We have seen already the accusation that it is damaging to the family and family responsibility. There are also the more specific charges that public provision induces dependency, demoralisation, and irresponsibility and saps initiative, self-reliance and other desirable Victorian values and virtues. The capacity of the beneficiaries of welfare programmes for independence and for making their own decisions, Friedman asserts, 'atrophies through disuse'. The end result of the whole miserable business is 'to rot the moral fabric that holds a decent society together' (Friedman and Friedman, 1980: 149).

It remains to say a little about anti-collectivist attitudes to individual social services.

Anti-collectivists agree that the state has a duty to relieve poverty but see that as the limit of state responsibility. They therefore favour minimum benefits based on means tests. Public schemes aimed at income maintenance in sickness, old age or unemployment are an illegitimate extension of this duty. So too are benefits paid to all irrespective of need and schemes aimed at egalitarian redistribution.

Anti-collectivists condemn the insurance principle as fraudulent, as a mechanism used to introduce backdoor socialism and as a way of imposing higher rates of taxation without proper debate. In practice, they argue, contributions are a tax on employment. They therefore discourage employers from hiring workers and increase unemployment. Government schemes of social insurance are virtual monopolies with all that means for inflexibility and inefficiency. This means that they are an assault on freedom. They both deprive us 'of control over a sizeable fraction of our income' (Friedman, 1962: 189) and give us no choice over the type and level of benefits we wish to purchase.

Friedman's summary of the blessings which would accrue from a winding down of public social security provision is comprehensive. In his view it

> would eliminate its present effect of discouraging employment and so would mean a larger national income currently. It would add to personal saving and so lead to a higher rate of capital formation and a more rapid rate of growth of income. It would stimulate the development and expansion of private pension schemes and so add to the security of many workers (Friedman, 1962: 155).

In housing, there is general agreement among anti-collectivists that government intervention has worsened rather than improved the situation. Rent control and subsidy are the two chief villains. In Powell's words – and Hayek makes the same point – 'You have only to reduce the price of anything below the point at which current supply and demand balance to create shortages in the present and repress production in the future' (Lejeune, 1970: 32). Hayek and Friedman also stress the individually and socially damaging effects of public housing. As Hayek puts it, people 'become subject to arbitrary decisions of authority in their daily affairs and accustomed to looking for permission and direction in the main decisions of their lives' (Hayek, 1960: 344). Anti-collectivist policy will therefore be directed to the rejuvenation of the private market in housing through the abolition of rent control and subsidy and the running down of the public sector.

Anti-collectivists accept the case for state provision of a compulsory minimum of education because it is better for all if all are educated and because a minimum of education is a necessary precondition for democratic government. The basis for anti-collectivists' anxiety about the state's role in provision beyond a minimum is that the major beneficiary is the individual and not society. There is therefore no case for state subsidies to vocational education which increase the earning power of the recipient. On the other hand, there may be a case for subsidies to non-vocational education because such education benefits the community at large as much, if not more, than the recipients.

The most distinctive contribution which the anti-collectivists have made to the debate about education provision is their advocacy of educational vouchers to be cashed by parents at government-approved schools of their choice. The argument for vouchers is based on the belief that the recreation of a market situation in education – schools supplying and parents buying – will increase parental choice, raise standards, through competition between schools and reduce inequality (Friedman, 1962: 107).

Anti-collectivists are firmly opposed to the public provision of free health care. They see health care as a commodity, no different in essence from other goods and services which the market system supplies more efficiently than any other mechanism. By definition, a publicly provided service will be inferior because of people's reluctance to pay the taxes to finance it; it will be inefficient because not stimulated by competition; it will offer individuals little or no choice; it will be cluttered by bureaucracy. However prodigal the public provision, resources will still have to be rationed and rationing in public services is less fair than rationing by price. In the British National Health Service, rationing, according to Seldon, is 'by influence and bully power' (Bosanquet, 1983: 150).

The anti-collectivists' attitudes to individual services can generally be predicted from their values, their attitudes to society and the state and their views on the proper role of government. Their concern for freedom predisposes them against public provision. So too does their confidence in the superiority of market provision in terms of quality, price, efficiency of production, flexibility of response to need and demand. Their commitment to freedom and the market underpins their apprehensions about any extension of the range of government activity.

Understandably, the anti-collectivists are depressed that misconceived notions about the beneficence and superiority of state welfare provision have gained such a hold in so many countries. But history, they are confident, is on their side. Seldon is confident that the move from the welfare state to welfare provided primarily by the market is just round the corner. Market forces are stronger than political power just as good is ultimately stronger than evil.

Seldon's sources of hope are numerous. Rising incomes, he believes, will mean people will want more responsive services than the state can supply. The improved position of women in society will give a boost to provision through the market because women have a clearer appreciation of the advantages of competition from their experience of its benevolent impact on their supermarket shopping. The inequities of the welfare state will become more apparent. Technical innovation will expand to provide substitutes for state services. There will be an increasing rejection by minority groups of standardised state services. Increased tax evasion and avoidance will make the financing of acceptable levels of services increasingly problematic (Seldon, 1981: 12–14). With such grounds of hope the anti-collectivists wait confidently for the collapse of the walls of the welfare state.

# References

Barry, N. P. (1979) *Hayek's Social and Economic Philosophy*. Basingstoke: Macmillan.

Bosanquet, N. (1983) *After the New Right*. London: Heinemann.

Friedman, M. (1962) *Capitalism and Freedom*. Chicago: University of Chicago Press.

Friedman, M. and Friedman, R. (1980) *Free to Choose*. Harmondsworth: Penguin.

Harris, R. and Seldon, A. (1979) *Overruled on Welfare*. London: Institute of Economic Affairs.

Hayek, F. A. (1960) *The Constitution of Liberty*. London: Routledge & Kegan Paul.

Hayek, F. A. (1976) *Law, Legislation and Liberty, Volume 2*. London: Routledge & Kegan Paul.

Hayek, F. A. (1978) *New Studies in Philosophy, Politics and Economics and the History of Ideas*. London: Routledge & Kegan Paul.

Hayek, F. A. (1979) *Law, Legislation and Liberty, Volume 3*. London: Routledge & Kegan Paul.

Lees, D. S. (1961) *Health through Choice*. London: Institute of Economic Affairs.

Lejeune, A. (ed.) (1970) *Enoch Powell*. London: Stacey.

Seldon, A. (1967) *Taxation and Welfare*. London: Institute of Economic Affairs.

Seldon, A. (1981) *Wither the Welfare State*. London: Institute of Economic Affairs.

Thatcher, M. (1977) *Let Our Children Grow Tall*. London: Centre for Policy Studies.

# Chapter 30

## The slow birth of New Labour Britain

*David Coates*

[...]

## The social legacy

[...] The Labour government in 1945 inherited a society at war. It was one used to the discipline of military effort, its people sealed from the full force of market processes by labour direction and rationing. The Labour government of 1997 inherited a society at peace. The restrictions of wartime were all long gone. If they figured at all in the society's collective memory at the century's end, they did so only in the recollections of the very old. By 1997 you had to be at least 50, and male, to have experienced even the vestigial national service of the 1950s.

New Labour inherited a society in which the vast majority of potential voters were used to the high and rising standards of personal consumption of the long post-war boom. In 1997 people bought and spent freely, and they spent in volume: using a system of credit cards unknown in 1945 and personal bank accounts that at the end of the Second World War had been the status symbol of the few. They spent on commodities unimaginable a generation before, and on things which in 1945 had been beyond the grasp of most of the Labour electorate. By 1997, the majority of Labour voters expected to own their own home, to drive their own car, to take their own vacation, to settle each night in front of their own multichannel television set, and to be free to settle their own private earning and spending priorities. By 1997 too, the capacity of most potential Labour voters to sustain the lifestyle that they desired required that both adult members of the UK's conventional nuclear families brought in a wage or salary, for by then one of the new ways to be

From: D. Coates (2005) *Prolonged Labour: The Slow Birth of New Labour Britain*. Basingstoke: Palgrave Macmillan, pp. 11–20.

excluded from this generalized affluence was to be trapped in a single-parent family unit split asunder by divorce. And by 1997, there was a lot of divorce. Four marriages in ten ended that way in 1997. In 1947 it had been less than one in ten. Whatever 1997 was, in social terms it was not 1945 at all.

# A society transformed

As the old industries of the UK's Victorian heyday faded in the post-war period, the men and women who had worked in them had been obliged to work elsewhere. To remain in those industries, or to remain where they had once been, was to miss out on the rising productivity (and so on the growing wages and living standards) of the New Britain. The old working class was slow to vanish entirely. Its members remained locked in the river valleys of the English North and on the coalfields of the Celtic fringe, as industrial power shifted south into the English Midlands in the 1950s and 1960s, and then later into the Scottish lowlands and the English South East. A new working class emerged around those Midland and South Eastern industries: a new working class which, in the Midlands and the car industry, remained unionized and Labour, but a new working class which everywhere was more private and family-focused in its ambitions and social habits than had been the Northern and Celtic working class of the generations before. In 1945 Old Labour had appealed to a sense of solidarity in a working class which had sustained a distinct sense of community: with its own traditions of working men's clubs, workers' libraries, Saturday football and May Day parades. It had been, in a real sense, a class apart from the middle-class world of the then small English suburbs. The rise and fall of the new manufacturing industries, and the Thatcherite assault on trade unionism, had changed much of that. So New Labour, by contrast, faced a working class whose members largely shared the concerns of middle England. It faced a working class less likely than in 1945 to be unionized, more likely to own its own home and transport, more likely to enjoy untrammelled access to credit (and so to consumption), and less comfortable with self-definitions that emphasized its shared proletarian condition. Such individualized ambitions had never been entirely absent from previous generations of the UK working class: but by 1997 they were central in ways that had not been true before.

In part, that was because, alongside this changing working class a new and wider middle class has also emerged. In fact, two new middle classes had emerged. One – based in the private sector – had emerged as … a new stratum of technocrats: men (and they were mainly men) who supervised production, planned marketing, supervised accounts and managed corporate divisions. Such men did not actually own the companies they helped to run. They still earned a wage (which they normally called a salary). But it was a wage that was inflated to match their managerial function and elevated industrial status, and accordingly they acquired with it many of the attitudes and self-definitions traditionally associated with the owners of capital. By 1997 the UK had had its managerial revolution. A whole generation of self-made managers had embedded itself. It had embedded itself industrially, setting itself apart from ordinary factory and office workers by differentiations in pay, hours, conditions and facilities. It had embedded itself socially, setting itself apart from ordinary workers by the quality and location of its housing, and by its … consumption of private education and health care. And it had set itself apart politically, by giving the Conservative Party its loyalty as the party of business.

That new private sector middle class had been staffed by the brightest boys of the first post-war generation of English workers, filtered out from the rest through the new selective education system set up in 1944 and organized around the 11+[test]. Initially (and that means until the mid-1960s) this was a middle class that in the main was recruited directly from the new grammar schools. The brightest and the best went straight into industry at 18, trained there and were promoted internally. But progressively from the 1960s, that route of short-term social mobility was itself abandoned, replaced instead by the 'milk round': the selection of bright graduates generated by and through the expanded university system ... . With the rise of education and the new universities, the UK acquired a second middle class: one based not in the private sector but in the public. By 1997 New Labour faced ... an electorate in which the largest group of unwavering Labour supporters worked in the schools and offices of the greatly expanded welfare state. Those supporters worked as teachers. They worked as social workers. They worked as nurses. They worked as hospital administrators. Not all of these new public service semi-professionals were Labour supporters, but the majority of them certainly were; and they too took home a salary, lived in the suburbs, and owned their own cars. In fact, one of the great differentiators between these two new middle class blocs by 1997 was precisely car ownership. In general, the private sector-based middle class received their cars as part of their package of benefits. They paid tax on those cars but they did not actually own them. The public sector middle class, in general and by contrast, did: and of course, because they did, they tended to drive smaller and older cars. The ... nuances of the new social structure faced by New Labour were as class-inflected as they had ever been.

So when New Labour surveyed its potential electorate in 1997, it faced a mixture of the old and the new. There were definite continuities with the past. In Scotland and Wales in particular, the older industries remained entrenched, and older class patterns and attitudes remained entrenched with them. The small business sector and the traditional professions: they too were still in place, and still largely closed to the Labour Party in electoral terms. But the old was overlaid with the new; and the old and new alike enjoyed a prosperity that was historically unprecedented. With that prosperity, and with the confidence in consumption that accompanied it, other cultural changes had come as well. Traditional patterns of deference had all but ebbed away by 1997. The monarchy was significantly less popular than it had been in 1945 (or indeed 1953), and religious commitments (and the social impact of the clergy) had been largely marginalized: except in the new ethnic communities and in Northern Ireland, where a different politics still prevailed. A new youth culture was now a whole generation old. Indeed the youth culture of the 1960s had been transformed into a middle-age commodity and repackaged by 1997: no longer radical, but challenged itself by the musical preferences and lifestyle of the baby boomers' own children. And by then the patriarchal and racist elements of the culture that had been widely taken for granted in 1945 were no longer acceptable ... . By 1997 there was a new political correctness. Patriarchy and racism were still there: but in a much more subterranean form.

For by 1997 the public world of gender and immigration had been reset in the UK by a half-century of major social change. Women had entered the public domain on an unprecedented scale in the years after 1945. Women, of course, had always provided the bulk of the unpaid labour on which UK society rested. They had always borne and raised the children, fed the men and cared for the sick and the old, and most of that was still firmly intact in 1997, for all the talk of 'new men' and the resetting of gender divisions. But those same women had increasingly joined the paid labour force as well, so taking on double burden of work … (Walby, 1997). By 1995, for every 100 men with higher education qualifications in the UK, there were 115 women. The numbers of men and women in employment were also approaching parity as New Labour took office, though women continued to be disproportionately employed in part-time work … (Desai et al., 1999). At work, women still met a series of glass ceilings – barriers to equal access to high wages and promotion – but at least by 1997 the immediate port-war notion of a society built around the male breadwinner was well and truly gone (Creighton, 1999). New Labour in 1997 inherited a society in which, in affluent households, two-income families were increasingly the norm, and in which women – and to a lesser extent, their men – therefore juggled the conflicting demands of family and work. It also inherited a society in which, as a new group among the poor, there were at least a million homes in which divorce and desertion had left women raising children alone. […]

The UK was also, by 1997, far more of a multicultural society than it had been in 1945. Before the Second World War, the UK had experienced only two major immigrations in the modern period: one from Ireland from the 1840s (a migration that was formally internal to the UK until 1922) and an Eastern European Jewish migration from the 1890s. After 1945, however, it experienced a third. For with full employment, many UK-based firms (particularly in the older industries now in decline) turned outwards for new sources of labour, and waves of migrants arrived (initially single men in the main, followed later by their families) mainly from the Caribbean and South Asia. Political persecution added Ugandan Asians to the mix in the late 1960s. By 1997 two or three generations of such immigrant families were settled in the UK, and ethnic minority numbers were rising faster than natural population growth for the first time since the war. By then, the 4 million members of ethnic minority communities in the UK made up 7% of the total population, but they were not randomly scattered through that population, either socially or geographically. On the contrary, immigrant communities had largely been ghettoized by the strength and ubiquity of English racism, predominantly obliged to settle and work in decaying sections of the industrial towns and cities of the English Midlands and the North, and initially locked there (and in equivalent areas in the capital) in conditions of urban poverty. Over time, however, these ghettoized communities had developed their own internal social differences, as an immigrant business and professional class had emerged and flourished, particularly so in the various Asian communities now established in major English cities. […] So New Labour entered office facing a difficult cocktail of issues set in motion by the way in which urban decay and immigration, class and race had all interlocked in the years of the Thatcherite ascendancy. New Labour may have inherited a young country in May 1997, but it also inherited one riddled with tensions of gender change and ethnic division.

# A society in need of reform

In fact, the social agenda waiting for New Labour ran wider even than this, and was a considerable one. It was an agenda partly rooted in the problems of affluence, and partly in the problems of the poor. …

New Labour inherited a social fabric in which the results of systematic underinvestment by public bodies over a long period of time were increasingly difficult to ignore. This was particularly so in the areas of education and health care, housing and transport. As early as

1991 the European Commission had issued figures showing capital expenditure rates on education per head of the population in Germany and France running twice as high as in the UK,[1] and through the 1990s a whole string of reports had documented significant shortfalls in the quality of the education and training being provided by those undercapitalized schools, when compared to the performance of equivalent institutions elsewhere in the advanced capitalist world. Likewise, the health system was in serious difficulty. New Labour inherited growing public disquiet with the length of hospital waiting lists, the quality of medical service and the regional disparities in its availability … . Moreover, New Labour inherited a public sector labour force whose job conditions and employment security had been systematically eroded by the privatization initiatives of the Conservatives, and whose wage range remained limited when set against that available in the private sector. Demographics too were not helping New Labour here. Instead, an ageing population, a low productivity manufacturing base and an electorate trained by Thatcherism in the desirability of low rates of personal taxation were by 1997 combining to present the incoming government with a welfare dilemma of unprecedented proportions.

If that was not enough, New Labour also inherited serious weaknesses in the UK transport systems and housing market. The public provision of low-cost housing had been stopped by the Conservatives in the 1980s, and towards the end of that decade declining interest rates and a slowly growing housing stock had triggered an explosion in house prices. … particularly marked in the English South East where, during the recession in jobs and house prices of the early 1990s, many homeowners had found themselves trapped into negative equity. But only temporarily, for by 1997 the house price explosion was on again: with, in consequence, in significant sections of the country, whole tranches of low-paid workers unable to afford the cost of housing. … There was probably not a single nurse in London by then who could afford, on her NHS salary alone, to buy even the most modest house close to her place of work.

The resulting retreat into the suburbs, and the associated lengthening of people's daily commuter runs, then added a generalized transport crisis to the emerging housing one as New Labour came to power. The typical British commuter added a remarkable 17% to the length of his/her daily commute during the 1990s (Doward, 2003): partly by travelling further, and partly by travelling more slowly on public systems that were overcrowded and along road networks that were increasingly jammed. In 1950 there had been just 2 million cars on UK roads. By 1997 that number was approaching 24 million, and 120 people were being killed or injured on UK roads every day. It was generally understood in government circles by then that road traffic in England was likely to grow, unless regulated, … rais[ing] the possibility of generalized gridlock around major UK cities within a lifetime. […] Britain's transport infrastructure, New Labour's transport watchdog would later report to ministers, was suffering from 'two generations of neglect' which had left the UK with 'the worst transport record in Europe, with the most congested roads, highest prices and neglected networks starved of investment'. (Walters, 2001)

# Patchwork Britain

These resource pressures applied to all of us in varying ways by 1997, and coloured daily life everywhere, but they were particularly acute in certain regions and among certain groups. Regional disparities in the quality and cost of social capital were a particularly marked feature of the Conservatives' legacy to New Labour. The housing stock left behind from the Victorian creation of Northern towns and cities remained in generalized need of renovation by 1997. In fact, across whole swathes of the English North West and Midlands, and ageing housing stock, a scarcity of new building land and an associated propensity to squeeze new and small houses between old and dilapidated ones, had combined by 1997 to leave those parts of the UK with a dense patchwork of inadequate housing. A special report commissioned by the *Guardian* later reported:

> Nowhere is this seen more clearly than in the northern conurbations. Despite the welcome city centre developments in places like Leeds and Manchester, go half a mile away from the new penthouses, restaurants, offices and multi-screen cinemas and you will be in the land of the forgotten – the endless rows of impoverished (private) terraces and half empty council housing...where unemployment levels are horrendous, where houses sell – if at all – for less than £10,000, where crime or the fear of crime traps people in their homes ... where drugs are common currency.[2]

These 'forgotten' houses were increasingly the dwellings of the poor: isolated from a more affluent Britain by the middle-class flight into the suburbs. Travel in 1997 through the Lancashire cotton towns and then out into the Cheshire countryside, or leave inner London in search of the commuter towns served by the M25, and you could not avoid seeing the new and socially unequal society that New Labour would inherit. And it was unequal: more unequal by 1997, in fact, than at any time since records began in the 1880s.

It was regionally unequal, and increasingly so. [...] On unemployment, on wealth and poverty, on health and the length of life, on education and on skills, regional inequalities intensified after 1979, so that New Labour inherited a genuine and an entrenched North–South divide. It also inherited a large and widening disparity in incomes ... . Between 1979 and 1993 the poorest fifth of the UK's population had seen its income rise by at most 6–13% (the income of the bottom tenth had actually fallen by 17% during that period), against a rise of more than 60% for the richest fifth of the population.[3] [...]

In April 1997, when the average hourly wage rate for male workers in the UK had reached £8.24, there were 1.5 million workers earning less than £3.00 an hour, and 6 million (one worker in four) earning less than £4.50 (Stewart, 1999). Moreover and as early as 1991, the income of 3.4 million state pensioners in the UK had slipped below the official poverty line of half average income, as had that of 2 million recipients of other state benefits (for disability, single-parenting and long-term unemployment). In consequence, the Child Poverty Action Group (CPAG) as early as 1987 had been able to locate 10 million people living at or just above Supplementary Benefit level in the UK. By 1990, one-third of all UK workers earned less than the decency threshold set by the Council of Europe; and by 1994 one child in three in the UK (4.1 million in total) was living below the official poverty line. In 1979 poverty had been the condition of only one child in ten. In the Thatcher years, income inequality had grown faster in the UK than in any comparable industrial country. In just two decades of predominantly Conservative rule, the proportion of the population with access to less than half the average income had actually trebled.[4]

The result was that New Labour inherited a patchwork Britain. It inherited a country, part of whose social geography looked Second World rather than First: a society of run-down and crime-ridden housing estates, closed factories and long-term unemployment.

Yet New Labour also inherited a country, part of whose social geography stood at the tip of that banana-shaped wedge of land – stretching from London in the north through the eastern parts of France, the Low Countries and the western part of Germany, down into northern Italy – where living standards were as high as anywhere in the Western world.[5] Market forces and individual self-interest continued through the 1990s to set those two worlds increasingly apart. New Labour faced more than a two-speed economy. It also faced the two-speed society which that economy had created and sustained, and it would have to design policies to deal with them both.

# Notes

1   *Observer*, 5 November 1995, p. 18.
2   Quoted in the *Guardian*, 1 March 2001, p. 15.
3   *Financial Times*, 20 May 1997, p. 15; figures from the Joseph Rowntree Foundation.
4   Cited in the *Guardian*, 10 February 1995, p. 7.
5   *Guardian*, 14 August 1998, p. 4.

# References

Creighton, C. (1999) 'The rise and decline of the "male breadwinner family" in Britain', *Cambridge Journal of Economics*, 23: 519–541.
Desai, T., Gregg, P., Steer, J. and Wadsworth, J. (1999) 'Gender and the labour market', in P. Gregg and J. Wadsworth (eds), *The State of Working Britain*. Manchester: Manchester University Press, p. 170.
Doward, J. (2003) 'Jam tomorrow', *Observer*, 3 July, p. 12.
Stewart, M. (1999) 'Low pay in Britain', in P. Gregg and J. Wadsworth (eds), *The State of Working Britain*. Manchester: Manchester University Press, p. 225.
Walby, S. (1997) *Gender Transformations*. London: Routledge, p. 27.
Walters, J. (2001) 'Gridlocked UK: now it's official', *Observer*, 25 November, p. 16.

# Chapter 31

## The Positive Care Law

*Mary Shaw and Danny Dorling*

The 'inverse care law' was first suggested by Julian Tudor Hart in 1971, stating that medical services were distributed inversely to population health needs and, moreover, that this law operates more completely where medical care is most exposed to market forces:

> In areas with most sickness and death, general practitioners [GPs] have more work, larger lists, less hospital support, and inherit more clinically ineffective traditions of consultation, than in the healthiest areas; and hospital doctors shoulder heavier case-loads with less staff and equipment, more obsolete buildings, and suffer recurrent crises in the availability of beds and replacement staff. These trends can be summed up as the inverse care law: that the availability of good medical care tends to vary inversely with the need of the population served. (Hart, 1971)

This inverse care law has subsequently been found to apply to a range of health service provision; for example, the uptake of childhood immunisations, the use of child health services, the provision of coronary artery revascularisation and waiting times for cardiac surgery, transport accessibility in rural areas, the management of depression in primary care, the provision of health promotion clinics, GP consultation times in relation to the presence of psychological symptoms, advice giving in community pharmacies, and the take-up of annual health checks for the elderly. As Julian Tudor Hart himelf commented in 2000: 'You name it, there's now some inverse law for it, or soon will be. The world never runs out of injustice'. (Hart, 2000).

Three decades on from the original paper, as the debate over the role of market forces in the National Health Service (NHS) intensifies, this observation continues to ring true. Here we consider the inverse care law in a new context: a) with data covering the whole of England and Wales, and b) considering not only medical care but also informal care. We ask the question 'does empirical evidence support the notion that those most in need receive the least care?'

Originally published in the *British Journal of General Practice*, (2004), 54: 899–903 [abridged].

# Method

Our analysis is based on data for England and Wales from the 2001 census, (ONS, 2003), aggregated to county, unitary, or former metropolitan authority level. These areas were used in this analysis to minimise the influence of cross-border commuting. For the first time, the census in 2001 asked questions on general health status as well as limiting long-term illness, on the qualifications and current employment status of healthcare workers (nurses, qualified medical practitioners, dentists, and other health professionals and therapists), and on the care provided by the population as a whole (those providing 50 or more hours of unpaid care per week). We calculated unweighted and weighted (for population size) correlation coefficients for these variables, to investigate the relationship between health and care.

# Results

In England and Wales in 2001, 7.6% of the population stated that their health was not good and that they also lived with a limiting long-term illness (defined by the census as an 'illness, health problem, or disability which limits your daily activities or the work you can do') (ONS, 2003). Although these are self-reported and hence subjective assessments of health, and some of these answers will have been imputed from forms that were not completed, the 2001 census is the most accurate and comprehensive source of information on this topic to date (Dorling and Rees, 2003). For the purposes of this article we consider this group as being those most in need of health care. Of this group of almost 4 million people, 54% are women (women make up 51% of the population as a whole), 54% live north [of the Severn–Wash divide] compared with 44% of the population, one-third are aged over 70 years, a sixth are over 85 years, but 10% are aged under 40 years. Other than mothers giving birth, children in the first few months of life, and adults suffering an accident or injury, this group clearly includes the bulk of healthcare need in England and Wales.

Over 1 million people in England and Wales stated on their census form that they provided at least 50 hours a week of unpaid care. This care was principally for people's health needs and included looking after and giving help or support to family members, friends, neighbours or others because of long-term physical or mental ill-health or disability or health problems relating to old age. Of these million carers, [31.4%] were aged over [65] years; 60% were women; 21% were not in good health themselves but provided care to someone else in spite of that.

[There is a] remarkably close relationship, at the ecological level, between the provision of unpaid care and the need for that care. On average, one person provided 50 or more hours of unpaid care a week for every 3.58 people with the health needs described above. This ratio hardly varies at all across England and Wales. Clearly, some individuals in need of care will find that friends and family are more generous with their time than others, and this care is more likely to be provided by women. On a population level, however, there is no evidence that people are more or less altruistic in their care, when given for free, within any particular area of the country – it is provided (geographically) on the basis of need.

We term this the 'positive care law', whereby informal care is provided in direct proportion to the degree that care is needed; the correlation coefficient for these two variables is 0.97 ($P<0.001$). …Obviously, many [qualified health professionals] commute, and so any disparity between need and care might be caused by commuting patterns. However, the vast majority of the disparities shown occur over the north–south divide. Doctors and nurses do not live in Oxford and Bristol and commute to Easington or Salford to work. The health professionals shown are, respectively: nurses, medical practitioners, dentists, and other health professionals with a professional qualification. Of these four groups only nurses (the largest in number and predominantly female) are geographically distributed roughly in proportion to need ($r = 0.31$, $P = 0.001$). Weighting the correlations for population size does not alter their rank order. An inverse care law applies … to the distribution of people working in all of the more highly paid forms of healthcare. [The correlation coefficients are $-0.22$ ($P = 0.022$) for medical practitioners, $-0.42$ ($P<0.001$) for dental practitioners and $-0.48$ ($P<0.001$), the strongest,] for the fourth group – the group most likely to be providing private services (such as chiropractors and osteopaths).
[…]

# Discussion

The census reveals that a considerable amount of care is provided by the friends and families of those in need. This care is provided at no cost to the state save the benefit payments and allowances that are paid to some carers. This care is provided in almost direct and exact proportion to need – defined here as the geographical distribution of people both suffering poor health and living with a limiting long-term illness. The observation of the 'inverse care law', as originally stated, can thus now be supplemented with additional data referring to the provision of informal care. We propose that an additional regularity, observed from analysis of the 2001 census data, can be stated as a 'postive care law', a law that takes into account not only medical care in the formal sector of paid work, but health care in its broadest sense. We suggest that the 'positive care law' can be stated thus:

> In contemporary society, both informal and professional care are provided to those in need. When we consider these very different types of care, informal and formal, we observe that in those areas with most people in need, people disproportionately receive even more care from the informal, unpaid sector – the least skilled form of care. This is also the cheapest form of care (for the state) and constitutes a group of carers without power or representation. Conversely, those people living in areas least in need of care (as defined here) receive the most specialised and skilled medical care through the formal paid sector. Between these two extremes there is a continuum. Formal medical care is thus distributed inversely to need whereas informal care is positively related to need – where care is most needed it is informal care that is most likely to be provided. Where market forces are allowed to intervene in the relationships between the need for care and its provision, the more likely the inverse care law is found to apply.

These findings concern the motivations that underpin human actions, and the value that we ascribe to the services that we provide for each other. A key motivation for the provision of personal or medical care is traditionally considered to be altruism. The issue of whether the fundamental basis of human relationships operates through altruism or exchange, and the consequences of that, was central to the analysis in *The Gift Relationship* (Titmuss, 1970). Titmuss' analysis of the donation of human blood in the United Kingdom and the selling of human blood in the United States, has relevance for understanding 'gift relationships' – or how and why people help one another – more generally. When someone gives their blood to another person the act is altruistic, unselfish and unconditional. When a donor sells their blood, however, then the relationship is mechanical, impersonal and responsive to pressure of demand and supply.

However, they truly altruistic act, such a the gift relationship of giving blood, appears to be rare and is not easily measured, as Murray (2003) points out. Altruism implies a lack of connection and lack of reciprocation between the carer and the cared for, which characterises the giving of blood, and to some extent the provision of medical services, but is unlikely to be the case with informal care. In fact, it may be because people are connected, because they experience reciprocation, that they care for each other. Conversely, there are many collective actions that suggest that the population may be more altruistic than this simple reciprocal model would suggest, and that altruism is partly learnt behaviour. In the north … more middle-class people tend to vote for left-wing politicians advocating redistributive policies, despite the implementation of these policies being to their direct immediate disadvantage. Perhaps the more you can see the benefits of altruistic behaviour, the more likely you are to act altruistically. On the other hand, the greater the role of the market, the more likely people are to be driven by motives other than altruism; the contrast between nurses and doctors, in terms of their altruism; the contrast between nurses and doctors, in terms of their choice of occupation, their salaries and in our results presented here, are an example of this.

It is important to note that this paper is only concerned with ecological data: the number of medical practitioners per head of the population as they vary between areas, the number of informal carers as a proportion of the population and the number in need of medical care. Within any area it is almost certainly the case that those most in need of care will be cared for by medical practitioners more than those who are in less need of care. It is important not to invoke the ecology fallacy and suggest that the sickest people in England and Wales are not cared for by paid carers. Nevertheless, this analysis does reveal that where there are more ill people there are fewer people, per head, being paid to provide medical care. There are also very large geographical distances between the areas where more doctors and dentists live and where the population is most in need of their services. Thus it is certainly the case that, by area, there is less paid care available where it is most needed, and most paid care available where it is least needed. Conversely, and everywhere in England and Wales, almost exactly the same proportions of people give up 50 or more hours per week of their time to care for those in need, unpaid. Altruism is found everywhere, but in greatest quantities where it is most needed.

This geographical division of England and Wales revealed through the data used in this paper is a division familiar to those who have studied the human geography of these countries over the last century. As the land rises to the north and west of Gloucestershire, Warwickshire, Leicestershire, and Lincolnshire, more people are ill and fewer medical professionals (other than nurses) are in work. People of all professions are more likely to live in the southeast of England; they are more likely to have achieved access to university from there, to return there if they trained in the north, or to move there later in their working lives. What is unusual about medical professionals is that, as a group, they manage to achieve this same south-eastern bias despite the majority of their most needy client group living in the north and despite the large majority of them working for the NHS, which partly allocates resources in relation to the needs of area populations. The 2001 census figures would suggest that a greater proportion of those resources are used to employ nurses in the north and doctors in the south of England.

# References

Dorling, D. and Rees, P. (2003) 'A nation still dividing: the British census and social polarisation 1971–2001', *Environment and Planning A*, 35(7): 1287–1313.

Hart, J. T. (1971) 'The inverse care law', *Lancet*, 1: 405–412.

Hart, J. T. (2000) 'Commentary: three decades of the inverse care law', *British Medical Journal*, 320: 18–19.

Murray, T. H. (2003) 'Are we better than we can say? Altruism in general practice', *British Journal of General Practice*, 53: 355–357.

Office for National Statistics (ONS) (2003) *Census 2001: National Report for England and Wales*. London: HMSO.

Titmuss, R. M. (1970) *The Gift Relationship: From Human Blood to Social Policy*. Harmondsworth: Penguin.

# Acknowledgements

We thank Julian Tudor Hart, Helena Tunstall, and two anonymous referees for their constructive comments on earlier drafts of this paper. Mary Shaw is funded by the South West Public Health Observatory, Bristol.

# Index